Nutrition and Diet Therapy

Nutrition and Diet Therapy

Fourth Edition

Carolynn E. Townsend

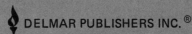

DELMAR PUBLISHERS INC. ®

NOTICE TO THE READER

Cover photo: United States Department of Agriculture

Delmar Staff
    Administrative Editor: Adele Morse O'Connell
    Project Editor: Karen Lavroff

For information address Delmar Publishers Inc.,
2 Computer Drive West, Box 15-015,
Albany, New York 12212

Printed in the United States of America
Published simultaneously in Canada
by Nelson Canada.
a division of International Thomson Limited

10 9 8 7 6 5 4

Library of Congress Cataloging in Publication Data

Townsend, Carolynn E.
    Nutrition and diet therapy.

    Includes bibliographies.
    1. Nutrition. 2. Diet. 3. Cookery. 4. Diet therapy. I. Title.
TX354.T7 1985   613.2   84-19975
ISBN 0-8273-2422-7
ISBN 0-8273-2423-5 (instructor's guide)

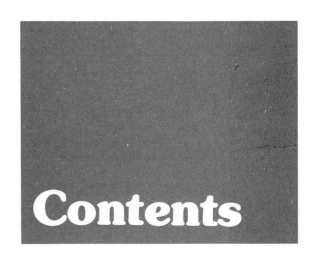

Contents

Preface/*vii*
Acknowledgments/*ix*

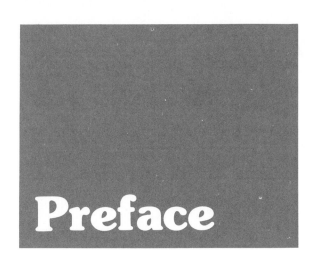

Preface

Nutrition and Diet Therapy was written for practical and vocational nursing students, beginning students in other health care professions, and students enrolled in food service and dietetic technician/assistant programs. Formerly entitled *Nutrition and Diet Modifications,* the book has proved successful as an introduction to or a review of the fundamentals of nutrition and diet therapy. This fourth edition has been substantially revised and updated to reflect the increasing awareness of the positive correlation between nutrition and health status, and the latest findings in the nutrition field.

Section 5, now entitled *Therapeutic Diets*, has been completely reorganized and extensively rewritten to include information that is typically emphasized in the curricula of a variety of health care programs. Chapters are organized by diseases or disorders and cover the therapeutic diets that are pertinent to a number of specific conditions. Case Studies give students an opportunity to apply theory and to prepare for state licensing or certification examinations. Information on diet therapy for ulcers and diabetes has been completely updated, and the most recent Exchange Lists from the American Diabetes Association have been included in the Appendix.

Section 4, now entitled *Nutrition During Life Stages* contains new chapters on nutrition and the elderly, diet during young adulthood and middle age, and diet during childhood and adolescence. Material on nutrition for athletes, the nutritional value of fast foods, fad diets, and anorexia nervosa have been added to this section.

Sections 1 through 3 have been thoroughly updated. Additional information on dietary customs and the influence of ethnicity, religion, and philosophy is presented, as well as the U.S. government's dietary guidelines.

As in previous editions, extensive learning aids are provided. Lists of key terms and learning objectives are located at the beginning of each chapter. Chapter summaries, suggested activities, and discussion and review questions reinforce learning. Extensive tables, charts, and photos present important material in a comprehensible and accessible manner. A bibliography and glossary (new to this edition) provide opportunities for further study and research.

The instructor's guide contains answers to the chapter review questions, reproducible section review questions that may be used as test material, and answers to the section review questions.

Acknowledgments

The author wishes to express her appreciation to the members of her family for their patience and understanding during the writing of this revision. Appreciation is also expressed to the following persons and organizations:

American Diabetes Association Inc.
American Dairy Association
American Heart Association
Black Hawk College
Bureau of Nutrition, Department of Health, New York, NY
Chesebrough-Ponds, Inc., Hospital Products Division
Food and Drug Administration, U.S. Department of Health, Education, and Welfare
Food and Nutrition Board, National Academy of Sciences, National Research Council
Gerber Products Company
Lea and Febiger
Metropolitan Life Insurance Company
National Bureau of Standards, U.S. Department of Commerce
National Canners Association
National Dairy Council
National Education Association
National Institute of Health
National Live Stock and Meat Board
Dr. R.L. Nemir
Parent's Magazine
Tupperware
Upjohn Company
United Nations
United States Department of Agriculture
World Health Organization

Reviewers of the third edition and the revised manuscript for the fourth edition:

Dorothy M. Born, Coordinator of Patient Education of the American Diabetes Association Inc.
Mary Ann Chaney, Allegheny Community College
Harriet Goldberg, Clara Barton High School
Jackie Hartgrove, Howard College
Marilyn Hutchins, Crowder College
Dorothy Kohn, Washington Irving High School
Christine Neff, Muskegon Area J Vocational School
Louise Parker, Muscle Shoals Technical School
Aileen Rowand, Decatur School of Practical Nursing

Kathy Yarbrough, Pines Vocational-
   Technical School
Lois West, Del Castle Technical High
   School

Adele Morse O'Connell, Ann Drylewski,
   and Karen Lavroff of Delmar Publishers
   Inc.

Section 1
Basic
Nutrition

1

Chapter 1

INTRODUCTION TO NUTRITION

OBJECTIVES

After studying this chapter, you should be able to

- List the essential nutrients and identify their primary functions
- Identify common characteristics of well-nourished people
- Identify symptoms of malnutrition
- Identify at least four hollow calorie foods

Most people enjoy food. Although they eat primarily because they are hungry, they also find eating pleasant because of the memories it may invoke, the social climate it promotes and because the taste of the food is pleasing to them. Unfortunately, many people make their food selections only on these bases and are not aware of their bodies' food needs.

There is an old saying, "You are what you eat." This statement has great significance when the results of good or poor nutrition are considered. *Nutrition* is the result of those processes whereby the body takes in and uses food for growth, development, and the main-tenance of health. Nutrition helps determine the height and weight of an individual. Nutrition also may affect the body's ability to resist disease, the length of one's life, and the state of one's physical and mental well-being.

Good nutrition enhances one's appearance and is commonly exemplified by shiny hair, clear skin, clear eyes, erect *posture* (body position), alert expressions, and firm flesh on well-developed bone structures. Good nutrition aids emotional adjustments, provides *stamina* (one's resistance to fatigue or illness), and promotes a healthy appetite. It also helps establish regular sleep and elimination habits.

ESSENTIAL NUTRIENTS

Nutrients are chemical substances found in food that are necessary for good health. For the body to be *well nourished* (provided with materials necessary to promote and sustain life), foods containing the essential nutrients must be eaten regularly.

These essential nutrients are

- Carbohydrates
- Fats
- Proteins
- Minerals
- Vitamins
- Water

A nutrient must accomplish at least one of three functions

- Supply heat and energy to the body
- Build and repair body tissues
- Regulate body processes

Carbohydrates and fats primarily furnish heat and energy. Proteins are used mainly to build and repair body tissues with the help of vitamins and minerals. Proteins also provide energy when carbohydrate and fat reserves are low. Vitamins, minerals, and water help regulate the various body processes such as circulation, respiration, digestion, and elimination.

Water comprises about 58 percent of body weight and is found in all body tissues. Water aids in the *digestion* (breakdown) of food. It makes up most of the *blood plasma* (fluid part of the blood), which carries nutrients to all parts of the body and removes wastes. Water helps the body tissues absorb nutrients. Food that is not used becomes waste and is excreted. Water helps move the waste through the body and prevents constipation. Because of its importance in maintaining body

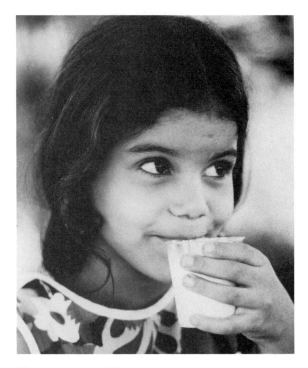

Figure 1-1 A child's general appearance is enhanced when she is well-nourished. (Courtesy of the United Nations/Guthrie)

processes, the average person needs to drink the *equivalent* (equal amount) of six to eight glasses of water each day.

MALNUTRITION

Malnutrition (poor nutrition) is a condition that results when the cells do not receive an adequate supply of the essential nutrients because of poor diet or poor utilization of food. Sometimes it occurs because people do not or cannot eat enough of the foods that provide the essential nutrients to satisfy body needs. Other times people may eat full, well-balanced diets, but suffer from diseases that

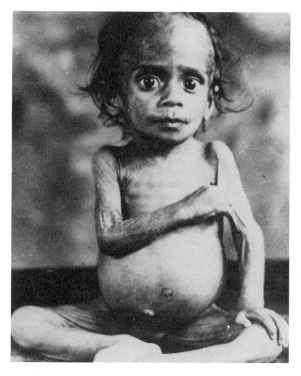

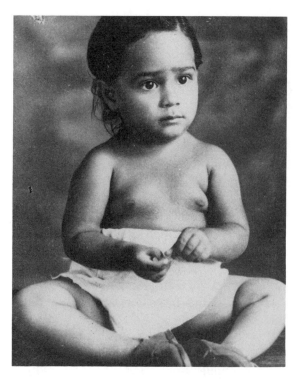

A. Signs of malnutrition (swollen abdomen, sagging skin, and sunken eyes) are easily seen in this two-year-old girl.

B. After ten months of diet therapy, improvements in nutritional status are evident.

Figure 1-2 A proper diet can produce great improvement, even after severe malnutrition. (Courtesy of World Health Organization)

prevent normal usage of the nutrients. Treatments such as drug therapy or surgery sometimes create changes that prevent food from being used normally.

Some characteristics of people suffering from malnutrition are: dull, lifeless hair; greasy, pimpled facial skin; dull eyes; slumped posture; fatigue and depression shown in spiritless expressions and behavior. Malnourished persons may be underweight or overweight and skeletal growth may be stunted. Resistance to disease is reduced, and recovery from disease or surgery may be slower than in well-nourished people. Appetite may be poor or excessive, resulting in underweight or overweight. Sleep may be affected because malnutrition influences the nervous system, just as it affects all body systems. Irritability and nervousness may result. The attention span is reduced. Constipation is common. Mental retardation, disease, and even death can result from severe malnutrition.

A disease that directly results from a lack of a certain nutrient is called a *deficiency disease*. Beriberi is an example of a deficiency disease. Beriberi affects the nervous system, causing weakness, paralysis, and sometimes death. It is due to a lack of a vitamin B (thiamin) in the diet.

Iron deficiency is a common form of malnutrition in the United States, particularly among children and women of all ages. *Iron* is a mineral component of the blood and therefore is lost during each menstrual period. In addition, there is an increased need for iron during pregnancy.

Persons most prone to malnutrition are infants, preschool children, adolescents, the elderly, and pregnant women (especially if they are adolescents). If mothers do not know about proper nutrition, their children will suffer. Infants and preschool children depend on their mothers' selection of foods. Preschool children may face an additional hazard since they are usually particular about what they eat.

Adolescents may eat often, but at unusual hours. They may miss regularly scheduled meals, become hungry, and satisfy this hunger with snacks of essentially *hollow calorie foods* such as potato chips, cakes, sodas, and candy. Hollow calorie foods provide an abundance of calories, but the nutrients are primarily carbohydrates and fat with very limited amounts of proteins, vitamins, and minerals. Adolescents are subject to *peer pressure*; that is, they are influenced by the opinions of their friends. If friends favor the hollow calorie foods, it is difficult for an adolescent to differ with them. Crash diets, which unfortunately are common among adolescents, sometimes result in a form of malnutrition. This condition occurs because some essential nutrients are eliminated from the diet when the types of foods allowed are severely restricted.

Pregnancy increases a woman's appetite and the need for certain nutrients, especially proteins, minerals, and vitamins. Pregnancy during adolescence requires extreme care in food selection. The young mother-to-be requires a diet that provides sufficient nutrients for the developing fetus, as well as for her own still-growing body.

The elderly are often alone and unwell. Their living conditions are not always conducive to forming a healthy appetite. Part of the joy of eating is sharing one's food in pleasant company. Lack of companionship or illness can make eating unpleasant and difficult.

THE STUDY OF NUTRITION

A detailed study of nutrition and its relationship to body functions, general health, and specific illnesses is essential for the nurse or homemaker. Patients, family members, and friends frequently ask questions regarding nutrition. An understanding of nutrition is useful when helping others whose eating habits require improvement.

Sometimes patients undergo *diet therapy*, which means that their medical treatment includes eating prescribed foods in specified amounts. The nurse must be able to check a patient's tray quickly to see that it actually contains the correct foods for the diet prescribed.

Patients frequently have questions and complaints about a diet that is new to them. Their anxieties can be relieved by the nurse's clear and simple explanation. Anyone who plans and prepares meals should have knowledge of the value of sound nutrition and should be able to apply the principles of it.

Parents must have a good, basic knowledge of nutrition for the sake of their personal health, the health of their children, and to instruct the children in proper dietary habits. Greater knowledge of nutrition would help eliminate many health problems caused by malnutrition.

SUMMARY

Nutrition is the process by which the body uses food for growth, development, and the maintenance of health. Signs of good nutrition include shiny hair, clear skin and eyes, erect posture, a well-developed body, an alert expression, a pleasant disposition, a healthy appetite, and regular habits of sleep and elimination. Nutrition helps determine a person's height, weight, resistance to disease, and length of life.

To be well-nourished, one must eat foods that supply heat and energy, build and repair body tissue, and regulate body functions. To accomplish these functions, foods must contain the six essential nutrients—carbohydrates, fats, proteins, minerals, vitamins, and water.

Discussion Topics

1. Why is eating pleasant?
2. What is the relationship of nutrition and heredity to each of the following?
   a. the development of physique
   b. the ability to resist disease
   c. the lifespan
3. How may nutritional status affect personality?
4. What health habits, in addition to good nutrition, contribute to making a person healthy?
5. What are the six essential nutrients? What are their three basic functions?
6. Of what value is water to the body?
7. Why are women prone to iron deficiency?
8. Why are some foods called hollow calorie foods? Give examples of these foods.
9. If anyone in the class has been on a crash diet to lose weight, discuss its effects on the individual.
10. What is meant by the saying, "You are what you eat?"
11. Why are people in the following age groups sometimes prone to malnutrition?
    a. young children
    b. adolescents
    c. the elderly

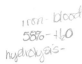

Suggested Activities

1. List ten signs of good nutrition and ten signs of poor nutrition.
2. Write an essay discussing your personal nutrition. List possible improvements.

3. List the foods you have eaten in the past 24 hours. Underline the hollow calorie foods.
4. Using a biology or anatomy textbook as your source, describe one or more of the following body processes: circulation, respiration, elimination.
5. Write a brief description of how you feel at the end of a day when you know you have not eaten wisely.
6. Write sentences using all of the words in the vocabulary list correctly. Read them to the class and discuss them.

Review

A. Multiple choice. Select the *letter* that precedes the best answer.

1. The result of those processes whereby the body takes in and uses food for growth, development, and maintenance of health is called
   a. respiration
   c. nutrition
   b. diet therapy
   d. digestion
2. Nutrition is important in helping to determine a person's
   a. height and weight
   c. physical and mental well-being
   b. ability to resist disease
   d. all of the above
3. To nourish the body adequately, one must
   a. keep warm at all times
   c. sleep 10 hours each night
   b. eat the essential nutrients
   d. resist all disease
4. Nutrients used primarily to provide heat and energy to the body are
   a. water, vitamins, and minerals
   c. none of these
   b. carbohydrates and fats
   d. all of these
5. Nutrients used mainly to build and repair body tissues are
   a. proteins, minerals, and vitamins
   c. water and fats
   d. iron and fats
   b. carbohydrates and fats
6. Foods such as potato chips, cakes, sodas, and candy are called
   a. dietetic foods
   c. hollow calorie foods
   b. essential nutrient foods
   d. nutritious foods
7. An inadequate supply of essential nutrients in the diet may result in
   a. stamina
   c. indigestion
   b. malnutrition
   d. diabetes
8. Beriberi is caused by lack of a
   a. protein
   c. vitamin
   b. carbohydrate
   d. fat

9. The nutrient that comprises about 58 percent of the body weight is
   a. protein   c. carbohydrate
   b. vitamin A   d. water
10. In the United States, a common form of malnutrition is
   a. iron deficiency   c. scurvy
   b. lactation   d. diabetes

B. Match the term listed in column I with its definition in column II.

	Column I		Column II
a	1. posture	a.	body position
d	2. stamina	b.	physical change that may be due to malnutrition.
g	3. nutrients		
e	4. blood plasma	c.	deficiency disease caused by lack of thiamin
k	5. protein		
c	6. beriberi	d.	deficiency disease caused by lack of iron
h	7. peer pressure		
j	8. diet therapy	e.	fluid part of blood
i	9. iron	f.	one's resistance to fatigue or illness
b	10. swollen abdomen	g.	chemical substances found in food and essential for nourishing the body
		h.	influence by the opinions of friends
		i.	mineral that is a component of the blood
		j.	eating prescribed foods in specified amounts
		k.	a basic nutrient that is essential for building and repairing body tissue

References

Bland, Jeffrey, ed. 1983. *Medical Applications of Clinical Nutrition*. New Canaan, Ct.: Keats Publishing Co.

Green, Marilyn L., and Joann Harry. 1981. *Nutrition in Contemporary Nursing Practice*. New York: John Wiley & Sons.

Howard, Roseanne B., and Nancie H. Herbold. 1982. *Nutrition in Clinical Care*, 2nd ed. New York: McGraw Hill Book Company.

Long, Patricia J., and Barbara Shannon. 1983. *Focus on Nutrition*. Englewood Cliffs, N.J.: Prentice-Hall Inc.

Poleman, Charlotte M., and Christine Locastro Capra. 1984. *Shakelton's Nutrition Essentials and Diet Therapy*, 5th ed. Philadelphia: W.B. Saunders Co.

Robinson, Corinne H. 1980. *Basic Nutrition and Diet Therapy,* 4th ed. New York: Macmillan Publishing Company.

Whitney, Eleanor Noss, and Eva May Nunnelley Hamilton. 1984. *Understanding Nutrition*, 3rd ed. St. Paul: West Publishing Co.

Williams, Sue Rodwell. 1984. *Mowry's Basic Nutrition and Diet Therapy*, 7th ed. St. Louis: C.V. Mosby Co.

Chapter 2

THE BODY'S USE OF FOOD

VOCABULARY

absorption	feces	obesity
adipose tissue	food residue	oxidation
amylase	fundus (of	pancreas
anabolism	stomach)	pancreatic amylase
basal metabolism	gastric juices	pancreatic protease
rate (BMR)	gastic lipase	pepsin
bile	gastrointestinal	peptidases
caloric	system	peristalsis
requirement	hormone	protease
caloric value	hydrochloric acid	ptyalin
calorie	hydrolysis	pylorus
calorimeter	hyperthyroidism	rennin
capillary	hypothyroidism	saliva
catabolism	joule	salivary amylase
chemical digestion	kilocalorie	sucrase
chyme	kilojoule	thyroid gland
digestion	lactase	thyroxine
duodenum	lacteals	triiodothyronine
emulsified fats	maltase	(T$_3$)
endocrine glands	mechanical	villi
enzyme	digestion	
esophagus	metabolism	

OBJECTIVES

After studying this chapter, you should be able to

- Explain the processes of digestion, absorption, and metabolism

- Label the organs and glands in the digestive system

- List enzymes or digestive juices secreted by each organ and gland in the digestive system

- State one function of the thyroid gland

- Define calorie

- Calculate individual minimum caloric requirements

Although the body is infinitely more complex than the automobile engine, it may be compared to the engine because both require fuel to run. The body's fuel is, of course, food. For the body to use its fuel, the food must first be prepared by the body and appropriately distributed. This is done through the processes of digestion and absorption. The actual use of the food as fuel, resulting in energy, is called *metabolism*.

DIGESTION

The body's preparation of its food begins with *digestion*. Digestion is the process whereby food is broken down into smaller parts, chemically changed, and moved through the gastrointestinal system. The *gastrointestinal* or *digestive system* consists of the body structures that participate in digestion. As the process of digestion is discussed, refer to figure 2-1, and note the locations of the structures that perform the functions of digestion.

Digestion occurs through two types of action—mechanical and chemical. With mechanical action, food is broken up by the teeth. It is then moved along the gastro-intestinal tract through the esophagus, stomach, and intestines. This movement is caused by a rhythmic contraction of the muscular walls of the tract called *peristalsis*.

During chemical digestion, the composition of food is changed. Chemical changes occur through the addition of water, and the resulting splitting, or breaking down of the food molecules. This process is called *hydrolysis*. Food is broken down into nutrients that the tissues can absorb and use. Hydrolysis also involves *enzymes*, which are organic substances that cause chemical changes in other substances. Digestive enzymes are secreted by the mouth, stomach, pancreas, and the small intestine. (See table 2-1.) An en-

Table 2-1 Enzymes and Foods Acted Upon

	Enzyme	Food Acted Upon
Mouth	Ptyalin	Starch
Stomach	Pepsin	Proteins
	Rennin	Proteins in milk
	Gastric lipase	Emulsified fat
Small Intestine	Pancreatic amylase	Starch
	Pancreatic proteases (trypsin) (chymotrypsin) (carboxypeptidases)	Proteins
	Pancreatic lipase (steapsin)	Fats
	Lactase	Lactose
	Maltase	Maltose
	Sucrase	Sucrose
	Peptidases	Proteins

zyme is usually named for the substance on which it acts. For example, the enzyme *sucrase* acts on sucrose, and the enzyme *maltase* acts on maltose.

Digestion in the Mouth

Digestion begins in the mouth where the food is broken up by the teeth and mixed with saliva. *Saliva* is a secretion of the salivary glands that contains a digestive enzyme called *ptyalin* (also called *salivary amylase*), which acts on starch. However, because food is normally held in the mouth for such a short time, very little starch is chemically changed there. The final chemical digestion of starch occurs in the small intestine.

Digestion in the Stomach

Peristalsis and gravity transfer food from the mouth to the stomach via the esophagus.

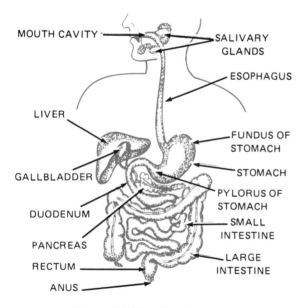

MOUTH CAVITY

SALIVARY GLANDS

ESOPHAGUS

LIVER

FUNDUS OF STOMACH

STOMACH

GALLBLADDER

PYLORUS OF STOMACH

DUODENUM

SMALL INTESTINE

PANCREAS

LARGE INTESTINE

RECTUM

ANUS

Figure 2-1 The digestive system

The *esophagus* is the tube connecting the mouth and the stomach. The stomach has three main functions in digestion. It serves to

- temporarily store food
- mix food with gastric juices
- provide a slow, controlled emptying of food into the small intestine

The stomach consists of the upper portion known as the *fundus*, the middle area known as the *body*, and the end nearest the intestine called the *pylorus*.

Food accumulates in the fundus and moves to the body where it mixes with the gastric juices. *Gastric juices* are digestive secretions of the stomach. The gastric juices contain hydrochloric acid and the enzymes, pepsin, rennin, and gastric lipase. *Hydrochloric acid* breaks the food down, so the enzymes can work on the food, helps to dissolve some minerals, and destroys much of the bacteria present on food. *Pepsin* changes proteins into smaller forms. *Rennin* acts on the protein in milk, causing it to curdle. *Gastric lipase* acts on emulsified fats such as are found in cream and egg yolk. An emulsified fat is a fat finely divided and held in suspension by another liquid.

Digestion in the Small Intestine

After the food has been thoroughly mixed with gastric juices, it becomes a semiliquid mass called *chyme* (pronounced kime). In this

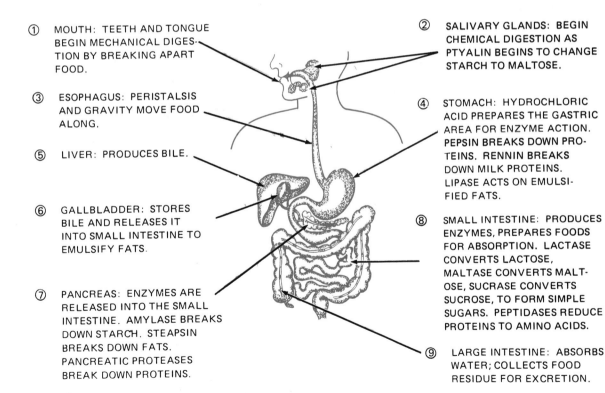

① MOUTH: TEETH AND TONGUE BEGIN MECHANICAL DIGESTION BY BREAKING APART FOOD.

③ ESOPHAGUS: PERISTALSIS AND GRAVITY MOVE FOOD ALONG.

⑤ LIVER: PRODUCES BILE.

⑥ GALLBLADDER: STORES BILE AND RELEASES IT INTO SMALL INTESTINE TO EMULSIFY FATS.

⑦ PANCREAS: ENZYMES ARE RELEASED INTO THE SMALL INTESTINE. AMYLASE BREAKS DOWN STARCH. STEAPSIN BREAKS DOWN FATS. PANCREATIC PROTEASES BREAK DOWN PROTEINS.

② SALIVARY GLANDS: BEGIN CHEMICAL DIGESTION AS PTYALIN BEGINS TO CHANGE STARCH TO MALTOSE.

④ STOMACH: HYDROCHLORIC ACID PREPARES THE GASTRIC AREA FOR ENZYME ACTION. PEPSIN BREAKS DOWN PROTEINS. RENNIN BREAKS DOWN MILK PROTEINS. LIPASE ACTS ON EMULSIFIED FATS.

⑧ SMALL INTESTINE: PRODUCES ENZYMES, PREPARES FOODS FOR ABSORPTION. LACTASE CONVERTS LACTOSE, MALTASE CONVERTS MALTOSE, SUCRASE CONVERTS SUCROSE, TO FORM SIMPLE SUGARS. PEPTIDASES REDUCE PROTEINS TO AMINO ACIDS.

⑨ LARGE INTESTINE: ABSORBS WATER; COLLECTS FOOD RESIDUE FOR EXCRETION.

Figure 2-2 Basic functions of the digestive system

form it moves through the pylorus by peristalsis into the *duodenum*, the first section of the small intestine.

When food reaches the small intestine, the gallbladder is triggered into releasing a substance called *bile*. Bile is produced in the liver but stored in the gallbladder. Bile emulsifies fats after it is secreted into the small intestine. This action enables the enzymes to digest the fats more easily.

Chyme also triggers the pancreas to secrete its juice into the small intestine. Juice secreted from the pancreas contains the following enzymes:

- *Trypsin, chymotrypsin*, and *carboxypeptidases*, which split proteins into smaller substances. These are called pancreatic proteases because they are protein-splitting enzymes produced by the pancreas.
- *Pancreatic amylase*, which converts starches (polysaccharides) to simple sugars. Small intestine
- *Steapsin*, a lipase that reduces fats to fatty acids and glycerol.

The small intestine itself produces an intestinal juice that contains the enzymes *lactase, maltase,* and *sucrase*. These enzymes split lactose, maltose, and sucrose, respectively, into simple sugars. The small intestine also produces enzymes called *peptidases* that break down proteins into amino acids.

ABSORPTION

After digestion, the next major step in the body's preparation of its food is absorption. *Absorption* is the passage of nutrients into the body fluids and tissues. To be absorbed, nutrients must be in their simplest forms. Carbohydrates must be broken down to the simple sugars (glucose, fructose and galactose), proteins to amino acids, and fats to fatty acids and glycerol. Most absorption of nutrients occurs in the small intestine, although some occurs in the large intestine. Water is absorbed in the mouth, stomach, small intestine, and large intestine.

Absorption in the Small Intestine

The small intestine is approximately twenty-two feet long. Its inner surface contains many fingerlike projections called *villi*. Each villus contains numerous blood *capillaries* (tiny blood vessels) and *lacteals* (lymphatic vessels). The villi absorb nutrients from the chyme by way of these blood capillaries and lacteals which eventually transfer them to the bloodstream. Glucose, fructose, galactose, amino acids, minerals, and water-soluble vitamins are absorbed by the capillaries. Fructose and galactose are subsequently carried to the liver where they are converted to glucose. Lacteals absorb glycerol and *fatty acids* (end products of fat digestion), in addition to the fat-soluble vitamins.

Absorption in the Large Intestine

When the chyme reaches the large intestine, most digestion and absorption (except of water) have already occurred. However, some digestive juices are carried into the large intestine in the chyme where they continue their work for a time.

The major tasks of the large intestine are to absorb water and collect *food residue*. Food residue is that part of food body enzyme action cannot digest and consequently cannot absorb. Such residue is also called *fiber* or *bulk*. Examples of fiber include the outer hulls of corn kernels and grains of wheat, celery strings, and apple skins. It is important that the diet contain some bulk since it promotes the health of the large intestine by helping to produce softer stools and more frequent bowel movements.

Undigested food is excreted as feces by way of the rectum. In healthy people, 99 percent of carbohydrates, 95 percent of fat, and 92 percent of protein is absorbed.

METABOLISM

After digestion and absorption, nutrients are carried by the blood to the cells of the body. Within the cells, nutrients are changed into energy through a complex process called metabolism. During metabolism, nutrients are combined with oxygen within each cell. This is known as oxidation. Oxidation reduces carbohydrates and fats ultimately to carbon dioxide and water; proteins are reduced to carbon dioxide, water, and nitrogen.

As nutrients are oxidized, energy and its by-product, heat, are released. When this released energy is used to build new substances from simpler substances, the process is called anabolism. An example of anabolism is the formation of new body tissues. When released energy is used to break down substances into simpler substances, the process is called catabolism. Catabolism occurs in the breakdown of tissue associated with surgery, burns, and during periods of high fever. This building up and breaking down of substances (metabolism) is a continuous process within the body and requires a continuous supply of nutrients. Whenever the body performs work, it uses energy. It does not matter whether the work is voluntary, such as walking and swimming, or involuntary, such as breathing and digesting food. More energy is needed to perform work that is difficult than to perform

work that is easy. The body usually stores an excess of nutrients and is able to use these stores during times of need.

Metabolism and the Thyroid Gland

Metabolism is governed primarily by the secretions of the thyroid gland. These secretions are thyroxine and triiodothyronine (T_3). When the thyroid gland secretes too much of these hormones, a condition known as hyperthyroidism may result. In such a case, the body metabolizes its food too quickly, and weight is lost. When too little thyroxine and T_3 are secreted, the condition called hypothyroidism may occur. In this case, the body metabolizes food too slowly and the patient tends to become sluggish and accumulate fat.

BASAL METABOLISM RATE

Energy is needed for maintenance of body tissue and temperature, for growth and for physical and mental activity. The rate at which energy is needed just for body maintenance is called the basal metabolism rate (BMR). Medical tests can determine a person's BMR. When a BMR test is given, the body is at rest and performing only necessary involuntary functions. Respiration, circulation, cell activity, and maintenance of body temperature are examples of these functions. Voluntary activity is not measured in a BMR test.

DETERMINING ENERGY NEEDS

The unit used to measure the fuel value of foods is the kilocalorie or kcal, commonly known as the "large calorie" or "calorie". In the metric system it is known as the kilojoule.

One kcal is equal to 4.184 kilojoules, but this may be rounded off to 4.2 kilojoules. A kcal is the amount of heat needed to raise the temperature of one kilogram of water one degree Celsius (°C).

The number of kcal in a food is its *caloric value*. Caloric values of foods vary greatly because foods contain varying amounts of nutrients. In addition, nutrients differ in the number of calories they contain. One gram of carbohydrate yields 4 kcal or 17 kilojoules; one gram of protein yields 4 kcal or 17 kilojoules; and one gram of fat yields 9 kcal or 38 kilojoules. The caloric or energy values of foods are scientifically determined by a device known as the *bomb calorimeter*. As a reference, the number of calories in average servings of common foods are listed in Table A-7 of the Appendix.

Calculating Caloric Requirements

A person's average daily *caloric requirement* is the number of kcal needed by an individual in a twenty-four hour period. Caloric requirements of people differ, depending upon basal metabolism rate, age, size, sex, physical condition, activity, and climate.

Children, in proportion to their weight, require more calories than adults because they are growing and are usually more active than adults. As people age, their basal metabolism rates decline and their physical activities are usually reduced. These reductions cause their caloric requirements to be lowered as well.

Tall people with large body frames require more calories than short people with small body frames. Larger people have more body mass to maintain and to move around than do smaller people. Men usually require more food than women. Someone whose physical condition includes pregnancy or lac-

tation, for example, requires more calories than when she is not in such condition. Conversely, someone recuperating with a broken leg requires fewer calories than she or he normally would. People living and working in extremely cold or extremely warm climates require more calories to maintain normal body temperature than they would in a more temperate climate. Activity, however, is the greatest single factor determining energy needs as can be seen in table 2-2.

The Food and Nutrition Board of the National Research Council has made recommendations of energy intakes that meet the average needs of people in categories based on sex, size, and age. See Table 2-3. Obese people and those who are engaged in very sedentary occupations may require fewer kcal than this table indicates.

To determine one's minimum caloric requirement, first determine the basal metabolic rate (BMR). The BMR equals one kcal, per kilogram of body weight, per hour. The BMR, plus 50 percent of that total, equals the person's minimum caloric requirement. To obtain the minimum caloric requirement

1. Change body weight from pounds to kilograms by dividing the body weight by 2.2 (2.2 pounds = 1 kilogram)
2. Multiply the number of kilograms of body weight times 24 (hours per day).
3. Multiply the answer in step 2 by .50 (50 percent).
4. Add the answers in steps 2 and 3. The sum is the daily minimum caloric requirement.

For example, assume a woman weighs 110 pounds.

1. One kilogram equals 2.2 pounds. Therefore, 110 pounds must be divided by 2.2.

Table 2-2 Energy Expenditure in Daily Activities

Activity Category*	Time (hr)	Man, 70 kg		Woman, 58 kg	
		Rate (kcal/ min)	Total [kcal (k J)]	Rate (kcal/min)	Total [kcal (k J)]
Sleeping, reclining	8	1.0-1.2	540(2270)	0.9-1.1	440(1850)
Very light	12	up to 2.5	1300(5460)	up to 2.0	900(3780)
Seated and standing activities, painting trades, auto and truck driving, laboratory work, typing, playing musical instruments, sewing, ironing					
Light	3	2.5-4.9	600(2520)	2.0-3.9	450(1890)
Walking on level 2.5-3 mph, tailoring, pressing, garage work, electrical trades, carpentry, restaurant trades, cannery workers, washing clothes, shopping with light load, golf, sailing, table tennis, volleyball					
Moderate	1	5.0-7.4	300(1260)	4.0-5.9	240(1010)
Walking 3.5-4 mph, plastering, weeding and hoeing, loading and stacking bales, scrubbing floors, shopping with heavy load, cycling, skiing, tennis, dancing					
Heavy	0	7.5-12.0		6.0-10.0	
Walking with load uphill, tree felling, work with pick and shovel, basketball, swimming, climbing, football					
Total	24		2740(11,500)		2030(8,530)

Source: Food and Nutrition Board, National Academy of Sciences, National Research Council, 1980.

* Data from Durnin and Passmore, 1967.

Table 2-3 Mean Heights and Weights and Recommended Daily Energy Intake

Category	Age (years)	Weight (kg)	Weight (lb)	Height (cm)	Height (in.)	Energy Needs (with range) (kcal)		Energy Needs (with range) (MJ)
Infants	0.0–0.5	6	13	60	24	kg × 115	(95–145)	kg × 0.48
	0.5–1.0	9	20	71	28	kg × 105	(80–135)	kg × 0.44
Children	1–3	13	29	90	35	1300	(900–1800)	5.5
	4–6	20	44	112	44	1700	(1300–2300)	7.1
	7–10	28	62	132	52	2400	(1650–3300)	10.1
Males	11–14	45	99	157	62	2700	(2000–3700)	11.3
	15–18	66	145	176	69	2800	(2100–3900)	11.8
	19–22	70	154	177	70	2900	(2500–3300)	12.2
	23–50	70	154	178	70	2700	(2300–3100)	11.3
	51–75	70	154	178	70	2400	(2000–2800)	10.1
	76+	70	154	178	70	2050	(1650–2450)	8.6
Females	11–14	46	101	157	62	2200	(1500–3000)	9.2
	15–18	55	120	163	64	2100	(1200–3000)	8.8
	19–22	55	120	163	64	2100	(1700–2500)	8.8
	23–50	55	120	163	64	2000	(1600–2400)	8.4
	51–75	55	120	163	64	1800	(1400–2200)	7.6
	76+	55	120	163	64	1600	(1200–2000)	6.7
Pregnancy						+300		
Lactation						+500		

Source: Food and Nutrition Board, National Academy of Sciences—National Research Council, 1980

The woman weighs 50 kilograms.

2. Multiply the 50 kilograms by 24 hours. This gives a total of 1200 kcal, the estimated basal metabolism rate.
3. Multiply the 1200 kcal by .50 (50 percent). The total is 600 kcal.
4. Add 1200 kcal plus 600 kcal for a minimum daily caloric requirement of 1800 kcal.

A person who takes in fewer kcal than she or he burns usually becomes thinner. If a person takes in more kcal than she or he burns, the body stores them as *adipose tissue* (fat). Some adipose tissue is necessary to protect the body and support its organs. Adipose tissue also helps to regulate body temperature, just as insulation helps regulate the temperature of a building. An excess of adipose tissue, however, leads to obesity, which can endanger health.

SUMMARY

The body is comparable to an automobile engine because it too requires fuel. Food acts as the fuel, but to be usable it must undergo a series of processes which include digestion, absorption, and metabolism. Digestion is the process whereby food is broken down into smaller parts, chemically changed, and moved along the gastrointestinal tract. Mechanical digestion refers to that part of the process performed by the teeth and muscles of the

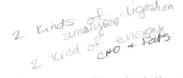
2 Kinds amalyses digestion
2 Kind of energy CHO + Fats

digestive system. Chemical digestion refers to that part of the process wherein food is broken down to nutrients that the blood can absorb. Chemical changes are performed mainly by enzymes. Following digestion, food is absorbed by the blood, primarily in the small intestine, and then carried to all body tissues. After absorption, food is metabolized. During metabolism, food is combined with oxygen in a process called oxidation. Energy released during oxidation is measured by the kcal or kilojoule. Caloric values of foods vary as well as people's caloric (energy) requirements. Requirements vary according to a person's age, size, sex, activity, physical condition, and climate.

Discussion Topics

1. Describe the process of digestion.
2. Of what value are enzymes to digestion? Name 5 enzymes and the nutrients on which they act.
3. Describe absorption of nutrients.
4. Of what value is indigestible residue in the diet? What are some examples of foods that provide it?
5. Describe metabolism.
6. What is the BMR? If anyone in the class has undergone a BMR test, ask her or him to describe it.
7. Explain why the body requires food even during sleep. p.15
8. Why is it incorrect to say, "He ate 2000 calories today"? What did he eat? What are calories? What are joules? How are they comparable?
9. Explain the differences between the terms *caloric value* and *caloric requirement*.
10. What does it mean to be overweight? What is the most common cause faulty diet of overweight? What reasons do people give for being overweight? inherit, gland How can one prevent excessive weight gain? How can overweight people reduce? How may overweight endanger health? balance diet + exercise   mental outlook, motivation

X Ch. 25

Suggested Activities

1. Trace figure 2-1. On the traced figure, insert the names of the body structures without referring back to the original illustration.
2. Using the method of calculating a person's minimum caloric requirement as given in this chapter, calculate your minimum caloric requirement. Convert it to kilojoules.
3. Using table 2-3, and table A-7 (in the Appendix), plan a menu for one

day that would satisfy the caloric requirement of a 40-year-old woman who weighs 120 pounds.

4. Adapt the preceding menu to the needs of a 22-year-old man who weighs 147 pounds.

5. Using table 2-3, and A-7 (in the Appendix), compile a list of foods, especially vegetables, fruits, milk, eggs, and meat, that would satisfy the daily caloric requirement of a woman who is nursing her baby. She is 30 years old and weighs 120 pounds. Compute the grams of protein included.

6. Adapt the preceding menu to the needs of the woman after weaning her baby.

7. Write definitions of the words listed under "Vocabulary".

Review

A. Complete the following statements.
1. Food is broken down for body use during the process known as _digestion_ .
2. Food is combined with oxygen during the process called _oxidation_
3. The tube connecting the mouth and the stomach is the _esophagus_
4. The two kinds of digestive action are _mechanical_ and _chemical_.
5. The rhythmic contraction of the muscular walls of the digestive tract is called _peristalsis_ .
6. Protease, lipase, and amylase are examples of _enzymes of D.I._ .
7. Saliva contains the digestive enzyme called _ptyalin/salivary amylase_
8. Hydrochloric acid, pepsin, and rennin are all secretions of the _stomach_ .
9. The semiliquid mass of food that has been mixed with gastric juices is called _chyme_ .
10. The passage of nutrients into the body fluids and tissues is called _absorption_ .
11. Metabolism is primarily governed by the secretions of the _thyroid gland_ .
12. The unit used to measure the fuel value of food is the _kcal_ or the _kilocalorie_ .
13. The average daily total of calories needed by an individual is called the _caloric requirement_ .
14. A condition of extreme overweight is called _____ .
15. The rate of energy that is needed just for body maintenance is called the _BMR_ .

B. Label the structures on the following diagram.

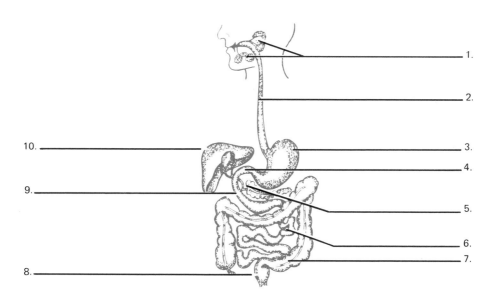

1.

2.

3.

4.

5.

6.

7.

8.

9.

10.

C. In the space opposite each enzyme or secretion, name the structure that *secretes* it.

1. ptyalin — mouth
2. hydrochloric acid — stomach
3. pepsin — stomach
4. rennin — stomach
5. trypsin — small intestine
6. steapsin — small intestine
7. lactase — small intestine
8. maltase — small intestine
9. peptidases — small intestine
10. bile — produce in liver, stored gallbladder

D. Briefly answer the following questions.

1. Name the four steps in computing an individual's minimum caloric requirements.

1 pound to kilogram
2 kilogram × 24
3 × by .50
4 add 2 & 3 together

2. Where does most absorption of nutrients take place?

Small intestines

3. How does an enzyme get its name?

for the substance on which it acts

References

Biology book of choice

Gray, Henry. 1977. *Gray's Anatomy*. New York: Bounty Books.

Green, Marilyn L., and Joann Harry. 1981. *Nutrition in Contemporary Nursing Practice*. New York: John Wiley & Sons.

Howe, Phyllis Sullivan. 1981. *Basic Nutrition in Health and Disease*. Philadelphia: W.B. Saunders Co.

Robinson, Corinne H., and Marilyn R. Lawler. 1982. *Normal and Therapeutic Nutrition*, 16th ed. New York: MacMillan Publishing Company

Suitor, Carol W., and Merrily F. Crowley. 1984. *Nutrition Principles and Application in Health Promotion*. Philadelphia: J.B. Lippincott Co.

Whitney, Eleanor Noss, and Corinne Balog Cataldo. 1983. *Understanding Normal and Clinical Nutrition*. St. Paul: West Publishing Co.

Williams, Sue Rodwell. 1982. *Essentials of Nutrition and Diet Therapy*, 3rd ed. St. Louis: C.V. Mosby Co.

Chapter 3

CARBOHYDRATES AND FATS

OBJECTIVES

After studying this chapter, you should be able to

- Name six sources of carbohydrates and six sources of fat

- Identify the ways in which carbohydrates and fats are classified

- Identify the number of calories provided per gram of carbohydrate or fat

- State the functions of carbohydrates and fats

Energy foods are those that can be rapidly oxidized by the body to release heat and energy. In this chapter, the two major sources of energy (carbohydrates and fats) will be discussed.

CARBOHYDRATES

Carbohydrates are the least expensive and most abundant of the energy nutrients. Foods rich in carbohydrates grow easily in most climates. They keep well and are generally easy to digest. Carbohydrates provide the major source of calories for people all over the world. They provide approximately half the calories for people living in the United States. Carbohydrates are named for the chemical elements they are composed of—carbon, hydrogen, and oxygen.

Functions

Providing energy and heat is the major function of carbohydrates. Each gram of carbohydrate provides 4 kcal (17 kJ). This is the same number of calories provided

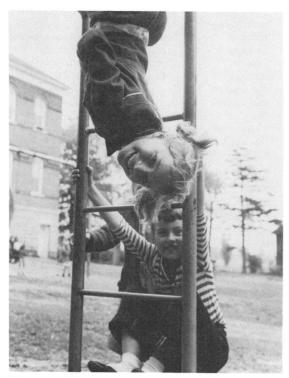

Figure 3-1 Vigorous play is important for children to develop strong muscles and good coordination. They must be supplied with sufficient carbohydrates and fats in their diets to provide adequate energy. (Courtesy of the National Education Association)

by proteins. When carbohydrates provide energy, they spare proteins for another essential use—building and repairing body tissues. This function is known as the *protein sparing action* of carbohydrates. Carbohydrates are also essential for the metabolism of fats.

Food Sources

The principal sources of carbohydrates are plants. Examples of foods rich in carbohydrates are bread, cereals, crackers, macaroni products, rice, potatoes, corn, peas, beans, bananas, apples, pears, sweet desserts, sugars, syrups, honey, and candy.

Classification

Carbohydrates may be divided into three groups: monosaccharides, disaccharides, and polysaccharides.

Monosaccharides (also known as simple or single sugars) are the simplest form of carbohydrates. They are sweet, require no digestion, and can be absorbed directly into the bloodstream from the small intestine. They include *glucose, fructose*, and *galactose. Glucose*, also called dextrose, is the form of carbohydrate to which all other forms are converted for eventual metabolism. *Fructose*, also called levulose and fruit sugar, is found with glucose in many fruits and vegetables, and in honey. It tastes especially sweet. *Galactose* is a product of the digestion of milk. It is not found naturally.

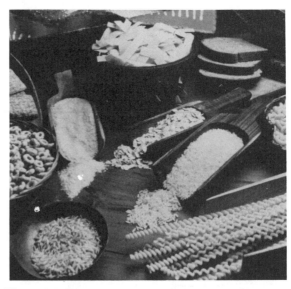

Figure 3-2 Good sources of carbohydrates. (Courtesy of Tupperware)

Table 3-1 Carbohydrates

BEST SOURCES	FUNCTIONS	DEFICIENCY SYMPTOMS
Sugars (monosaccharides and disaccharides) sugars candy, syrups jams and jellies honey molasses cakes and cookies	Furnish heat and energy Aid in metabolism of fats	Loss of weight; fatigue
Starch (polysaccharides) flour macaroni products bread crackers cereals potatoes corn lima beans green peas bananas, pears, apples	Furnish heat and energy Aid in metabolism of fats The fruits and vegetables also provide bulk and some vitamins and minerals	Loss of weight; fatigue

Cellulose (polysaccharide)
bran, whole grain cereals
green and leafy vegetables
fruits, especially
   apples, pears, oranges
   grapefruit
	Provides bulk necessary for peristalsis	Possible constipation

Disaccharides are sometimes called double sugars. They are sweet and must be changed to simple sugars by hydrolysis before they can be absorbed. Disaccharides include *sucrose, maltose,* and *lactose. Sucrose* is the form of carbohydrate present in granulated, powdered and brown sugar, and molasses. It is one of the sweetest and least expensive sugars. Its sources are sugar cane, sugar beets, and the sap from maple trees. *Maltose* is an intermediate product in the digestion of starch within the body. It is manufactured from starch by enzyme action and is not found naturally. *Lactose* is the sugar found in milk. It is distinct from most other sugars because it is not found in plants. Lactose is less sweet than the other single or double sugars. For this reason, it is sometimes added to beverages to increase their caloric value while not greatly changing the flavor.

Polysaccharides are complex compounds of monosaccharides. Their solubility and

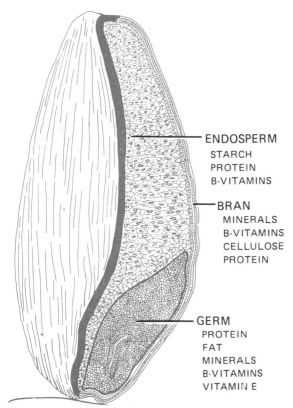

ENDOSPERM
STARCH
PROTEIN
B-VITAMINS

BRAN
MINERALS
B-VITAMINS
CELLULOSE
PROTEIN

GERM
PROTEIN
FAT
MINERALS
B-VITAMINS
VITAMIN E

Figure 3-3 A grain of wheat has three parts. All parts are used in whole wheat flour; only the endosperm is used in white flour.

Wheat germ is included in products made of whole wheat. It may also be purchased and used in baked products or as an addition to breakfast cereals. Wheat germ is a rich source of vitamin B complex, vitamin E, minerals, and protein.

Before the starch in grain can be used for food, the bran must be broken down. The heat and moisture of cooking break this outer covering, making the food more flavorful and more digestible. Although bran itself is indigestible, it is important that some be included in the diet because of the fiber it provides.

Dextrins are digestible polysaccharides that are the intermediate products of the hydrolysis of starch by enzymes or cooking. They form, for example, during the toasting of bread.

Glycogen is sometimes called animal starch because animals store carbohydrates in the form of glycogen. Glucose is converted to glycogen for storage. Glycogen is converted back to glucose when the body requires fuel for heat and energy.

Cellulose, also called roughage, is a fibrous form of carbohydrate that makes up the framework of plants. Cellulose has no energy value and is insoluble and indigestible. It provides bulk for the intestines. Cellulose aids in carrying food along the digestive tract by providing the fiber necessary for normal peristalsis. This action helps to prevent constipation.

The major sources of cellulose are bran, whole grain cereals, and fibrous fruits and vegetables. These foods leave a high residue of cellulose after digestion. Highly processed or refined foods such as white bread, macaroni products, and pastries leave little or no residue because cellulose has been removed during processing.

digestibility vary. They include starch, dextrins, cellulose, and glycogen.

Starch is a polysaccharide found in grains and vegetables. Vegetables contain less starch than grains because vegetables have a higher moisture content. The starch in grain is found mainly in the *endosperm* (center part of the grain). This is the part from which white flour is made. The tough outer covering of grain kernels is called the *bran*, figure 3-3. The bran is used in coarse cereals and whole wheat flour. Although the *germ* is the smallest part of the cereal grain, it is the life center.

Digestion and Absorption

The monosaccharides, (*glucose, fructose,* and *galactose*), are single or simple sugars that may be absorbed from the intestine directly into the bloodstream. They are subsequently carried to the liver where fructose and galactose are changed to glucose.

The disaccharides, *sucrose, maltose,* and *lactose* require an additional step of digestion. They must first be converted to the simple sugar, glucose, before they can be absorbed into the bloodstream.

The polysaccharides are more complex and their digestibility varies. After the cellulose wall is broken down, starch is changed to an intermediate product called *dextrin*; it is then changed to maltose and finally to glucose. Cooking can change starch to dextrin. For example, when bread is toasted, it turns golden brown and tastes sweeter because the starch has been changed to dextrin.

The digestion of starch begins in the mouth where the enzyme ptyalin begins to change starch to dextrin. The second step occurs in the stomach where the food is mixed with gastric juices. The final step occurs in the small intestine where the digestible carbohydrates are changed to simple sugars and subsequently absorbed by the blood.

Metabolism and Elimination

All carbohydrates are changed to the simple sugar glucose before metabolism can take place. After the blood has carried the glucose to the cells, it can be oxidized. Frequently, the volume of glucose that reaches the cells exceeds the amount the cells can use. In these cases, glucose is converted to glycogen and is stored in the liver and muscles. Glycogen is broken down and released as glucose is needed for energy or heat. This process is controlled mainly by the hormone insulin, secreted by the islets of Langerhans in the pancreas. When the secretion of insulin is impaired or absent, as in diabetes, either insulin or a hypoglycemic agent, which stimulates the production of insulin in the pancreas, must be provided. When insulin is given, the diabetic patient's intake of carbohydrates must be carefully controlled to balance the prescribed dosage of insulin.

Oxidation of glucose results in energy and its by-product, heat. With the exception of cellulose, the only waste products of carbohydrate metabolism are carbon dioxide and water. It is a very efficient nutrient.

Dietary Requirements

While there is no specific daily dietary requirement for carbohydrate, the Food and Nutrition Board of the National Research Council recommends that people have at least 50 to 100 grams of digestible carbohydrate each day. A diet seriously deficient in carbohydrate could cause *ketosis* (excessive breakdown of tissue protein) and dehydration. The American Heart Association recommends that 50% of kcal be in the form of carbohydrate. This is also the estimated average amount of carbohydrate in current U.S. diets. Because overweight is a major health problem in the United States, it should be noted that eating an excess of carbohydrates is one of the most common causes of obesity. Although some of the surplus carbohydrate is changed to glycogen, the major part of any surplus becomes adipose tissue. Also, an excess of carbohydrate in the form of sugar can spoil an appetite for other nutrients that are more important. Too many carbohydrates may cause tooth decay, and may irritate the lining

Table 3-2 Fats

BEST SOURCES	FUNCTIONS	DEFICIENCY SYMPTOMS
Butter	Furnish heat and energy	Loss of weight
Lard or lard substitutes	Carry fat-soluble vitamins	Retarded growth
Margarine	Supply essential	Abnormal skin
Meat fats	fatty acids	
Bacon	Give satiety to meals	
Oils		
Nuts		
Cheese		
Cream		
Egg yolk		

of the stomach causing flatus. A deficiency of carbohydrate usually results in loss of weight and possible metabolic problems.

FATS

Fats or lipids furnish the most concentrated form of energy. They are oily substances that are not soluble in water. Each gram of fat provides 9 kcal or 38 kJ. Most foods high in fat are more expensive than those high in carbohydrates. Like carbohydrates, fats are composed of carbon, hydrogen, and oxygen, but in different proportions.

Functions

In addition to providing energy and heat, fats are important in the function and structure of body tissues. Some fats act as carriers of essential fatty acids and vitamins. Fats give a feeling of *satiety* (satisfaction) after meals.

The satisfaction that fats provide is due partly to the flavor they give other foods and partly to their slow rate of digestion, which prevents hunger.

Food Sources

Fats are present in both plants and animals. Examples of foods rich in fat are butter, margarine, cooking oils, mayonnaise, cream, rich pastries, fatty meats, and egg yolk.

Classification

Fats may be classified as visible fats and invisible fats. The *visible fats* are the foods that are purchased and used as fats such as butter, margarine, and cooking oils. *Invisible fats* (hidden fats) are those found in meats, milk, cheese, eggs, and pastries. Fats are further classified as saturated, monounsatu-

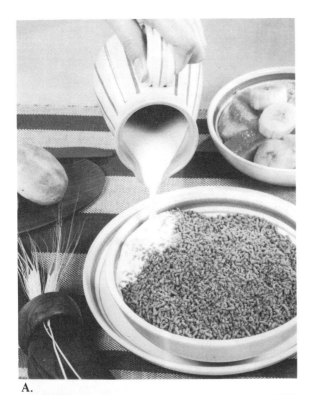

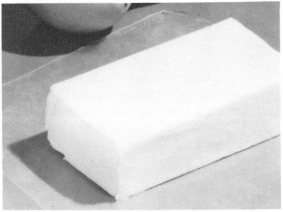

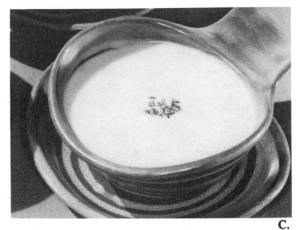

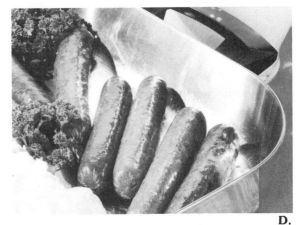

A.

B.

C.

D.

Figure 3-4 A fat may be hidden in other foods or used as a food itself. A. Cream B. Margarine C. Creamed Soup D. Sausage

rated, or polyunsaturated, according to their chemical composition. Fats are composed of fatty acids that can be divided into these three groups.

When a fat is *saturated*, each carbon atom in the fatty acid carries all the hydrogen atoms possible. Examples of saturated fats are the fats in meat, eggs, whole milk, whole milk cheeses, cream, ice cream, butter, hydrogenated fats, and chocolate

If a fat is *monounsaturated*, there is one place among its carbon atoms where there are

Table 3-3 Types of Fat in Common Foods

High in Saturated Fats	High in Polyunsaturated Fats	High in Monounsaturated Fats
Meat—beef, veal*, lamb, pork, and their products, such as cold cuts, sausages	Liquid vegetable oils corn, cottonseed, safflower, soybean	Olive oil
Eggs	Margarines containing	Olives
Whole milk	substantial amounts of the above oils	Avocados
Whole milk cheese	in liquid form	Cashew nuts
Cream, sweet and sour	Fish	
Ice cream	Mayonnaise, salad dressing	
Butter and some margarines	Nuts—walnuts, filberts, pecans, almonds,	
Lard	peanuts	
Hydrogenated shortenings	Peanut butter	
Chocolate	Products made from or with the above	
Coconut and coconut oil		
Products made from or with the above		

Source: Bureau of Nutrition, Dept. of Health, City of New York
*Lean veal is low in total fat

fewer hydrogen atoms attached than in saturated fats. Examples of monounsaturated fats are olive oil, avocados, and cashew nuts.

If a fat is *polyunsaturated*, there are two or more places among its carbon atoms where there are fewer hydrogen atoms attached than in saturated fats. Examples of polyunsaturated fats include vegetable oils, margarines containing liquid vegetable oils, mayonnaise, fish, and peanuts.

Saturated fats are usually solid at room temperature. Polyunsaturated fats are usually soft or oily. Manufacturers add hydrogen to the oily vegetable fats to make them solid. This process, called *hydrogenation*, turns vegetable oils into saturated fats. Margarine is made from the inexpensive vegetable oils in this way. The margarine is churned with milk to enhance its flavor. Vitamin A, and sometimes vitamin D, are added to make it nutritionally equal to butter. When it has been enriched with these vitamins, it is called *fortified* margarine.

A fatty substance called *cholesterol* exists in saturated fats and in body cells. A certain amount of cholesterol is essential for health, and the body manufactures (synthesizes) it from food. There is evidence, however, that an excess of saturated fats in the diet raises the blood cholesterol level which, in turn, increases the probability of heart disease. For this reason, it is advisable to use foods containing the polyunsaturated fats as much as possible, rather than those containing saturated fats.

Digestion and Absorption

The chemical digestion of fats occurs mainly in the small intestine. Fats are not digested in the mouth. They are digested only slightly in the stomach where gastric lipase acts on emulsified fats such as those found in cream and egg yolk. Fats must be mixed well with the gastric juices before entering the small intestine. In the small intestine, bile emulsifies the fats and the enzyme steapsin (pancreatic lipase) reduces them to fatty acids and glycerol, which the body subsequently absorbs. Ninety-five percent of the fats eaten are digested. However, the digestion of fats is very complex. Usually soft fats, or fats that melt at low temperatures, are easier to digest than the hard fats in meats.

Fats are insoluble in water, which is the main component of blood. Because of this, special carriers must be provided for the fats to be absorbed and transported by the blood to body cells. In the initial stages of absorption, bile joins with the products of fat digestion to carry fat. Later, protein combines with the final products of fat digestion to form special carriers called *lipoproteins*. The lipoproteins subsequently carry the fats to the body cells by way of the blood.

Lipoproteins are classified as Very Low Density Lipoproteins (VLDL), Low Density Lipoproteins (LDL) and High Density Lipoproteins (HDL), according to their mobility and density. LDL carry most of the blood cholesterol and are thought to contribute to a heart disease called atherosclerosis (See Chapter 26). HDL carry much less cholesterol and a type that is not thought to contribute to heart disease. The VLDL also carry cholesterol., but it is not known if their cholesterol contributes to heart disease.

Metabolism and Elimination

Fats are carried by way of lipoproteins to body cells where metabolism occurs. Fatty acids are broken down to carbon dioxide and water, releasing energy. The portion of fat that is not needed for immediate use is stored as adipose tissue. Carbon dioxide and water are

waste products that are removed from the body by the circulatory, respiratory, and excretory systems.

Dietary Requirements

Although there is no specific daily dietary requirement for fats, the American Heart Association suggests that people limit their fat intake. They suggest that no more than 30 percent of the total calories should come from fats.

Certainly an excess of fat should be avoided in the diet. Each gram of fat yields more than twice the energy of one gram of carbohydrate or protein, and therefore, an excess can easily cause overweight.

SUMMARY

Energy foods are those that can be rapidly oxidized to release energy and heat. The two major sources of energy are carbohydrates and fats. They are both composed of carbon, hydrogen, and oxygen, but in different amounts. One gram of carbohydrate provides 4 kcalories (17kJ) and one gram of fat provides 9 kcalories (38 kJ). Carbohydrates are less expensive and more abundant than fats.

The principal sources of carbohydrates are plant products such as sugars, breads, cereals, pasta, rice, potatoes, and bananas. In addition to providing energy, carbohydrates are essential for fat metabolism. Digestion of carbohydrates begins in the mouth, continues in the stomach and is completed in the small intestine.

Fats are found in both plants and animals. Specific sources include butter, margarine, cooking oils, mayonnaise, cream, and fatty meats. Besides providing energy, fats are important in the function and structure of body tissues. Some fats are carriers of fatty acids and vitamins. They also give satiety to meals.

Digestion of fats occurs mainly in the small intestine where they are reduced to fatty acids and glycerol. Eating an excess of either fats or carbohydrates can result in obesity.

Discussion Topics

1. What are the three basic groups of carbohydrates? Name several foods in each group.
2. Discuss the effects of regularly eating an excess of carbohydrates.
3. Which polysaccharides (starches) might be considered a dietary staple for the following nationalities?
   - Italian
   - American Indian
   - Mexican
   - French
   - Chinese
4. Why should people eat roughage? Name three sources of roughage.
5. Describe the digestion and metabolism of carbohydrates.
6. Of what value are fats to the body? What are some good food sources of fats.
7. Classify each of the following fats, indicating if they are saturated, monounsaturated, or polyunsaturated. Are they visible or invisible?
   - lard
   - butter
   - vegetable shortening
   - margarine
   - vegetable oil
   - chocolate
8. Describe the digestion and metabolism of fats.
9. Compare the energy yields of carbohydrates and fats. Why does fat provide a more concentrated form of energy than carbohydrate?
10. Which of the two energy nutrients studied in this chapter is generally more expensive to supply through food items? Give reasons why you believe this is true.

Suggested Activities

1. Hold a soda cracker in your mouth until you notice the change in flavor as the starch changes to dextrin.
2. Toast a slice of bread and describe the change in appearance and flavor that occurred in the carbohydrate.

3. Make a chart of the six sugars and their sources discussed in this chapter. Indicate whether they are single or double sugars.
4. Using hospital sources, find out how glucose may be given to patients too weak to take food. Under what circumstances may glucose or sugar foods be given? In what emergencies must the diabetic patient be given sugar?
5. Visit a grocery store. Compare the costs of six foods that are good sources of carbohydrates with six foods that are good sources of fats.
6. Make a list of the foods you have eaten in the past 24 hours. Circle the carbohydrate-rich foods and underline the fats. Approximately what percentage of your calories were in the form of carbohydrate? In the form of fats? Could your diet be improved? If so, how?
7. Trace figure 2-1 in chapter 2. Use it to explain the digestion of carbohydrates using words and arrows.
8. Trace figure 2-1 in chapter 2. Use it to explain the digestion of fats using both words and arrows.
9. Role play a situation between a diet counselor and a teenage girl who has placed herself on an extremely low-calorie diet. She refuses to eat anything that she believes contains fat and will take very little carbohydrate. Explain to her the functions of carbohydrates and fat in the human body.
10. Make a list of foods that contain large amounts of saturated fats. Beside each food listed, write the name of another food that could be used as a substitute, but which contains largely polyunsaturated fats.

Review

A. Multiple choice. Select the *letter* that precedes the best answer.
   1. The three main groups of carbohydrates are
      a. fats, proteins, and minerals
      b. glucose, fructose, and galactose
      c. monosaccharides, disaccharides, and polysaccharides
      d. sucrose, cellulose, and glycogen
   2. Galactose is a product of the digestion of
      a. milk   c. breads
      b. meat   d. vegetables
   3. A simple sugar to which all forms of carbohydrates are ultimately converted is
      a. sucrose   c. galactose
      b. glucose   d. maltose

4. Wheat germ is a source of vitamins
   a. B complex and D
   c. B complex and E
   b. B complex and C
   d. none of these

5. A fibrous form of carbohydrate that cannot be digested is
   a. glucose
   c. cellulose
   b. glycogen
   d. fat

6. Glycogen is stored in the
   a. heart and lungs
   c. pancreas and gallbladder
   b. liver and muscles
   d. small and large intestines

7. Fats may be classified as
   a. visible and invisible
   b. saturated, monounsaturated, and polyunsaturated
   c. neither of the above
   d. both a and b

8. Fats are sometimes called
   a. lipids
   c. lactose
   b. lipoproteins
   d. lacteals

9. Two foods that contain large amounts of saturated fats are
   a. lamb and ice cream
   c. mayonnaise and peanut butter
   b. margarine and jam
   d. chocolate and fish

10. The digestion of fats occurs mainly in the
    a. small intestine
    c. stomach
    b. large intestine
    d. mouth

B. Match the term listed in column II with its definition in column I.

Column I		Column II
C	1. least expensive energy nutrient	a. body fat
a	2. adipose tissue	b. endosperm
j	3. carbohydrate as stored in the liver	c. carbohydrate
l	4. disaccharide	d. four
b	5. center part of grain	e. six
i	6. outer covering of grain	f. nine
d	7. number of calories per gram of carbohydrate	g. glucose
		h. saturated
f	8. number of calories per gram of fat	i. bran
h	9. fats that are solid at room temperature	j. glycogen
k	10. fats that are liquid or soft at room temperature	k. polyunsaturated
		l. sucrose

References

Corbin, Cheryl. 1980. *Nutrition*. New York: Holt Rinehart & Winston.

Eschleman, Marian M. 1984. *Introductory Nutrition and Diet Therapy*. Philadelphia: J. B. Lippincott Company.

Long, Patricia J., and Barbara Shannon. 1983. *Focus on Nutrition*. Englewood Cliffs, New Jersey: Prentice-Hall Inc.

Suitor, Carol W., and Merrily F. Crowley. 1984. *Nutrition Principles and Application in Health Promotion*. Philadelphia: J. B. Lippincott Company.

U. S. Department of Agriculture. 1963, 1975. *Composition of Food*.

Whitney, Eleanor Noss, and Corinne Balog Cataldo. 1983. *Understanding Normal and Clinical Nutrition*. St. Paul: West Publishing Co.

Whitney, Eleanor Noss. 1982. *Nutrition Concepts and Controversies*, 2nd ed. St. Paul: West Publishing Co.

Chapter 4
PROTEINS

VOCABULARY

amino acids	marasmus
coagulate	nitrogen
complete protein	nutritional edema
incomplete protein	proteins
kwashiorkor	textured protein

OBJECTIVES

After studying this chapter, you should be able to

- State the functions of protein in the body
- Identify the elements of which proteins are composed
- Describe the effects of protein deficiency
- State the energy yield of proteins
- Identify at least six food sources of complete proteins and six food sources of incomplete proteins

Body cells are constantly wearing out; as a result, they are continuously in need of replacement. Protein is the basic material of every body cell. It is the only nutrient that can make new cells and rebuild tissue. Therefore, an adequate amount of protein in the diet is essential for normal growth and development and for the maintenance of health. Protein is appropriately named. It is a word of Greek derivation that means "of first importance."

PROTEINS

Like carbohydrates and fats, proteins contain carbon, hydrogen, and oxygen, but in different proportions. In addition, proteins contain nitrogen. Some contain sulfur, phosphorus, iron, and iodine as well. Each gram of protein provides 4 kcal (17 KJ).

Proteins coagulate (thicken) when heated or when acid is added to them. For example, when an egg is cooked, it becomes thick and firm. Meat, eggs, and cheese cooked at too high a temperature become tough. When lemon juice is added to milk, the protein in the milk coagulates, and the milk appears curdled.

Functions

The primary function of protein is to build and repair body tissues. Proteins are important components of hormones and enzymes and as such they play major roles in the regulation of the body processes of digestion and metabolism. They can provide energy if and when the supply of carbohydrates and fats is insufficient.

Classification

Proteins are composed of chemical compounds containing nitrogen that are known as amino acids. These amino acids are sometimes called the building blocks of proteins. Scientists have identified 22 amino acids but found only eight of them to be essential to adult humans and nine necessary for infants, table 4-1. An essential amino acid is one that is necessary for normal growth and development, and must be provided in the diet. A nonessential amino acid can be produced by the body if an adequate supply of nitrogen is provided in the diet.

The quality of a protein depends on the number and types of amino acids it contains. Proteins containing all essential amino acids

Table 4-1 Amino Acids

Essential	Nonessential
Histidine*	Alanine
Isoleucine	Arginine
Leucine	Asparagine
Lysine	Aspartic acid
Methionine	Cysteine
Phenylalanine	Cystine
Threonine	Glutamic acid
Tryptophan	Glutamine
Valine	Glycine
	Hydroxyproline
	Proline
	Serine
	Tyrosine

*Histidine is only known to be essential for infants.

are complete proteins. A complete protein can build and repair tissue. The best sources of complete proteins are animal products.

Incomplete proteins are those that lack one or more of the essential amino acids. Consequently, incomplete proteins cannot build tissue without the help of other proteins. The value of each is increased when it is eaten in combination with another incomplete protein at the same meal. This way one incomplete protein may provide the essential amino acids missing in the other. The combination may thereby provide all nine essential amino acids. Incomplete proteins are found in plant foods.

Food Sources of Proteins

Proteins are found in both animal and plant foods. The animal food sources provide the highest quality, or complete proteins. They include meats, fish, poultry, eggs, milk, and cheese.

Proteins found in plant foods are called incomplete proteins and are of a lower quality than those found in animal foods. Even so, plant foods are important sources of protein. Examples of plant foods containing protein are corn, grains, nuts, sunflower seeds, sesame seeds, and legumes such as soybeans, navy beans, pinto beans, split peas, chick peas, and peanuts.

Plant proteins can be used to produce textured protein products, also called analogs. These products are made by extracting the protein from plants (usually soybeans), and spinning it into fibers of nearly pure protein. The fibers are colored, flavored, and shaped into a product that resembles and tastes like meat. Textured protein can also be used as a filler in other foods, such as ground meat. Textured protein increases the protein content

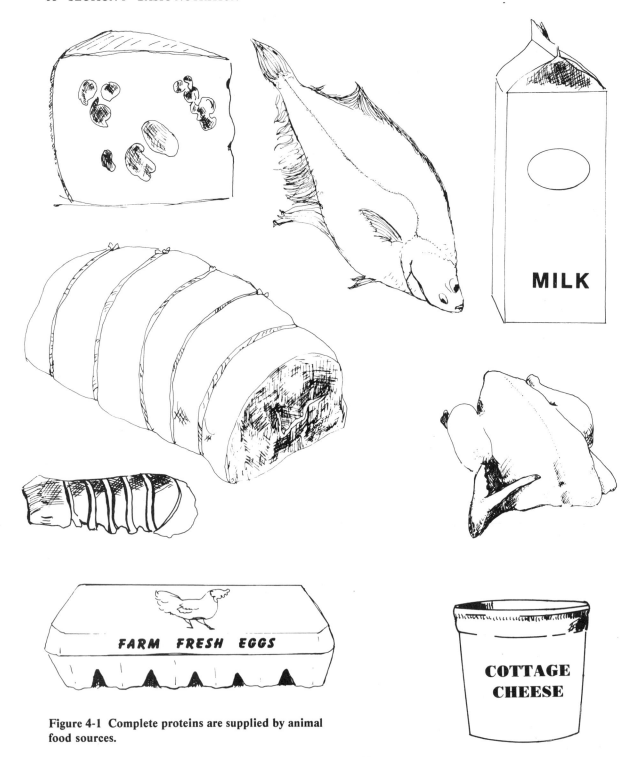

Figure 4-1 Complete proteins are supplied by animal food sources.

of the food to which it is added. It may be used as an economical meat replacement.

Digestion and Absorption

The mechanical digestion of protein begins in the mouth where the teeth grind the food into small pieces. Chemical digestion begins in the stomach. Hydrochloric acid prepares the stomach so the enzyme pepsin can begin its task of reducing proteins to polypeptides. In young children, the enzyme rennin coagulates milk in the stomach, which prevents the milk from passing through the stomach too quickly. Adults do not produce rennin.

After the partially digested proteins (polypeptides) reach the small intestine, three pancreatic enzymes (trypsin, chymotrypsin, and carboxypeptidase) continue chemical digestion. Two intestinal peptidases finally reduce the proteins to amino acids.

After digestion, the amino acids in the small intestine are absorbed by the blood and carried to all body tissues.

Metabolism and Elimination

All essential amino acids must be present to build and repair the cells as needed. Surplus amino acids are sent back to the liver where they are dismantled by splitting off the nitrogen. The remaining parts are used for energy or converted to carbohydrate or fat and stored as glycogen or adipose tissue. The end products of the metabolism of amino acids are carbon dioxide, water, and nitrogen. The excess nitrogen is sent to the kidneys and excreted in urea. Urea is the main end product of human protein metabolism.

Table 4-2 Daily Protein Requirements

	Age (years)	Weight		Height		Protein (g)
		(kg)	(lb)	(cm)	(in)	
Infants	0.0–0.5	6	13	60	24	kg × 2.2
	0.5–1.0	9	20	71	28	kg × 2.0
Children	1–3	13	29	90	35	23
	4–6	20	44	112	44	30
	7–10	28	62	132	52	34
Males	11–14	45	99	157	62	45
	15–18	66	145	176	69	56
	19–22	70	154	177	70	56
	23–50	70	154	178	70	56
	51+	70	154	178	70	56
Females	11–14	46	101	157	62	46
	15–18	55	120	163	64	46
	19–22	55	120	163	64	44
	23–50	55	120	163	64	44
	51+	55	120	163	64	44
Pregnant						+30
Lactating						+20

Source: Food & Nutrition Board, National Academy of Sciences, Washington, D.C. 1980

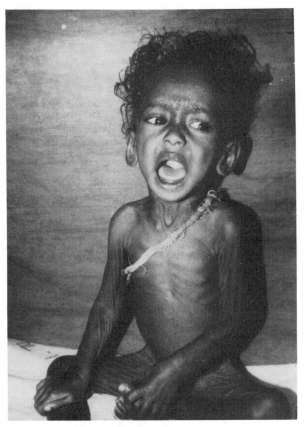

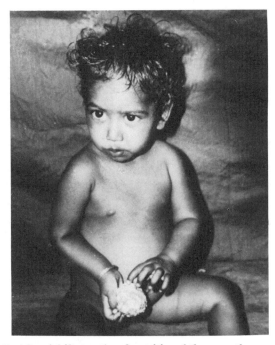

A. Visible signs of marasmus include extreme wasting, wrinkled skin, and irritablity.

B. After 4 1/2 months of nutritional therapy, the same child shows great improvement.

Figure 4-2 A child with marasmus may not recover completely but is greatly helped by nutritional therapy. (*World Health Organization*)

Dietary Requirements

A person's daily protein requirement depends on his size, age, sex, and physical condition. A large person has more body cells to maintain than a small person. A growing child, a pregnant woman, or a woman who is breastfeeding needs more protein per pound of body weight than an average adult. When digestion is inefficient, fewer amino acids are absorbed by the body, consequently raising the protein requirement. In addition, extra protein is usually required after surgery and for patients with severe burns. The Food and Nutrition Board of the National Academy of Sciences has compiled a chart of recommended daily protein allowances for average groups of people, table 4-2.

Nutritional edema may occur when people are unable to obtain an adequate supply of protein. They may lose appetite, strength and weight, and wounds may heal very

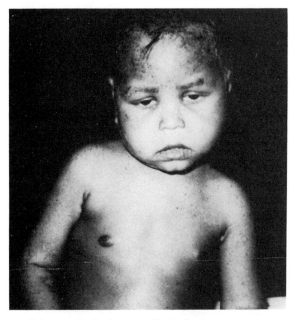

A. Edema, skin lesions, and hair changes are common signs of kwashiorkor.

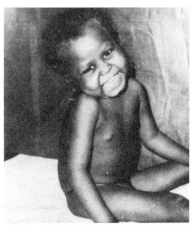

B. Only one month after receiving a proper diet, hunger, discomfort, and visible signs of disease are greatly reduced.

Figure 4-3 Effects of kwashiorkor can be partly eliminated by putting protein back into the diet. (*World Health Organization*)

slowly. Patients suffering from nutritional edema become lethargic and depressed. *Edema* is the retention of fluids in body tissues, resulting in an extremely swollen appearance. This water is excreted when sufficient protein is eaten.

Children who lack sufficient protein do not grow to their potential size. Babies born to mothers eating insufficient protein during pregnancy may have permanently impaired mental capacities. There are two deficiency diseases caused by a grossly inadequate supply of protein that affect children. *Marasmus,* a condition resulting from severe malnutrition, afflicts very young children who lack both protein and energy foods. The infant with marasmus appears emaciated, but does not have edema. Hair is dull and dry, and the skin is thin and wrinkled, figure 4-2. The other protein deficiency disease that affects children is *kwashiorkor.* Kwashiorkor causes fat to accumulate in the liver and results in edema, painful skin lesions, and changes in the pigmentation of skin and hair, figure 4-3. The mortality rate for kwashiorkor patients is high.

SUMMARY

Protein is the only nutrient containing nitrogen, an element that is necessary for growth and the maintenance of health. In addition to building and repairing body tissues, proteins regulate body processes and supply energy. Each gram of protein provides 4 kcalories (17 kJ). Proteins are composed of

Table 4-3 Protein in an Average Diet for One Day

Breakfast Menu	Serving Size	Protein (Grams)	KCAL
Orange Juice	1/2 cup	1	45
Cornflakes	3/4 cup	1	75
with sugar	2 tsp.		30
Toast	2 slices	4	140
Butter	1 Tbsp.		65
Jelly	1 Tbsp		60
Skim Milk	1/2 cup	4	50
Lunch Menu			
Grapefruit Juice	1/2 cup	1	50
Tuna Salad Sandwich	2/3 cup tuna salad	20	220
on Bread	2 slices (bread)	4	140
c/ lettuce			
Carrot Sticks	1 carrot	1	25
Canned Pears	1/2 cup	1	100
Oatmeal Cookies	2	1	160
Skim Milk	1 cup	8	100
Dinner Menu			
Chicken Breast	1/2 (3 oz.)	26	160
Baked Potato	1	4	145
Asparagus	1/2 cup		25
Sliced Tomato Salad	1 tomato	1	25
Roll	1	1	100
with butter	1 Tbsp.		65
Ice Cream	2/3 cup	3	200
Skim Milk	1 cup	8	100
		89	2080

amino acids, nine of which are essential for growth and repair of body tissues. Complete proteins contain all of the essential amino acids and can build tissues. The best sources of complete protein are animal foods such as meat, fish, poultry, eggs, milk, and cheese. Incomplete proteins do not contain all of the essential amino acids and cannot build tissues. The best sources of incomplete proteins are legumes, corn, grains, and nuts. The nutritional value of incomplete protein foods may be increased by eating two or more incomplete protein foods at the same meal. Chemical digestion of proteins occurs in the stomach and small intestine. Proteins are reduced to amino acids and ultimately absorbed into the blood through the small intestine.

A severe deficiency of protein in the diet may cause marasmus or kwashiorkor in children, and may result in impaired physical and mental development.

Discussion Topics

1. Why are proteins especially important to children, pregnant women, and people who are ill?
2. What is the composition of proteins?
3. What functions do proteins perform in the body?
4. After having read chapters 3 and 4, discuss why it may be unwise to use protein foods as energy foods.
5. Discuss protein deficiency and the effects it may have on children and pregnant women.
6. Describe the digestion of proteins.
7. Describe the metabolism of proteins.
8. Tell what amino acids are and explain their importance. Tell where they are found.
9. Describe textured protein products. If anyone in class has eaten textured protein, ask her or him to describe the taste, color, appearance, and cost of the food.
10. Discuss why foods rich in complete proteins are usually more expensive than foods containing incomplete proteins.

Suggested Activities

1. Cook an egg at a low temperature and another at a high temperature. Observe, taste, and discuss the differences. Do the same with two portions of ground meat, being careful not to burn them. What characteristics of protein foods do these demonstrations indicate?
2. Keep a record of the foods you eat in a 24-hour period. Using table A-7 in the Appendix, compute the grams of protein consumed. Did your diet provide the recommended amount of protein as indicated in table 4-2 of this chapter?
3. Make a chart for display in the classroom showing complete and incomplete protein foods.
4. Add 1 teaspoon of lemon juice to 1/2 cup of milk. Observe, taste, and discuss the result.
5. Plan a day's menu for yourself. Include foods especially rich in complete proteins.
   a. Alter your planned menu; replace some of the complete protein foods with those containing incomplete proteins.
   b. Visit a local supermarket and compute the cost of the menu that contains complete proteins. Compute the cost of the menu that contains the incomplete proteins. Which is less expensive? Why?
   c. Adapt the planned menu to suit a 30-year-old pregnant woman, weighing 120 pounds.

Review

A. Multiple Choice. Select the *letter* that precedes the best answer.

1. The building blocks of proteins are
   a. ascorbic acids
   b. amino acids
   c. nitrogen and sulphur only
   d. meat and fish
2. Proteins can
   a. provide energy and heat
   b. build body tissue
   c. repair body tissue
   d. perform all of these functions
3. Corn, peas, and beans
   a. are complete protein foods
   b. are incomplete protein foods
   c. contain no protein
   d. lose proteins during cooking
4. A person's daily protein requirement depends on
   a. current physical condition
   b. height and weight
   c. age and sex
   d. all of these factors
5. Protein deficiency may result in
   a. beriberi   c. nutritional edema
   b. goiter   d. leukemia
6. Good sources of complete protein foods are
   a. eggs and ground beef   c. butter and margarine
   b. breads and cereals   d. legumes and nuts
7. One gram of protein provides
   a. 4 kcal   c. 19 kilojoules
   b. 9 kcal   d. 37.8 kilojoules
8. The chemical digestion of protein occurs in
   a. the mouth and stomach
   b. the mouth and small intestine
   c. the stomach and small intestine
   d. all of these
9. Complete proteins contain all the essential
   a. nutrients   c. amino acids
   b. ascorbic acid   d. kcalories and kjoules
10. The *primary* function of protein is to
    a. build and repair body cells   c. digest minerals and vitamins
    b. provide heat and energy   d. none of these

HW
B. Arrange the following foods into two lists, one containing those that are the best sources of complete proteins and one containing those that are the best sources of incomplete proteins.

scrambled eggs C beefburgers C
lima beans I baked navy beans I
corn on the cob I filet of sole C
hot chocolate milk C fried chicken C
chick peas and rice I peanuts I
skim milk C Swiss cheese C

C. Match the term in column I with its definition in column II.

Column I		Column II
D	1. rennin	a. chemical element in an amino acid
G	2. amino acids	b. disease of severe protein deficiency
I	3. corn	c. reduces proteins to smaller sub-stances in the stomach
C	4. pepsin	
J	5. roast beef	d. coagulates milk
H	6. legumes	e. retention of body fluids
B	7. kwashiorkor	f. carbohydrate
E	8. edema	g. 22 building blocks of protein
A	9. nitrogen	h. lima beans
K	10. textured protein	i. example of incomplete protein
		j. example of complete protein
		k. meat substitute

References

Corbin, Cheryl. 1980. *Nutrition.* New York: Holt Rinehart & Winston.

Eschleman, Marian M. 1980. *Introductory Nutrition and Diet Therapy.* Philadelphia: J. B. Lippincott Company.

Kerschner, Velma L. 1983. *Nutrition and Diet Therapy.* Philadelphia: F. A. Davis Co.

Robinson, Corinne H., and Marilyn R. Lawler. 1982. *Normal and Therapeutic Nutrition,* 16th ed. New York: Macmillan Publishing Company.

U. S. Department of Agriculture. *Composition of Food.* 1963, 1975.

Whitney, Eleanor Noss, and Corinne Balog Cataldo. 1983. *Understanding Normal and Clinical Nutrition.* St. Paul: West Publishing Co.

Whitney, Eleanor Noss. 1982. *Nutrition Concepts and Controversies,* 2nd ed. St. Paul: West Publishing Co.

Chapter 5
MINERALS

OBJECTIVES

After studying this chapter, you should be able to

* List at least two food sources of given mineral elements

* List one or more functions of given mineral elements

* Describe the recommended method of avoiding mineral deficiencies

Chemical analysis shows that the human body is made up of specific chemical elements. Four of these elements—oxygen, carbon, hydrogen, and nitrogen—make up 96 percent of body weight. All the remaining elements, called *mineral elements* or just *minerals*, represent only four percent of body weight. Nevertheless, these minerals are essential for good health.

A *mineral* is an *inorganic* (nonliving) element that is necessary for the body to build tissues, regulate body fluids, or assist in various body functions. Minerals are found in all body tissues. They cannot provide energy by themselves, but in their role as body regulators, they contribute toward the production of energy within the body.

Minerals are found in water and in *natural* (unprocessed) foods, together with proteins, carbohydrates, fats, and vitamins. Minerals in the soil are absorbed by growing plants. Humans obtain minerals by eating plants grown in mineral-rich soil, or by eating animals that in turn have eaten such plants. The specific mineral content of food is determined by burning the food and then chemically analyzing the remaining ash.

Highly processed or refined foods such as sugar and white flour contain almost no minerals. Iron is added to some flour and baked products, which are then labelled *enriched*. foods to which nutrients have been added to improve its nutritional value

Minerals may be divided into two groups. One group contains the major or *macro-*

Table 5-1 Macrominerals and Microminerals

Macrominerals	Microminerals (Trace Elements)
Calcium	Iron
Phosphorus	Copper
Magnesium	Iodine
Sodium	Manganese
Potassium	Zinc
Chlorine	Fluorine
Sulfur	Cobalt
	Chromium
	Molybdenum
	Selenium
	Vanadium
	Tin
	Silicon
	Nickel

minerals, which are required in large amounts. The second group contains the *microminerals* or trace elements. This group is so named because the minerals within it are required in very small amounts. Table 5-1 names the macrominerals and microminerals (trace elements).

Some of these minerals may be referred to as *electrolytes* when they are found in chemical compounds such as salts, acids, and bases. Electrolytes are chemical compounds that break up into separate particles in water. These separate particles are called *ions*. Sodium, potassium, and chloride are often called electrolytes. See Table 5-2.

Scientists lack exact information on some of the trace elements although they do know that trace elements are essential to good health. The study of these elements continues to discover their specific relationships to human nutrition. It must be noted that precisely because of the lack of specific know-

Table 5-2 Estimated Safe and Adequate Daily Dietary Intakes of Minerals

	Age (years)	Trace Elements						Electrolytes		
		Cooper (mg)	Manganese (mg)	Fluoride (mg)	Chromium (mg)	Selenium (mg)	Molybdenum (mg)	Sodium (mg)	Potassium (mg)	Chloride (mg)
Infants	0–0.5	0.5–0.7	0.5–0.7	0.1–0.5	0.01–0.04	0.01–0.04	0.03–0.06	115–350	350–925	275–700
	0.5–1	0.7–1.0	0.7–1.0	0.2–1.0	0.02–0.06	0.02–0.06	0.04–0.08	250–750	425–1275	400–1200
Children and Adolescents	1–3	1.0–1.5	1.0–1.5	0.5–1.5	0.02–0.08	0.02–0.08	0.05–0.1	325–975	550–1650	500–1500
	4–6	1.5–2.0	1.5–2.0	1.0–2.5	0.03–0.12	0.03–0.12	0.06–0.15	450–1350	775–2325	700–2100
	7–10	2.0–2.5	2.0–3.0	1.5–2.5	0.05–0.2	0.05–0.2	0.10–0.3	600–1800	1000–3000	925–2775
	11+	2.0–3.0	2.5–5.0	1.5–2.5	0.05–0.2	0.05–0.2	0.15–0.5	900–2700	1525–4575	1400–4200
Adults		2.0–3.0	2.5–5.0	1.5–4.0	0.05–0.2	0.05–0.2	0.15–0.5	1100–3300	1875–5625	1700–5100

Source: Food and Nutrition Board, National Academy of Sciences—National Research Council, 1980

ledge concerning some of these minerals, it is important that people avoid ingesting large amounts of them. Some can produce toxic effects in the body when taken in large amounts. A balanced diet is the only safe way of including the appropriate amounts of minerals in amounts necessary to maintain health.

The Food and Nutrition Board of the National Academy of Sciences-National Research Council has recommended daily dietary allowances for minerals where research indicates knowledge is adequate to do so. See Table 5-3.

For those minerals where there remains some uncertainty as to amounts of specific human requirements, the Board has provided a table of Estimated Safe and Adequate Daily Dietary Intakes of Selected Minerals, see Table 5-2. The Board recommends that the upper levels of listed amounts not be exceeded habitually.

CALCIUM AND PHOSPHORUS

Calcium and phosphorus together are necessary for the formation of strong, rigid bones and teeth. Calcium also helps maintain normal clotting of the blood and the action of the heart, muscles, and nerves. Phosphorus is important in the metabolism of carbohydrates, fats, and proteins. It is a constituent of all body cells and is necessary for a proper acid-base balance of the blood.

Table 5-3 Recommended Daily Dietary Allowances, Revised 1980

| | | | | | | Minerals | | | | | |
| | | Weight | | Height | | Calcium (mg) | Phos-phorus (mg) | Mag-nesium (mg) | Iron (mg) | Zinc (mg) | Iodine (µg) |
	Age (years)	(kg)	(lb)	(cm)	(in)						
Infants	0.0–0.5	6	13	60	24	360	240	50	10	3	40
	0.5–1.0	9	20	71	28	540	360	70	15	5	50
Children	1–3	13	29	90	35	800	800	150	15	10	70
	4–6	20	44	112	44	800	800	200	10	10	90
	7–10	28	62	132	52	800	800	250	10	10	120
Males	11–14	45	99	157	62	1200	1200	350	18	15	150
	15–18	66	145	176	69	1200	1200	400	18	15	150
	19–22	70	154	177	70	800	800	350	10	15	150
	23–50	70	154	178	70	800	800	350	10	15	150
	51+	70	154	178	70	800	800	350	10	15	150
Females	11–14	46	101	157	62	1200	1200	300	18	15	150
	15–18	55	120	163	64	1200	1200	300	18	15	150
	19–22	55	120	163	64	800	800	300	18	15	150
	23–50	55	120	163	64	800	800	300	18	15	150
	51+	55	120	163	64	800	800	300	10	15	150
Pregnant						+400	+400	+150	h	+5	+25
Lactating						+400	+400	+150	h	+10	+50

Source: Food and Nutrition Board, National Academy of Sciences—National Research Council,

Table 5-4 Minerals

MINERALS	BEST SOURCES	FUNCTIONS	DEFICIENCY SYMPTOMS

Calcium	Milk & products
	Cheese
	Some dark green,
	   leafy vegetables
		Normal development and
		   maintenance of bones and
		   teeth
		Clotting of the blood
		Nerve irritability
		Normal heart action
		Normal muscle activity
		Activates enzymes
			Retarded growth
			Poor tooth and bone
			   formation
			Rickets
			Slow clotting
			   time of blood
			Tetany

Phosphorus	Milk and cheese
	Meat
	Poultry
	Fish
	Whole grain cereals
	Legumes
	Nuts
		Normal development and
		   maintenance of bones
		   and teeth
		Maintenance of normal acid-
		   base balance of the blood
		Constituent of all body cells
		Necessary for effectiveness
		   of some vitamins
		Metabolism of carbohy-
		   drates, fats, and proteins
			Retarded growth
			Poor tooth and bone
			   formation
			Rickets - babies + children
			Weakness
			Anorexia
			Pain in bones
			General malaise
			(Symptoms are rare)

Magnesium	Meat
	Nuts
	Milk
	Cereal grains
	Fresh green vegetables
	Legumes
		Constituent of bones,
		   muscles, and red blood
		   cells
		Necessary for healthy
		   muscles and nerves
		Metabolism
			Unusual heart action
			Mental, emotional, and
			   muscle disorders
			Kidney defects

Sodium	Salt Meat Poultry Fish Eggs Milk	Fluid balance Acid-base balance Osmosis Regulates muscle and nerve irritability Glucose absorption	Nausea Exhaustion Muscle cramps

Potassium	Meat
	Milk
	Vegetables
	Fruits, especially
	   oranges, bananas,
	   and prunes.
		Osmosis
		Fluid balance
		Regular heart rhythm
		Cell metabolism
			Muscle weakness
			Apathy
			Abnormal heartbeat

Chlorine	Salt
	Meat
	Milk
	Eggs
		Osmosis
		Fluid balance
		Acid-base balance
		Formation of hydrochloric
		   acid
			Very rare, but may occur
			   after prolonged vomiting
			Nausea
			Exhaustion

Table 5-4 *Continued*

MINERALS	BEST SOURCES	FUNCTIONS	DEFICIENCY SYMPTOMS
Sulfur	Protein Foods	For building hair, nails, and all body tissues Constituent of all body cells Metabolism	Unknown
Trace Minerals			
Iron	Liver Muscle meats Legumes Dried fruits Egg yolk Whole grain or enriched breads and cereals Dark green and leafy vegetables Potatoes	Essential for formation of hemoglobin of the red blood cells Constituent of cellular enzymes	Anemia characterized by weakness, dizziness, loss of weight, and pallor
Copper	Oysters Nuts Liver Kidney Legumes	Essential for formation of hemoglobin of the red blood cells Component of enzymes	Anemia (see iron) Bone disease
Iodine	Salt water fish Foods grown in soil bordering salt water Iodized salt	Formation of hormones in thyroid gland	Goiter
Manganese	Whole grains Legumes Nuts Vegetables Fruits	Component of enzymes Glucose utilization	Unknown
Zinc	Seafood, especially oysters Liver Meat Eggs Milk	Component of insulin and enzymes Wound healing Taste acuity Essential for growth	Thought to be dwarfism, hypogonadism, anemia Loss of appetite Skin changes Impaired wound healing Decreased taste acuity
Fluorine	Fluoridated water	Increases resistance to tooth decay	Tooth decay
Cobalt	Supplied in Vitamin B_{12}	A component of vitamin B_{12}, necessary for formation of the red blood cells	Unknown

Table 5-4 *Continued*

MINERALS	BEST SOURCES	FUNCTIONS	DEFICIENCY SYMPTOMS
Chromium	Meats Cheese Whole grains	Associated with glucose metabolism May influence protein and fat metabolism	Possibly disturbances of glucose metabolism
Molybdenum	Meats Poultry Cereal Legumes	Constituent of all body tissues and fluids	Unknown
Selenium	Seafood Kidney Liver Muscle meats	Constituent of all tissue	Muscle aches

The best sources of calcium are milk and milk products. Calcium is also found in some dark green leafy vegetables. Phosphorus is obtained from eating milk, cheese, meat, poultry, and fish.

Calcium and phosphorus deficiencies may result in rickets. *Rickets* is a disease that occurs in early childhood and results in poorly formed bone structure. It causes bowed legs and enlarged wrists or ankles. Severe cases can result in stunted growth. Insufficient calcium in the blood may cause a condition characterized by involuntary muscle movement, *tetany*.

After the age of 22 and except during pregnancy and lactation, the recommended allowance of calcium and phosphorus is 800 milligrams for both sexes. Until the age of 22, and during pregnancy and lactation, calcium and phosphorus requirements are higher. Milk and cheese provide large quantities of calcium in small servings. For example, one cup of milk provides 300 milligrams of calcium. One ounce of cheddar cheese provides 250 milligrams of calcium. Phosphorus is widely dis-

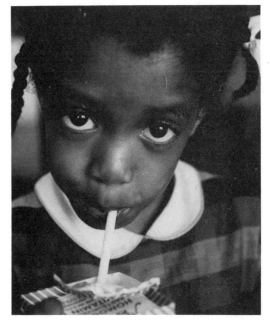

Figure 5-1 Milk is an important source of calcium and phosphorus. These minerals are essential for the normal growth and development of bones and teeth. *(Courtesy of the National Education Association)*

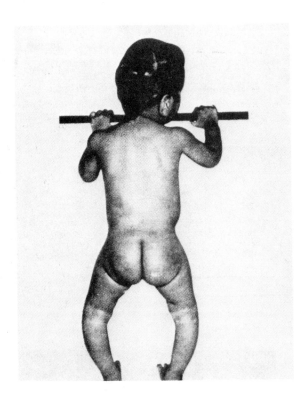

Figure 5-2 One of the symptoms of rickets is bowed legs, a symptom appearing after the child has learned to walk. *(Courtesy of the Upjohn Co., and Dr. R.L. Nemir)*

tributed in foods and therefore a deficiency is rare.

MAGNESIUM

Magnesium is vital to both hard and soft body tissues, and is essential for metabolism. Its deficiency is very rare, but a grossly inadequate diet, an unusual loss of body fluids, or faulty metabolism may cause such a deficiency. This deficiency can result in mental, emotional, and muscular disorders.

Eating a balanced diet is the best method of avoiding magnesium deficiency. See table

5-3 for the recommended daily dietary allowances. Although magnesium is found in nearly all foods, its best sources are meats, milk, cereals, green vegetables, and nuts.

SODIUM, POTASSIUM, AND CHLORIDE

Sodium, potassium, and chloride are essential for normal *osmosis* (the entering and leaving of materials through the body cell walls). These minerals also help maintain the acid-base balance and the fluid balance of the body. Upsets in this balance may result in *dehydration* (loss of body fluid) or edema (abnormal accumulation of body fluids). Edema is frequently associated with *cardio-*

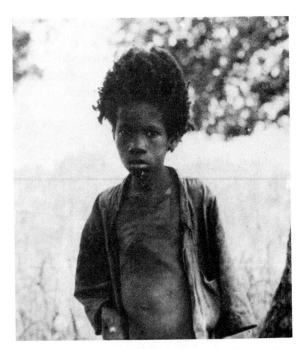

Figure 5-3 Calcium deficiency can cause bone malformation as seen in this child's chest. *(World Health Organization)*

vascular (heart) and *nephritic* (kidney) conditions. In such cases sodium may be restricted in the diet because it contributes to edema.

The metabolism maintains a constant acid-base balance in the body. Cells function best in a neutral or slightly *alkaline* (base) medium. Sodium, potassium, and chloride are essential for maintaining this balance, and deficiencies of these minerals can upset it. If too much acid is lost (which may happen during severe nausea), tetany due to *alkalosis* (too little acid) may develop. If the alkaline reserve is deficient due to starvation or faulty metabolism as in the case of diabetes, *acidosis* (too much acid) may develop.

SULFUR

Sulfur is necessary to all body tissues. It is a component of one of the amino acids and consequently is found in most protein foods. An adequate amount of protein in the diet ensures an adequate supply of sulfur. Its deficiency is unknown.

IRON AND COPPER

Iron and copper are both absolutely essential for healthy blood. Iron is a necessary part of *hemoglobin*, the coloring matter of red blood cells. Hemoglobin allows the red blood cells to combine with oxygen in the lungs and carry it to the body tissues. When red blood cells are worn out, the body collects the used iron and sends it to the *bone marrow* (the soft vascular tissue in the bone center) to be used in the manufacture of new red blood cells. Without copper, the body could not produce these cells.

Red meats (especially liver), egg yolks, dried fruits, whole grain cereals, and legumes are good sources of these minerals. Iron is also present to some extent in dark green leafy vegetables, enriched cereals, and potatoes.

Deficiencies in iron and copper can result in *nutritional anemia.* This is the lack of an adequate number of red blood cells or hemoglobin. Because the bloodstream cannot carry enough oxygen to the cells, the anemic person suffers from dizziness and weakness, which are two symptoms of a lack of oxygen. The person loses weight and has a lowered resistance to disease.

The recommended daily requirement for iron is increased for adolescent girls and women of childbearing age to prevent deficiencies resulting from the effects of menstruation and pregnancy. Women should make a special effort to include iron-rich foods in their diets, particularly during pregnancy and lactation. Iron deficiency is currently the most common nutritional deficiency in the United States.

IODINE

Iodine is necessary for the normal functioning of the thyroid gland. The thyroid gland determines the rate of metabolism. The best sources of iodine are seafood, plants grown in soil near the sea, and iodized salt. *Iodized salt* is common table salt that has had iodine added to it in an amount that, if used in normal cooking, provides sufficient iodine.

When the thyroid gland lacks sufficient iodine, it cannot function normally. This gland then grows larger than it should, forming a lump on the neck called a *goiter*, figure 5-4. If the lack of iodine is severe, it may retard the manufacture of thyroxine (T_4) and triodothyronine (T_3), the hormones secreted by the thyroid gland. This will lower the basal metabolism rate.

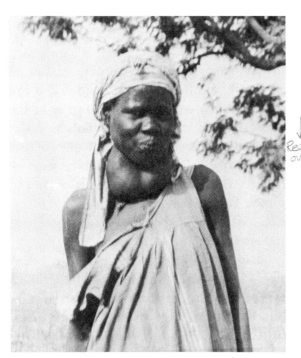

Figure 5-4 In goiter, which results primarily from iodine deficiency, the thyroid gland enlarges. *(Courtesy of the Food and Agriculture organization of the United Nations)*

MANGANESE

Manganese is a constituent of several enzymes and is necessary for glucose utilization. It is found in nuts, legumes, whole grains, vegetables and fruits. Effects of manganese deficiency are unknown.

ZINC

Zinc is a component of several enzymes. It is found in seafood, liver, meat, eggs, and milk. Deficiency symptoms are thought to include dwarfism, hypogonadism, anemia, loss of appetite, skin changes, and impaired wound healing.

FLUORINE

Fluorine increases one's resistance to dental caries. Its principal source is water that contains fluorine. A deficiency of fluorine may result in tooth decay.

COBALT

Cobalt is a component of vitamin B_{12}, which is necessary for the formation of red blood cells. A balanced diet usually provides an adequate amount of this mineral. Effects of its deficiency are unknown.

CHROMIUM

Chromium is associated with glucose metabolism and may also affect protein and fat metabolism. Its principal sources include meats, cheese, and whole grains. Its deficiency symptoms may include disturbances in glucose metabolism.

MOLYBDENUM

Molybdenum is a constituent of all body tissues and fluids. Its primary sources include meats, poultry, cereals, and legumes. Its deficiency symptoms are unknown.

SELENIUM

Selenium is a constituent of all body tissues. Its best sources include seafood, kidney, liver, and muscle meats. Muscle aches are symptomatic of its deficiency.

ADDITIONAL TRACE ELEMENTS

Vanadium, tin, nickel, and silicon have all been identified as essential in laboratory animals, but the specific functions in humans have not yet been identified.

COOKING FOODS CONTAINING MINERALS

Most of the minerals in food occur as salts, which are soluble in water. Therefore, the minerals leave the food and remain in the cooking water. Foods should be cooked in as little water as possible and the cooking liquid saved to be used in soups, gravies, and white sauces. Using this liquid improves the flavor of foods to which it is added. If there is a considerable amount of fat in the liquid, chill the liquid until the fat accumulates on the top. The fat can then be easily removed.

SUMMARY

Minerals are necessary to promote growth and regulate body processes. They are found in soil and water and are ingested via food and drink. Deficiencies can result in conditions such as rickets, anemia, and goiter. A well-balanced diet can prevent these deficiencies. Because minerals are soluble in water, the water used in cooking mineral-rich foods should be saved and used in preparing other foods.

Discussion Topics

1. Discuss the special importance of calcium and phosphorus to children.
2. In class discussions, list ways of supplying an adequate amount of calcium in the diet of an adult who dislikes milk. Plan a day's menu for this adult.
3. Ask if any member of the class has suffered from anemia. If so, ask the class member to describe the symptoms and treatment. What measures are being taken to prevent a recurrence of the condition?
4. What is a goiter? Has anyone observed a goiter? If so, describe it. What causes goiter?
5. If a person were to decrease sodium in her or his diet, should animal foods be increased or decreased?

Suggested Activities

1. Ask a biology teacher to demonstrate the process of osmosis. Discuss its function in the body.
2. Ask a chemistry teacher to explain the properties of acids and alkalies to the class. Have the teacher relate these properties to the uses of minerals by the body.

3. Using outside sources, prepare a report on how sodium and potassium regulate the body's fluid balance.
4. Plan a day's menu. List the minerals found in the foods included.
5. List the foods you have eaten in the past 24 hours. Using Table A-7, list the minerals in these foods. Note whether there appear to be mineral deficiencies. Make a list of foods that could be added to your diet to make up for the mineral deficiencies.
6. Name four foods rich in at least three minerals.
7. Using other sources, write a report on at least one of the following:

Rickets	Hyperthyroidism
Tetany	Diabetes
Nutritional anemia	Edema
Goiter	Dwarfism
Hypothyroidism	Hypogonadism

Review

A. Multiple Choice. Select the *letter* that precedes the best answer.

1. Minerals are inorganic elements that
   a. help to build tissues
   b. are found in all body tissues
   c. regulate various body functions
   d. all of the above

2. The trace elements in the human body are defined as
   a. those minerals that cannot be detected in laboratory tests
   b. those essential minerals found in very small amounts
   c. those minerals that are not essential to health
   d. only those minerals that are found in the blood

3. Calcium is necessary for
   a. healthy bones and teeth
   b. normal clotting of the blood
   c. action of the heart and muscles
   d. all of the above

4. Phosphorus is found in
   a. poultry and fish   c. vegetable oils
   b. common table salt   d. leafy vegetables

5. The coloring matter of the blood is
   a. hemoglobin   c. marrow
   b. lymph   d. plasma

6. Some of the common symptoms of nutritional anemia are
   a. muscle spasms and pain in the liver
   b. bowed legs and an enlarged thyroid gland
   c. edema and loss of vision
   d. dizziness and weakness

7. Iodine is essential to health because it
   a. is necessary for red blood cells
   b. strengthens bones and teeth
   c. helps the blood to carry oxygen to the cells
   d. affects the rate of metabolism

8. Sodium is often restricted in cardiovascular and nephritic conditions because it
   a. causes the heart to beat slowly
   b. encourages the growth of the heart
   c. contributes to edema
   d. raises the blood sugar

9. Iron is known to be a necessary component of
   a. thyroxine   c. hemoglobin
   b. adipose tissue   d. amino acids

10. Liquid from cooking vegetables should be used in preparing other dishes because
    a. mineral salts are soluble in water
    b. the hydrogen and oxygen in water aid the digestion of minerals
    c. the amino acids are soluble in water
    d. none of the above

B. Complete the following statements.

1. This mineral is essential for healthy bones and teeth. Its best sources are milk and cheese. It works closely with phosphorus. It is calcium.

2. This mineral is essential for the formation of hemoglobin. Some of its best sources are meats, legumes, and whole grain cereals. It works closely with copper. It is iron.

3. This mineral is essential for a healthy thyroid gland. Its best natural sources are seafood and foods grown in soil bordering the sea. It is iodine.

4. This mineral is essential for osmosis, maintenance of body neutrality, and water balance. It is sometimes restricted in cardiovascular conditions. It works closely with chloride. It is sodium.

5. This trace mineral increases resistance to tooth decay. It is fluorine.

6. This mineral is essential for healthy muscles and nerves. It is found in meat, milk, cereal grains, and fresh green vegetables. Its deficiency

may result in mental, emotional, and muscular disorders. It is
magnesium .

7. This mineral is essential for regular heart rhythm. It is found in meats, oranges, bananas, and prunes. Its deficiency may result in an abnormal heartbeat. It is _potassium_ .

8. This mineral is essential in the production of red blood cells. It works closely with iron. It is found in organ meats. Its deficiency may result in anemia. It is _copper_ .

9. This mineral is essential for healthy bones and teeth. It is found in milk and meats. It works closely with calcium. It is _phosphorus_ .

10. This mineral, along with sodium and potassium, is essential for normal osmosis. It is found in table salt, meat, milk, and eggs. It is _chloride_.

C. Match the item in column I with its description in column II.

	Column I	Column II
E	1. nutritional anemia	a. red coloring matter in blood
H	2. bone marrow	b. the passing of materials through cell walls
A	3. hemoglobin	
K	4. goiter	c. involuntary muscle movement
J	5. iodized salt	d. disease resulting in poorly formed bones
B	6. osmosis	
C	7. tetany	e. lack of iron
D	8. rickets	f. dry from loss of water
G	9. trace element	g. essential mineral needed in very small amounts
F	10. dehydrated	h. soft tissue filling bone cavity
		i. salt with iodine removed
		j. salt with iodine added
		k. enlarged thyroid gland

References

Howe, Phyllis Sullivan. 1981. *Basic Nutrition in Health and Disease.* Philadelphia: W. B. Saunders Co.

Kerschner, Velma L. 1983. *Nutrition and Diet Therapy.* Philadelphia: F. A. Davis Co.

U. S. Department of Agriculture. *Composition of Food.* 1963, 1975.

Whitney, Eleanor Noss. 1982. *Nutrition Concepts and Controversies*, 2nd ed. St. Paul: West Publishing Co.

Whitney, Eleanor Noss, and Eva May Nunnelley Hamilton. 1984. *Understanding Nutrition*, 3rd ed. St. Paul: West Publishing Co.

Williams, Sue Rodwell. 1984. *Mowry's Basic Nutrition and Diet Therapy*, 7th ed. St. Louis: C. V. Mosby Co.

Winick, Myron. 1980: *Nutrition in Health and Disease*. New York: John Wiley & Sons.

Chapter 6
VITAMINS

VOCABULARY

amenorrhea	hemolysis	phylloquinone
anorexia	hemorrhage	pigmentation
anticoagulant	hormone	polyuria
ascorbic acid	hypercholesteremia	precursor
avitaminosis	hypervitaminosis	prohormone
azotemia	hypocalcemia	provitamin
beriberi	International Units	pyridoxine
biotin	(IU)	pyridoxal
carotene	megaloblastic	pyridoxamine
catalyst	anemia	retinol
cheilosis	menaquinones	Retinol Equivalent
cholecalciferol	mucous membrane	(RE)
coagulation	niacin	riboflavin
cobalamins	niacin equivalent	scurvy
coenzyme	osteomalacia	thiamin
collagen	osteoporosis	tocopherols
ergocalciferol	pantothenic acid	tryptophan
fat soluble	pellagra	vitamers
folic acid	perenteral	water soluble
glossitis	pernicious anemia	xerophthalmia

OBJECTIVES

After studying this chapter, you should be able to

* State one or more functions of each of the vitamins discussed

* Identify at least two food sources of each of the vitamins discussed

* Identify some symptoms of, or diseases caused by, deficiencies of the vitamins discussed

BACKGROUND

Vitamins are organic compounds that are essential for body processes. Vitamins themselves do not provide energy; they enable the body to use the energy provided by fats, carbohydrates, and proteins. The name *vitamin* implies their importance. *Vita* in Latin, means life.

The existence of vitamins has been known since early in the twentieth century. It was discovered that animals fed diets of pure proteins, carbohydrates, fats, and minerals did not thrive as did those fed normal diets that included vitamins.

Vitamins were originally named by letter. Subsequent research has shown that many of the vitamins that were originally thought to be a single substance were actually groups of substances doing similar work in the body. Vitamin B proved to be more than one compound—B_1, B_6, B_{12}, etc.—and consequently is now known as "B complex". Many vitamins are currently named according to their chemical composition or function in the body.

Vitamins are found in minute amounts in natural foods. The specific amounts and types of vitamins in foods vary.

HUMAN REQUIREMENTS

The Food and Nutrition Board, National Academy of Sciences-National Research Council has prepared a list of RDA (recommended daily allowances) for those vitamins for which it considers current scientific research adequate for such determinations. (See Table 6-1.) In addition, the Board has also prepared a list of estimated safe and adequate daily dietary intakes of selected vitamins for which current research is inadequate to allow them to propose RDA. (See Table 6-2.)

Vitamin allowances are given by weight, milligrams (mg.), or micrograms (mcg. or μg.) in most cases, as in the tables, but sometimes, as on food labels, amounts of A, D, and E are listed as I.U. (International Units).

Vitamin deficiencies can occur and can result in disease. However, a person who eats a well-balanced diet usually avoids vitamin deficiencies. The term *avitaminosis* means "without vitamins." This word followed by the name of a specific vitamin is used to indicate a serious lack of that particular vitamin. *Hypervitaminosis* is the excess of one or more vitamins. Either a lack or excess of vitamins can be detrimental to a person's health.

Extra amounts of vitamins taken beyond those received in the diet are called *vitamin supplements*. These are available in concentrated forms in tablets, capsules and drops. Vitamin concentrates are sometimes termed natural or *synthetic* (man made). Some people believe a meaningful difference exists between the two types and that the natural are far superior in quality to the synthetic.

However, according to the United States Federal Drug Administration (FDA), the body cannot in any way distinguish between a vitamin of plant or animal origin and one manufactured in a laboratory since once they have been dismantled by the digestive system, both types of the same vitamin are chemically identical.

Synthetic vitamins are frequently added to foods during processing. When this is done, the foods are described as *enriched* or *fortified*. Examples of these foods are enriched breads and cereals to which thiamin, niacin, riboflavin, and the mineral iron have been added. Vitamins A and D are added to milk, and vitamin A is added to fortified margarine. Occasionally vitamins are lost during food processing. In most cases, food producers can replace these vitamins with synthetic vitamins, making the processed food nutritionally equal to the natural, unprocessed food. Foods in which vitamins are replaced are called *restored* foods.

Because some vitamins are easily destroyed by light, air, heat, and water, it is important to know how to preserve the vitamin content of food during its preparation and cooking. To avoid vitamin loss, it is advisable to

- Buy the freshest, unbruised vegetables and fruits. Use them raw whenever possible.
- Prepare fresh vegetables and fruits just before serving.
- Heat canned vegetables quickly and in their own liquid.
- Follow package directions when using frozen vegetables or fruit.
- Use as little water as possible when

Table 6-1 Recommended Daily Vitamin Allowances

	Age (years)	Weight (kg)	(lb)	Height (cm)	(in)	Fat-Soluble Vitamins Vita-min A (µg RE)	Vita-min D (µg)	Vita-min E (mg α-TE)	Water-Soluble Vitamins Vita-min C (mg)	Thia-min (mg)	Ribo-flavin (mg)	Niacin (mg NE)	Vita-min B-6 (mg)	Fola-cin (µg)	Vitamin B-12 (µg)
Infants	0.0–0.5	6	13	60	24	420	10	3	35	0.3	0.4	6	0.3	30	0.5
	0.5–1.0	9	20	71	28	400	10	4	35	0.5	0.6	8	0.6	45	1.5
Children	1–3	13	29	90	35	400	10	5	45	0.7	0.8	9	0.9	100	2.0
	4–6	20	44	112	44	500	10	6	45	0.9	1.0	11	1.3	200	2.5
	7–10	28	62	132	52	700	10	7	45	1.2	1.4	16	1.6	300	3.0
Males	11–14	45	99	157	62	1000	10	8	50	1.4	1.6	18	1.8	400	3.0
	15–18	66	145	176	69	1000	10	10	60	1.4	1.7	18	2.0	400	3.0
	19–22	70	154	177	70	1000	7.5	10	60	1.5	1.7	19	2.2	400	3.0
	23–50	70	154	178	70	1000	5	10	60	1.4	1.6	18	2.2	400	3.0
	51+	70	154	178	70	1000	5	10	60	1.2	1.4	16	2.2	400	3.0
Females	11–14	46	101	157	62	800	10	8	50	1.1	1.3	15	1.8	400	3.0
	15–18	55	120	163	64	800	10	8	60	1.1	1.3	14	2.0	400	3.0
	19–22	55	120	163	64	800	7.5	8	60	1.1	1.3	14	2.0	400	3.0
	23–50	55	120	163	64	800	5	8	60	1.0	1.2	13	2.0	400	3.0
	51+	55	120	163	64	800	5	8	60	1.0	1.2	13	2.0	400	3.0
Pregnant						+200	+5	+2	+20	+0.4	+0.3	+2	+0.6	+400	+1.0
Lactating						+400	+5	+3	+40	+0.5	+0.5	+5	+0.5	+100	+1.0

Reproduced from: Recommended Dietary Allowances, 9th Edition (1980), with the permission of the National Academy of Sciences, Washington, D.C.

Table 6-2 Estimated Safe and Adequate Daily Dietary Intakes of Selected Vitamins

	Age (years)	Vitamin K (μg)	Biotin (μg)	Pantothenic Acid (mg)
Infants	0–0.5	12	35	2
	0.5–1	10–20	50	3
Children	1–3	15–30	65	3
and	4–6	20–40	85	3–4
Adolescents	7–10	30–60	120	4–5
	11+	50–100	100–200	4–7
Adults		70–140	100–200	4–7

Reproduced from: Recommended Dietary Allowances, 9th Edition (1980), with the permission of the National Academy of Sciences, Washington, D.C.

cooking and have it boiling when adding vegetables.

- Cover the pan (except for the first few minutes when cooking strongly flavored vegetables such as broccoli and cauliflower), and cook as short a time as possible.
- Save the cooking liquid for later use in soups, stews, and gravies.
- Store fresh vegetables and most fruits in a cool, dark place.

CLASSIFICATION

Vitamins are commonly grouped according to solubility. A, D, E, and K are fat soluble, and B complex and C are water soluble. In addition, vitamins A and D are sometimes classified as *hormones* (substances that produce specific biological effects) and the B complex group may be classified as *catalysts* or *coenzymes*. (Catalysts and enzymes are substances that cause chemical changes in other substances. A coenzyme is the active part of an enzyme.) When a vitamin has different chemical forms but serves the

same purpose in the body, these forms are sometimes called *vitamers*. Vitamin E is an example of this. Sometimes a *precursor*, or a *provitamin* is found in foods. This is a substance from which the body can *synthesize* (manufacture) a specific vitamin. Carotene in vitamin A is an example of this.

FAT-SOLUBLE VITAMINS

The fat-soluble vitamins, A, D, E, and K, are chemically similar. They are not lost easily in cooking and can be stored in the liver. Deficiencies are slower to appear than those caused by lack of the water-soluble vitamins. The use of mineral oil interferes with the absorption of fat-soluble vitamins and should be discouraged.

Vitamin A

Vitamin A consists of two basic dietary forms: preformed vitamin A, *retinol*, and provitamin A, *carotene*.

Vitamin A is essential for maintaining healthy eyes, skin, and bone growth. In addition, it aids in the prevention of infections by helping to maintain healthy *mucous membranes* (the lining of the nose and throat, the gastrointestinal tract, and genitourinary tract).

Preformed vitamin A or retinol is found in fat-containing animal foods such as fish liver oils, liver, butter, cream, whole milk, whole milk cheeses, and egg yolk. It is also found in foods such as margarine, lowfat milk products, and cereals that have been fortified with vitamin A. Provitamin A or carotene is found in yellow and dark green leafy vegetables, in yellow fruits, cream, and butter.

Some carotene is converted into retinol during absorption in the intestines. Some is converted in the liver, after being carried there by the blood, and some is stored in adipose tissue.

Deficiency symptoms of vitamin A include night blindness; dry, rough skin; and increased susceptibility to infections. Avitaminosis A can result in blindness or *xerophthalmia*, a condition characterized by dry, lusterless, mucous membranes of the eye.

A well-balanced diet is the preferred way to obtain the required amounts of vitamin A. The use of vitamin supplements should be discouraged as an excess of vitamin A can have serious consequences. Hypervitaminosis A can result in loss of appetite and hair, dry skin, unusual *pigmentation* (coloring of the skin), and bone pain.

Vitamin A values are commonly listed as IU on commercial food products in the United States, but the term *retinol equivalents* (RE) is becoming more common (See table 6-1). A retinol equivalent is equal to 3.33 IU of retinol, 1 μg retinol or 6 μg beta carotene (a particular type of carotene).

See table 6-1 for the recommended daily dietary allowances as prescribed by the Food and Nutrition Board of the National Research Council-National Academy of Sciences.

Vitamin D

Vitamin D exists in two forms—D_3 (*cholecalciferol*) and D_2 (*ergocalciferol*). Each is formed from a provitamin when irradiated with (exposed to) ultraviolet light. They are equally effective in human nutrition, but D_3 is the one that is formed in humans from cholesterol in the skin. D_2 is formed in plants. Vitamin D is considered a *prohormone* because it is converted to a hormone in the human body.

The major function of vitamin D is the regulation of calcium and phosphorus metabolism in the body. Vitamin D raises the concentration of calcium and phosphorus in the blood so that normal bone mineralization can occur and tetany is prevented. (Tetany can occur when there is too little calcium in the blood. This condition is called *hypocalcemia*.) Consequently, vitamin D is essential for strong bones and teeth.

The best source of vitamin D is the sun which, as previously discussed, changes a provitamin to vitamin D_3 in humans. It is sometimes referred to as "the sunshine vitamin". The amount of vitamin D that is formed depends on the individual's pigmentation and the amount of sunlight available. The best food sources of vitamin D are fatty fish, liver, eggs, cream, and butter. Because of the rather limited number of food sources of vitamin D and the unpredictability of sunshine, health authorities decided that the vitamin should be added to a common food. Milk was selected. Consequently, most milk available in the United States today has had 400 IU (10 mcg.) of vitamin D concentrate added per quart.

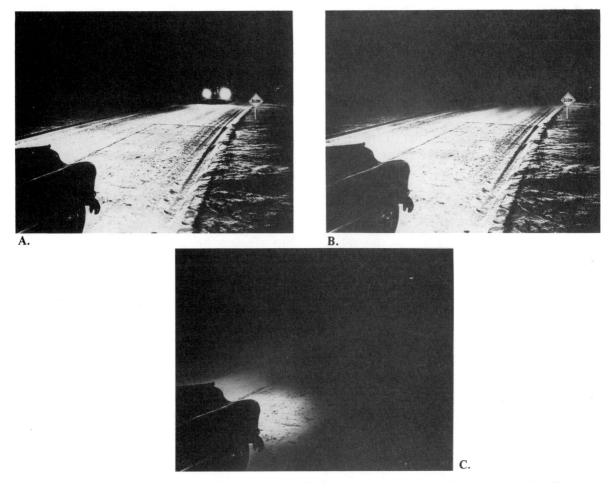

Figure 6-1 Both the normal individual and the person suffering from a deficiency of vitamin A see the headlights of an approaching car (A). After the car has passed, the normal individual sees a wide stretch of road (B). The vitamin-A deficient person cannot see the the road at all (C). This reaction to the contrast of light and dark at night is termed "night blindness." *(Courtesy of the Upjohn Company, Kalamazoo, Michigan)*

Vitamin D is heat stable and not easily oxidized so it is not harmed by storage, food processing, or cooking. It is absorbed through the intestines and is taken up by the liver and the kidney. Excess amounts of it are stored in the liver and in adipose tissue. Its deficiency may result in rickets (see Chapter 5) in children or *osteomalacia* (a softening of the bones because of a loss of calcium) in adults.

And it is thought that vitamin D may increase calcium absorption in patients with *osteoporosis*, a disease characterized by brittle, porous bones, which is common in people over 50 years of age, especially women.

Hypervitaminosis D must be avoided because it can cause calcium and phosphorus deposits in soft tissues of the body. Symptoms of hypervitaminosis D include nausea, weakness, *anorexia* (loss of appetite), weight loss, *polyuria* (excessive production of urine), *azotemia* (abnormally large amounts of nitrogen in the blood), kidney, heart, and aortic damage.

Vitamin D has commonly been measured in IU, but scientists are currently expressing its values in weight, specifically, micrograms of cholecalciferol. One IU equals .025 mcg. (μg) cholecalciferol.

While the vitamin D requirement has not been established, the Food and Nutrition Board, National Academy of Sciences-National Research Council has provided recommended daily dietary allowances. (See Table 6-1.) It is believed that the needs of most adults can be met by an average exposure to sunlight. People who are seldom outdoors should use dietary sources also. Drinking one quart of irradiated milk each day fulfills the recommended daily dietary allowance for people from birth to nineteen years of age and pregnant and lactating women over the age of 22, and more than fulfills the RDA for all others.

Vitamin E

Vitamin E consists of several chemical compounds of similar structure called *tocopherols* (these tocopherols may be referred to as vitamers). The precise function of vitamin E in humans has not been well defined, but it appears to be essential for the protection of cell structure, particularly of the red blood cell. Studies indicate that vitamin E is essential for normal reproduction in some animals, but there is no evidence that it is essential for human reproduction. Some people claim that vitamin E concentrate helps prevent or cure heart disease, cancer, muscular dystrophy, sterility, ulcers, burns, and other skin prob-

lems. These claims have not been substantiated by clinical evidence. Vitamin E has antioxidant properties and is used in commercial food products to retard spoilage.

While vitamin E is widely distributed in foods, wheat germ and vegetable and seed oils are some of its best sources. Other good sources include leafy vegetables, egg yolk, legumes, peanuts, and margarine. Animal foods are generally poor sources of vitamin E.

Vitamin E deteriorates when it is exposed to light and bleach so a great deal is lost during commercial food processing and cooking. Nevertheless, because of its wide availability, a deficiency of vitamin E is rare, but it is thought to have occurred in some premature infants. Clinical symptoms of vitamin E deficiency have not been observed, but laboratory studies have shown an increase in the rate of hemolysis (the destruction of red blood cells) and signs of muscle loss. The average American diet is thought to contain sufficient amounts of vitamin E. (See table 6-1 for the RDA.) Excess vitamin E is stored in adipose tissue. Toxic effects from overingestion have not been observed.

Vitamin E was previously measured in IU, but scientists now use milligrams of TE (tocopherol equivalent). One mg. TE may range from 1.1 to 1.49 IU, depending on the specific tocopherol.

Vitamin K

Vitamin K is found naturally in two forms—vitamin K_1 (*phylloquinone*) in green plants, and K_2 (*menaquinones*) in bacteria, animals, and humans.

Vitamin K is necessary for proper clotting of the blood. It may be given to newborns immediately after birth since their supply is naturally inadequate for a few days following birth. It may be given to patients who suffer from faulty fat absorption; to patients after extensive antibiotic therapy; as an antidote for an overdose of anticoagulant (blood thinner); or to treat cases of *hemorrhage* (bleeding).

Approximately half of the vitamin K in the body comes from food, in the form of phylloquinone. The other half is synthesized by bacteria in the intestines—menaquinones.

The best food sources of vitamin K are green leafy vegetables such as spinach, cabbage, or kale. Fruits, cereals, dairy products, and meats also provide some, but generally, the animal sources are the poorest.

Vitamin K is resistant to heat and air exposure, but it is destroyed by light, alkalis, and strong acids.

The only deficiency symptom found has been in animals, and is characterized by defective blood *coagulation* (clotting), which causes an increase in clotting time, making the patient more prone to hemorrhage. Human deficiency would be caused by faulty fat metabolism or extensive *antibiotic therapy* (ingestion of antibiotic drugs to combat infection), which interferes with the bacterial synthesis of vitamin K.

Vitamin K is absorbed like fats, but from both the small and large intestines. Although little is stored in the body, it is important that an excess be avoided as hypervitaminosis K can cause liver and kidney damage. It is considered so toxic in excessive amounts that its inclusion in supplements is carefully regulated.

Vitamin K is measured in micrograms. The Food and Nutrition Board, National Academy of Sciences-National Research Council provides an estimated daily requirement that averages two mcg. per kilogram of body weight, only half of which need be supplied in the diet since half is synthesized in the intestine by bacteria.

WATER-SOLUBLE VITAMINS

Water-soluble vitamins include B complex and C. These vitamins dissolve in water and are easily destroyed by air and cooking. They are not stored in the body to the extent that fat-soluble vitamins are stored.

Vitamin B Complex

Toward the end of the nineteenth century, a doctor in Indonesia discovered that chickens that were fed table scraps of polished rice developed symptoms much like those of his patients suffering from beriberi. When these same chickens were later fed brown (unpolished) rice, they recovered.

Some years later, this mysterious component of unpolished rice was recognized as an essential food substance and was named vitamin B. Subsequently, it was named vitamin *B complex* because the vitamin was found to be composed of several compounds. The B complex vitamins include thiamin (B_1), riboflavin, niacin, B_6, cobalamin (B_{12}), folacin, pantothenic acid, and biotin.

Thiamin

Thiamin, originally named vitamin B_1, is essential for carbohydrate metabolism. It is found in many foods, but generally in very small quantities. (See table A-7 in the appendix). Some of the best natural food sources of thiamin are dry yeast, wheat germ, pork, and organ meats. Most breads and cereals in the United States are enriched with thiamin so that the majority of people can and do easily fulfill their recommended daily dietary requirements (See table 6-1). Thiamin is measured in milligrams.

Thiamin is partially destroyed by heat and by alkalis, and is lost in cooking water. It is absorbed in the small intestine.

Symptoms of its deficiency include loss of appetite, fatigue, nervous irritability, and constipation. An extreme deficiency causes beriberi. Its deficiency is rare, however, occurring mainly among alcoholics whose diets include reduced amounts of thiamin while their requirements of it are increased and their absorption of it is decreased. Others at risk include renal patients undergoing long-term dialysis; patients fed intravenously for long periods; patients with chronic fevers; and people consuming large amounts of raw fish.

Riboflavin

Riboflavin is also called B_2. It is essential for carbohydrate, fat, and protein metabolism. It is also necessary for tissue maintenance, especially the skin around the mouth, and for healthy eyes.

It is widely distributed in both plant and animal foods, but in small amounts. Organ meats, milk, green leafy vegetables, and enriched breads and cereals are some of its richest sources. It is sensitive to light and unstable in alkalis.

Because of the small quantities of riboflavin in foods, deficiencies of riboflavin may develop. The generous use of milk in the diet is a good way of preventing a deficiency of this vitamin.

A deficiency of riboflavin can result in *cheilosis*, a condition characterized by sores on the lips and cracks at the corners of the mouth; dermatitis; and eye strain in the form of itching, burning, eye fatigue, and headache.

Riboflavin is absorbed from the small intestine. It is stored in very limited amounts in the body, and its toxicity is unknown. It is measured in milligrams (see table 6-1).

Niacin

Niacin is the generic name for nicotinic acid and nicotinamide. Niacin serves as a coenzyme in energy metabolism and consequently is essential to every body cell. In addition, niacin is essential for the prevention of *pellagra*. Pellagra is a disease characterized by sores on the skin, diarrhea, anxiety, and general irritability.

The best sources of niacin are meats, poultry, and fish. Enriched breads and cereals also contain some. Milk and eggs do not provide niacin per se, but they are good sources of its precursor, *tryptophan* (Tryptophan is an amino acid.). Vegetables and fruits contain very little.

Niacin is fairly stable in foods. It can withstand reasonable amounts of heat and acid and is not destroyed during food storage.

A deficiency of niacin is apt to appear if there is a deficiency of riboflavin. Symptoms of niacin deficiency include weakness, anorexia, indigestion, anxiety, and irritability.

Niacin is measured as Niacin Equivalents (NE). One NE equals one milligram of niacin or 60 milligrams of tryptophan. The general recommendation is a daily intake of 6.6 NE per 1,000 kcal. Because excessive amounts of niacin have been observed to adversely affect the heart and liver, self-prescribed doses of niacin concentrate should be discouraged.

Vitamin B_6

Vitamin B_6 is composed of three vitamers—*pyridoxine, pyridoxal*, and *pyridox-*

amine. It is essential for protein metabolism and affects the conversion of tryptophan to niacin.

Although information on the vitamin B_6 content of food is limited, some of its best sources appear to be pork, organ meats, legumes, bananas, and potatoes.

Vitamin B_6 is absorbed in the small intestine. It is stable to heat, but sensitive to light and alkalis.

Deficiency in adults can result in depression, confusion, convulsions, dermatitis, and anemia. In infants, deficiency can retard growth, cause weight loss, vomiting, anemia, convulsions, and general irritability.

It is measured in milligrams and the need varies with the protein intake. Generally, the requirement is .02 milligrams per gram of dietary protein.

Folacin

Folacin, also known as folic acid, is necessary for protein metabolism and the formation of hemoglobin.

Its best sources are green leafy vegetables, liver, kidney, fish, nuts, legumes, and whole grain cereals.

A deficiency of folacin can result in glossitis, gastrointestinal disburbances and *megaloblastic anemia*. Megaloblastic anemia is a condition wherein red blood cells are large and immature, and cannot carry oxygen properly.

Some forms of folacin are destroyed by storage, processing, heat or acids, and some are not. The addition of ascorbic acid during food processing appears to preserve the folacin content of food.

Folacin is measured in micrograms. During pregnancy, lactation, and periods of growth and stress, the regular requirement for folacin is increased.

Vitamin B_{12}

Vitamin B_{12} is a group of compounds called *cobalamins* that contain the mineral cobalt. It is thought to be involved with metabolism and is essential for healthy red blood cells and nerve tissue. It is given *parenterally* (by intravenous or intramuscular injections) as treatment for pernicious anemia. *Pernicious anemia* is a severe blood disease characterized by a decrease in the number of red blood cells. The anemia is caused by a body defect that inhibits red blood cell formation. The number of cells decreases but the size of the cells increases.

The best food sources of B_{12} are animal foods, especially meat, seafood, eggs, and dairy products. It is fairly stable in cooking, but can be destroyed by extremely high temperatures. It is stored in the liver.

Its deficiency is rare and is thought to be caused by problems of absorption, or from years of a strict vegetarian diet that contains no animal foods. Symptoms of vitamin B_{12} deficiency include sore mouth and tongue and *amenorrhea* (abnormal lack of menstruation).

Pantothenic Acid

Pantothenic acid is involved in the metabolism of carbohydrates, fats, and proteins. The word *pantothenic* is of Greek derivation and means "from many places". This is appropriate as this vitamin is found extensively in foods, especially animal foods. Its best sources are organ meats, salmon, eggs, yeast, whole grain cereals, and legumes. Deficiency symptoms of pantothenic acid include vomiting, abdominal cramps, cramping and weakness in the legs, and insomnia. Its recommended daily dietary allowances have not been established, but the Food and Nutrition Board has given an estimated intake in Table 6-2.

Biotin

Biotin participates as a coenzyme in human metabolism. Some of its best sources are liver, kidney, heart, mushrooms, and peanuts.

Deficiency symptoms include nausea, anemia, anorexia, depression, muscle pain, and *hypercholesteremia* (excessive amount of cholesterol in the blood.)

Biotin is measured in micrograms. Although RDA have not been established, the Food and Nutrition Board has provided suggested daily dietary intakes (see Table 6-2).

Vitamin C

Vitamin C is also known as *ascorbic acid*. It appears to have several functions in the human body, but they are not yet well understood. It is known that the absorption of iron is increased when iron and vitamin C are ingested at the same time, and that it prevents *scurvy*. Scurvy is a disease characterized by bleeding gums, loose teeth, sore joints and muscles, and weight loss. In extreme cases it can result in death. Vitamin C has an important role in the formation of *collagen*, a protein substance that holds body cells together, making it necessary for wound healing. It is thought to be essential for the metabolism of amino acids and folic acid. In addition, it is believed by some people to reduce the number and severity of colds. Some of the best sources of vitamin C are citrus fruits, tomatoes, potatoes, melon, and strawberries.

Vitamin C has anti-oxidant properties and so protects other foods from oxidation. However, it is readily destroyed by heat, air, and alkalis.

The clinical symptoms of scurvy include flesh that is easily bruised; tiny, pin-point hemorrhages of the skin, bones, and joints; easily-fractured bones; poor wound-healing and *gingivitis* (soft, bleeding gums, and loose teeth).

Vitamin C is measured in milligrams with the average adult in the United States requiring 60 milligrams per day under normal circumstances. In times of stress, this need is increased.

Vitamin C is absorbed in the small intestine.

It is generally considered non-toxic, but this has not been ascertained. It is known that an excess can cause diarrhea, nausea, cramps, and an excessive absorption of food iron.

SUMMARY

Vitamins are organic compounds that regulate body functions and promote growth. Each vitamin has a specific function or functions within the body. Food sources of vitamins vary, but generally a well-balanced diet provides sufficient vitamins to fulfill body requirements. Vitamin deficiencies can result from inadequate diets or from the body's inability to utilize vitamins. Vitamins are available in concentrated forms, but their use should be carefully monitored since overdoses can be detrimental to health. Vitamins A, D, E, and K are fat-soluble. Vitamin B complex

Table 6-3 Vitamins

VITAMINS	BEST SOURCES	FUNCTIONS	DEFICIENCY SYMPTOMS
Fat-Soluble Vitamins Vitamin A	Fish liver oils Liver Butter, margarine (fortified) Whole milk, cream, cheese Egg yolk Vegetables (leafy green and yellow) Fruits (yellow)	Growth Health of eyes Structure and functioning of the cells of the skin and mucous membranes	Functional disorders of the eye (night blindness) Increased susceptibility to infections Changes in skin and membranes Xerophthalmia
Vitamin D	Sunshine Fatty fish Milk (irradiated) Egg yolk Liver Cream Butter	Growth Regulating calcium and phosphorus metabolism Building and maintaining normal bones and teeth	Rickets Poor tooth development Osteomalacia
Vitamin E	Wheat germ and wheat germ oils Vegetable oils Margarine Legumes Peanuts Dark green, leafy vegetables Egg yolk	Considered essential for protection of cell structure, especially of red blood cell	Increased rate of hemolysis of the red blood cells
Vitamin K	Spinach Kale Cabbage Cereals	Normal clotting of blood	Defective blood clotting
Water-Soluble Vitamins Thiamine (B_1)	Wheat germ Lean pork Yeast Legumes Whole grain and enriched cereal products Liver Heart Kidney	Carbohydrate metabolism	Loss of appetite Irritability Fatigue Constipation Beriberi
Riboflavin	Milk, cheese Enriched bread and cereals Green, leafy vegetables Liver, kidney, heart	Carbohydrate, fat, and protein metabolism Health of the mouth tissue Healthy eyes	Cheilosis Eye sensitivity

Table 6-3 *continued*

VITAMINS	BEST SOURCES	FUNCTIONS	DEFICIENCY SYMPTOMS
Niacin	Meats (especially organ meats) Poultry and fish Enriched breads and cereals	Prevention of pellagra Carbohydrate, fat, and protein metabolism	Skin eruptions Diarrhea Nervous disorders Anorexia Pellagra
Vitamin B_6	Pork Organ meats Legumes Bananas Potatoes	Metabolism of proteins	Anemia Dermatitis Confusion Depression Convulsions Nausea
Vitamin B_{12}	Liver, kidney Muscle meats Milk, cheese Eggs	Metabolism Healthy red blood cells Treatment of pernicious anemia	Anemia Sore mouth & tongue Amenorrhea
Folacin	Dark green, leafy vegetables Liver Fish Whole grain cereals Legumes	Metabolism Formation of hemoglobin	Anemia Glossitis Diarrhea Gastrointestinal disturbances
Pantothenic Acid	Heart, liver, kidney Eggs, Salmon, Yeast Peanuts, Legumes Whole grain cereals	Metabolism of carbo-hydrates, fats and proteins	Vomiting Abdominal cramps Leg cramps Insomnia
Biotin	Organ Meats Mushrooms Peanuts	Metabolism	Nausea Muscle pain Depression Anorexia Hypercholesteremia Anemia
Vitamin C (Ascorbic Acid)	Citrus fruits, pineapple Melons Berries Tomatoes Cabbage Broccoli Green Peppers	Maintaining collagen Healthy gums Aids in wound healing Aids in absorption of iron	Sore gums Tendency to bruise easily Scurvy

and Vitamin C are water-soluble. Water-soluble vitamins can be destroyed during food preparation. It is important that care is taken during the preparation of food so as to preserve its vitamin content.

Discussion Topics

1. How do vitamins help to provide energy to the body?
2. Discuss possible times when avitaminosis of one or more vitamins may occur.
3. Discuss any vitamin deficiencies that class members have observed. What treatments were prescribed?
4. Discuss why it may be unwise for anyone but a physician to prescribe vitamin supplements.
5. Discuss the terms enriched, fortified, and restored. What do they mean in relation to food products? Name foods that are enriched, fortified, or restored.
6. Discuss the proper storage and cooking of foods to retain their vitamin content.
7. If any member of the class has experienced night blindness ask her or him to describe it. Discuss how this condition occurs, how it may be alleviated and how it can be prevented.
8. Ask if any class member has observed a child with rickets. Discuss the appearance of a child with rickets. Discuss how this disease can be prevented.
9. Why is it advisable to use liquids left over from vegetable cooking? How might these be used?
10. Why are fewer vitamins lost during cooking when the vegetables are cooked whole than when they are cooked in smaller pieces?
11. Explain the role of vitamin C in collagen formation and wound healing.
12. The addition of baking soda to green vegetables during cooking helps to maintain their color. Why is this not advisable?
13. If anyone in the class has taken concentrated vitamin C, ask why. If it was useful, ask why.
14. Why are some vitamins being called prohormones? Coenzymes?
15. What is a precursor? A prohormone? Give an example or two.
16. Discuss appropriate nutritional advice for a 60-year old woman whose doctor has suggested she drink one quart of milk per day, and she says she cannot.
17. What are vitamers? Give some examples.

18. Discuss appropriate nutritional advice for a young mother who is giving her four-year old 50 mcg. of vitamin D each day.
19. What are some possible reasons for a vitamin K deficiency?
20. If only half of the daily vitamin K requirement is supplied by the diet, how is the other half obtained?
21. What nutrients are commonly added to breads and cereals in the United States?
22. What is beriberi, and how can it be prevented?
23. Why should milk be sold in opaque containers?
24. Discuss appropriate nutritional advice for a young woman who has been on a very strict vegetarian diet for six months and says she intends to continue.

Suggested Activities

1. Prepare two packages of a frozen vegetable. Cook one package according to the directions on the package and the other in 2 cups of water for 30 minutes. Compare them for palatability. Discuss their probable vitamin and mineral content.
2. Many foods are described as enriched, fortified, and restored. Visit a supermarket and make lists of foods described by each term.
3. Write a menu for one day that is especially rich in the B-complex vitamins. Underline the foods that are the best sources of these vitamins.
4. Organize a "spelldown", asking the functions and sources of vitamins.
5. List the foods you have eaten in the past 24 hours. Write the name of a vitamin beside the food for which it is a rich source. What percentage of your day's food did *not* contain vitamins? Could this diet be nutritionally improved? How?
6. Plan a day's menu for a person who has been instructed to eat an abundance of foods rich in vitamin A.
7. Cut two slices of a peach. Leave one slice exposed to the air and pour lemon juice on the other. Set aside for five minutes. Describe what happened (or did not happen) to each slice and explain why.

Review

A. Multiple Choice. Select the *letter* preceding the best answer.

1. The daily vitamin requirement is best supplied by

a. eating a well-balanced diet
b. eating one serving of citrus fruit for breakfast
c. taking one of the many forms of vitamin supplements
d. eating at least one serving of meat each day

2. All of the following measures preserve the vitamin content of food except
    a. using vegetables and fruits raw
    b. preparing fresh vegetables and fruits just before serving
    c. adding, raw, fresh vegetables to a small amount of cold water and heating to boiling
    d. storing fresh vegetables in a cool place

3. Fat-soluble vitamins
    a. cannot be stored in the body
    b. are lost easily during cooking
    c. are dissolved by water
    d. are slower than water-soluble vitamins to exhibit deficiencies

4. Night blindness is caused by a deficiency of
    a. vitamin A
    b. thiamin
    c. niacin
    d. vitamin C

5. Good sources of thiamin include
    a. citrus fruits and tomatoes
    b. wheat germ and liver
    c. carotene and fish-liver oils
    d. nuts and milk

6. Water-soluble vitamins include
    a. A, D, E, and K
    b. A, B_6, and C
    c. thiamin, niacin, and retinol
    d. thiamin, riboflavin, niacin, B_6, B_{12}

7. Injections of vitamin B_{12} are given in the treatment of
    a. scurvy
    b. pernicious anemia
    c. pellagra
    d. beriberi

8. Blindness can result from a severe lack of
    a. vitamin K
    b. vitamin A
    c. thiamin
    d. vitamin E

9. Organ meats are good sources of the following vitamins:
    a. thiamin, riboflavin, B_{12}
    b. biotin, vitamin C
    c. vitamins E and K
    d. all of these

10. Irradiated milk is a good source of
    a. vitamin E
    b. vitamin D
    c. vitamin K
    d. vitamin C

11. Good sources of Vitamin C are
    a. meats
    b. milk and milk products
    c. breads and cereals
    d. citrus fruits

12. The vitamin that aids in the prevention of rickets is
    a. vitamin A   c. vitamin C
    b. thiamin   (d.) vitamin D
13. The vitamin that is necessary for the proper clotting of the blood is
    a. vitamin A   c. vitamin D
    (b.) vitamin K   d. niacin
14. The three vitamins that are commonly added to breads and cereals
    are
    a. vitamins A, D, and K
    (b.) thiamin, riboflavin, and niacin
    c. vitamins E, B_6, and B_{12}
    d. ascorbic acid, pantothenic acid, and folacin
15. The vitamin that is known to prevent scurvy is
    a. vitamin A   (c.) vitamin C
    b. vitamin B complex   d. vitamin D

B. Match the vitamins listed in column I with their characteristics listed in
   column II.

Column I	Column II
_F_ 1. vitamin A	a. also called vitamin C
_H_ 2. thiamin	b. also called amino acids
_L_ 3. riboflavin	c. essential for reproduction in some animals
_J_ 4. niacin	d. substance the body converts to vitamin A
_C_ 5. vitamin E	e. primarily found in polished rice
_I_ 6. vitamin D	f. deficiency causes night blindness
_G_ 7. vitamin B_{12}	g. best-known treatment for pernicious anemia
_A_ 8. ascorbic acid	h. extreme deficiency may cause beriberi
_K_ 9. vitamin K	i. severe deficiency may result in rickets
_D_ 10. carotene	j. deficiency may cause pellagra
	k. essential for proper clotting of the blood
	l. deficiency may cause cheilosis

C. Briefly answer the following questions.
   1. What vitamins are fat soluble? Name three characteristics of fat-
      soluble vitamins. A,D,E,K
      Not lost easily in cooking
      Can be stored in the liver
      Defencies are slower to appear than those
      caused by lack of H_2O soluble vitamins

2. What vitamins are water soluble? Name three characteristics of water-soluble vitamins. *dissolve in H₂O*

B complex + C   *easily destroyed by air and cooking*
not stored in the body to the same extent
that fat soluble vitamins are stored

References

American Dietetic Association. 1981. *Handbook of Clinical Dietetics*. Yale University.

Corbin, Cheryl. 1980. *Nutrition*. New York: Holt Rinehart & Winston.

Eschleman, Marian M. 1984. *Introductory Nutrition and Diet Therapy*. Philadelphia: J. B. Lippincott Company.

Long, Patricia J., and Barbara Shannon. 1983. *Focus on Nutrition*. Englewood Cliffs, N. J.: Prentice-Hall Inc.

U. S. Department of Agriculture. *Composition of Food*. 1963, 1975.

Whitney, Eleanor Noss. 1982. *Nutrition Concepts and Controversies*, 2nd ed. St. Paul: West Publishing Company.

Winick, Myron. 1980. *Nutrition in Health and Disease*. New York: John Wiley & Sons.

Section 2
Meal Planning

Chapter 7

DIETARY GUIDELINES

VOCABULARY

balanced diet

Basic Four food
groups

dietary guidelines

edible portion

hypertension

legumes

meat alternates

RDA

satiety

serving size

sweetbreads

OBJECTIVES

After studying this chapter, you should be able to

* List and explain the reasons for the U.S. Government's Dietary Guidelines

* Define a balanced diet

* Identify the Basic Four food groups

* Identify the chief nutrients provided by each of the four food groups

* Identify at least two foods contained in each of the four food groups

* State the recommended number of servings per day from each food group

The statement, "eat a balanced diet," has been repeated so many times that its importance is overlooked. Its value is so great, however, that it deserves serious consideration by people of all ages. A *balanced diet* is one that includes all the essential nutrients in amounts that preserve and promote good health.

THE BASIC FOUR FOOD GROUPS

The Food and Nutrition Board of the National Academy of Sciences-National Research Council has developed *recommended daily dietary allowances* (commonly known as the RDA) of the essential nutrients

Table 7-1 Recommended Daily Dietary Allowances

	Age (years)	Weight (kg)	Weight (lb)	Height (cm)	Height (in)	Protein (g)	Fat-Soluble Vitamins Vitamin A (µg RE)	Vitamin D (µg)	Vitamin E (mg α-TE)
Infants	0.0–0.5	6	13	60	24	kg × 2.2	420	10	3
	0.5–1.0	9	20	71	28	kg × 2.0	400	10	4
Children	1–3	13	29	90	35	23	400	10	5
	4–6	20	44	112	44	30	500	10	6
	7–10	28	62	132	52	34	700	10	7
Males	11–14	45	99	157	62	45	1000	10	8
	15–18	66	145	176	69	56	1000	10	10
	19–22	70	154	177	70	56	1000	7.5	10
	23–50	70	154	178	70	56	1000	5	10
	51+	70	154	178	70	56	1000	5	10
Females	11–14	46	101	157	62	46	800	10	8
	15–18	55	120	163	64	46	800	10	8
	19–22	55	120	163	64	44	800	7.5	8
	23–50	55	120	163	64	44	800	5	8
	51+	55	120	163	64	44	800	5	8
Pregnant						+30	+200	+5	+2
Lactating						+20	+400	+5	+3

Reproduced from: Recommended Dietary Allowances, 9th Edition (1980), with the permission of the National Academy of Sciences, Washington, D.C.

whose human requirements have been established (see Table 7-1). In addition, the nutritive values of the edible portions of foods have been determined and can be seen in Table A-7.

Daily review of these tables would certainly provide enough information to plan balanced diets. However, ordinary meal planning would be impossibly cumbersome and time-consuming if these tables had to be consulted each time a meal was planned. Fortunately, nutritionists have devised an elementary method that simplifies planning a balanced diet.

This simplified method of planning a balanced diet is based on the Basic Four food groups:

- vegetables and fruits
- milk and milk products
- breads and cereals
- meat and meat alternates

A thorough knowledge of these food groups makes planning nutritious meals fast and easy.

In using this simple guide, it is essential that the diet be selected primarily from these four broad food groups with additional foods included in amounts appropriate to one's energy requirements. The foods should be eaten as three meals plus snacks as desired. The body uses energy constantly and should be refueled at regular intervals.

Table 7-1 *Continued*

Water-Soluble Vitamins							Minerals					
Vitamin C (mg)	Thiamin (mg)	Riboflavin (mg)	Niacin (mg NE)	Vitamin B-6 (mg)	Folacin (μg)	Vitamin B-12 (μg)	Calcium (mg)	Phosphorus (mg)	Magnesium (mg)	Iron (mg)	Zinc (mg)	Iodine (μg)
35	0.3	0.4	6	0.3	30	0.5	360	240	50	10	3	40
35	0.5	0.6	8	0.6	45	1.5	540	360	70	15	5	50
45	0.7	0.8	9	0.9	100	2.0	800	800	150	15	10	70
45	0.9	1.0	11	1.3	200	2.5	800	800	200	10	10	90
45	1.2	1.4	16	1.6	300	3.0	800	800	250	10	10	120
50	1.4	1.6	18	1.8	400	3.0	1200	1200	350	18	15	150
60	1.4	1.7	18	2.0	400	3.0	1200	1200	400	18	15	150
60	1.5	1.7	19	2.2	400	3.0	800	800	350	10	15	150
60	1.4	1.6	18	2.2	400	3.0	800	800	350	10	15	150
60	1.2	1.4	16	2.2	400	3.0	800	800	350	10	15	150
50	1.1	1.3	15	1.8	400	3.0	1200	1200	300	18	15	150
60	1.1	1.3	14	2.0	400	3.0	1200	1200	300	18	15	150
60	1.1	1.3	14	2.0	400	3.0	800	800	300	18	15	150
60	1.0	1.2	13	2.0	400	3.0	800	800	300	18	15	150
60	1.0	1.2	13	2.0	400	3.0	800	800	300	10	15	150
+20	+0.4	+0.3	+2	+0.6	+400	+1.0	+400	+400	+150	+30	+5	+25
+40	+0.5	+0.5	+5	+0.5	+100	+1.0	+400	+400	+150	+30	+10	+50

The listed minimum number of servings is taken from each of the four food groups. Serving sizes vary according to the type of food and the individual eating the food. Pregnant women or mothers who are breast feeding require additional milk.

It is advisable to have some meat, poultry, fish, eggs, milk or a milk product at each meal. The protein that is generously provided in these foods gives satiety (satisfying fullness) to meals.

The Vegetable and Fruit Group

All vegetables and fruits are included in this group. Those vegetables and fruits that are especially rich sources of vitamins A and C are emphasized. Four or more servings of different fruits and vegetables should be eaten each day. Foods in this group provide sugar and cellulose in addition to vitamins A, E, K, B complex, and C, and the minerals iron, calcium, phosphorus, potassium, and magnesium. One-half cup of each is considered an average serving.

The best sources of vitamin C are the juicy fruits and the dark green vegetables. Fruits and vegetables that are dark green or yellow are good sources of vitamin A. Sometimes the same fruit or vegetable is an excellent source of both vitamins A and C. At least one serving from the fruit and vegetable group should be selected from those high in vitamin A and one from those high in vitamin C. The remaining two or more servings can be selected according to taste from other available

Table 7-2 Vegetable and Fruit Group

Vitamin C sources		Vitamin A sources
Oranges	Cantaloupe	Carrots
Lemons	Raw or lightly	Squash
Grapefruit	cooked cabbage	Spinach
Limes	Green peppers	Kale
Tomatoes	Turnip greens	Other greens
Raspberries	Broccoli	Apricots
Strawberries	Potatoes	Pumpkin
Pineapple	Brussels sprouts	Sweet potatoes
		Cantaloupe

Table 7-3 Milk and Milk Products Group

Whole fluid milk	Skim milk
Condensed milk	Dry milk
Evaporated milk	Cheese
Buttermilk	Ice cream

vegetables and fruits. It is important that care be taken during the preparation of these foods so as to minimize any nutrient loss.

Milk and Milk Products Group

All types of milk and milk products are included in this group except for butter which is excluded because of its very high fat content, and negligible protein and calcium content. This group provides proteins, fats, carbohydrates, calcium, phosphorus, vitamin A, riboflavin, and niacin. Fortified milk or fortified milk products also contain vitamin D.

The number of servings varies according to age and condition. The serving size is 8 fluid ounces of milk or its equivalent, according to calcium content. The following dairy foods contain calcium equal to that found in one cup of milk:

- 1½ ounces of cheddar cheese
- 1½ cups of cottage cheese
- 1½ cups of ice cream or ice milk

Milk used in making cream sauces, gravies, or baked products fulfills part of the requirement. A cheese sandwich would fulfill one of the serving requirements and a serving of ice cream or ice milk could fulfill half of one of the serving requirements. These examples show that drinking milk is not the only way to fulfill the milk requirement.

The Bread and Cereal Group

All whole grain, enriched, or restored breads and cereals are included in the bread and cereal group. This group provides carbohydrates, thiamin, niacin, B_6, iron, phosphorus, and magnesium.

The average person should have 4 or more servings daily from the bread and cereal group. Each of the following constitutes one serving: 1 slice of bread, 1 roll, 1 biscuit, about 2/3 cup cooked cereal, and 1 cup dry cereal.

The Meat Group

All meats, fish, poultry, eggs, and meat *alternates* (substitutes) are included in this group. Foods from the meat group provide protein, some fat, iron, copper, sodium, potas-

Table 7-4 Recommended Servings of Milk Per Day

Children	3 or more servings
Adolescents	4 or more servings
Adults over 19	2 or more servings
Pregnant women	4 or more servings
Mothers who are breast feeding	4 or more servings

Table 7-5 Bread and Cereal Group

breads	cereals
whole wheat	whole wheat
dark rye	rolled oats
enriched	brown rice
cornmeal, whole	converted rice
grain or enriched	other cereals, if
rolls or biscuits made	whole grain or
with whole wheat or	restored
enriched flour	noodles, spaghetti,
flour, enriched	macaroni
whole wheat, other	
whole grain	
oatmeal bread	
grits, enriched	

Table 7-6 Meat Group

MEATS	MEAT ALTERNATES
beef	dried beans
lamb	dried peas
veal	lentils
pork, except	nuts
bacon	peanuts
organ meats, such as	peanut butter
heart, liver, kidney,	soybean flour
brain, tongue,	soybeans
sweetbread	
poultry, such as	
chicken, duck,	
goose, turkey	
fish, shellfish	
lunch meats	
such as	
bologna	
liverwurst	

sium, chloride, magnesium, phosphorus, zinc, vitamins A, B complex, and D.

One should have 2 or more servings from this group each day. Approximately three ounces of boneless meat, poultry, fish, or meat alternate constitute one serving. Meat alternates such as beans and nuts can be good sources of protein and are usually less expensive than meats, fish, and poultry. *textured protein analogs – soybean*

Table 7-7 gives an analysis of the nutrients supplied by a day's menus based on the Basic Four food groups. These menus provide a balanced diet for a female between the ages of twenty-three and fifty years of age. Note that the nutrient values exceed the RDA, but that the caloric value closely follows the amount recommended. The total caloric value is very important. Both caloric value and nutrient content of the menu must be considered when planning meals.

THE GUIDELINES

The United States Departments of Agriculture and Health and Human Services have developed the following Guidelines to help people select and maintain healthy, balanced diets:

1. Eat a variety of foods
2. Maintain ideal weight
3. Avoid too much fat, saturated fat, and cholesterol *arteriosclerosis*
4. Eat foods with adequate starch and fiber
5. Avoid too much sugar
6. Avoid too much sodium
7. If you drink alcohol, do so in moderation

Eat a Variety of Foods

The first Guideline is intended to ensure that one's diet contains all the essential

Table 7-7 Nutrients Provided by the Sample Menu*

	1/2 cup prune juice	1 cup oatmeal	3 slices enriched bread	1 tablespoon butter	3 cups whole milk	3 ounces chicken	4 large lettuce leaves	1 tablespoon mayonnaise	1/2 carrot	1 medium banana	1/2 cup tomato juice	5.4 ounces lean roast beef	1 baked potato	1/2 cup green beans	3 fluid ounces ice cream	1 tablespoon "French" dressing	2 chocolate chip cookies	Total	Recommended Daily Allowances
Protein (g)	.5	5	6	Tr	27	20	2	Tr	.5	1	1	48	3	1	2	Tr	2	119	44
Calcium (mg)	18	22	63	3	864	8	68	3	9	10	9	20	9	31	73	2	8	122	800
Iron (mg)	5.2	1.4	1.8	0	.3	1.4	1.4	.1	.2	.8	1.1	6	.7	.4	Tr	.1	.4	21.3	18
Vitamin A (μgRE)	-	0	Tr	470	1050	80	1900	40	2750	230	970	Tr	Tr	340	220	-	20	8070	800
Thiamin (mg)	.015	.19	.18	-	.21	.05	.06	Tr	.015	.06	.06	.12	.1	.045	.02	-	.02	1.14	1.0
Riboflavin (mg)	.015	.05	.15	-	1.23	.16	.08	.01	.015	.07	.03	.36	.04	.055	.11	-	.02	2.39	1.2
Niacin (mg)	.5	.2	1.8	-	.6	7.4	.4	Tr	.15	.8	.95	8.6	1.7	.3	.1	-	.2	23.7	13
Vitamin C (mg)	2.5	0	Tr	0	6	-	18	-	2	12	20	-	20	7.5	1	-	Tr	89	60
Calories	100	130	210	100	480	115	20	100	10	100	23	250	90	15	95	65	100	2003	2000

* Menu selected from the Basic Four food groups.

† Daily allowance established for a female between the ages of 23 and 50 years, weighing 120 lbs.

Breakfast	Lunch	Dinner
Prune Juice	Chicken Sandwich with Lettuce and Mayonnaise	Tomato Juice
Oatmeal		Roast Beef
Buttered Toast	Carrot Sticks	Baked Potato
Milk	Milk	Green Beans
Coffee	Cookies	Lettuce Salad
		Milk
		Ice Cream
		Coffee

Figure 7-1 Menus based on the Basic Four food groups

nutrients. Because no one food contains all the nutrients necessary to humans, eating a variety of foods is the best insurance for a healthy diet.

Maintain Ideal Weight

Overweight increases one's risk of developing high blood pressure and diabetes, disorders which are associated with increased risk of heart attacks and strokes. As a general rule, *ideal weight* is thought to be the weight a person was between the ages of 20 and 25. See Table A-2 for acceptable body weights. As discussed in Chapter 2, energy needs of people differ, depending upon basal metabolism, age, size, sex, physical condition, activity, and climate. However, the bottom line remains this: the number of calories taken in must not exceed the number of calories burned by the body each day if the current weight is to be maintained.

If there is need to reduce one's weight, it should be done on a gradual basis of no more than one to two pounds per week. This may seem slow, but in fact from 26—52 pounds can be lost in a six-month period. This is the most effective method of weight loss because it is most conducive to affecting genuine change in eating habits, which helps one maintain the reduced weight afterward. This is also the safest method of weight loss. Diets of less than 1,000 calories per day or "crash" diets tend to limit the varieties of foods to such an extent that the nutrient intake may be reduced below the recommended daily allowances. This can damage one's health, and in extreme cases cause death.

Since one pound of body fat contains 3,500 calories, 3,500 calories need to be burned to lose one pound. If, for example, one takes in 500 calories less than one burns each day, there will be a one-pound weight loss at the end of one week. One way to speed weight loss is to increase physical activity, causing additional calories to be burned.

Conversely, it is important that weight loss does not continue beyond the acceptable range. Extreme weight loss may contribute to nutrient deficiencies, menstrual irregularities, infertility, hair loss, skin changes, intolerance to cold, constipation, psychological disturbances and even death. If there is unexplained weight loss, a physician should be consulted since it may be an indication of underlying disease.

Avoid too Much Fat, Saturated Fat, and Cholesterol

By reducing the amount of blood lipids, one's risk of heart attack can be reduced (refer to Chapter 3).

Because fats contain slightly more than twice the calories of carbohydrates, fats contribute to obesity, which increases the risk of heart attack. In addition, large amounts of saturated fat generally tend to raise blood cholesterol levels, which also increase the risk of heart attack. Consequently, it is considered advisable that one's total fat intake not exceed 30—35% of daily caloric intake. This can be done without sacrificing necessary nutrients or flavor. For example, lean meats, fish, poultry and *legumes* (various beans and peas) can be substituted for fatty meats. The fat on meats can be trimmed. Skim milk can be substituted for whole milk. Eggs, organ meats, butter, margarine, and cream can be used in moderation, and foods can be baked, broiled, or boiled rather than fried.

Eat Foods with Adequate Starch and Fiber

The fourth Guideline is included for several reasons. Starch is a complex carbo-

hydrate (polysaccharide) that provides energy. That energy total, however, is less than half that provided by fats—a useful fact that those who must watch their weight should know. Complex carbohydrates contain many essential vitamins and minerals and some of them also provide the fiber necessary for normal peristalsis. Whole grain cereals, nuts, fruits, and vegetables (especially raw), are all excellent sources of fiber (see Chapter 2).

Avoid too Much Sugar

Sugar is known to cause tooth decay (dental caries). In addition, sugar contributes to overweight since candies, desserts, and sweet beverages contain extremely large amounts of sugar in relation to their other ingredients, and consequently, large numbers of calories (see chapter 2).

Avoid too Much Sodium

Excessive amounts of sodium may contribute to *hypertension* (blood pressure that is over 140/90), which is known to increase one's risk of coronary heart disease (See Chapter 26).

If You Drink Alcohol, Do So in Moderation

Alcohol contains approximately 185 calories per ounce and no nutrients. In moderate drinkers, alcohol tends to increase the appetite which can contribute to weight gain. Conversely, heavy drinkers may lose their appetites, not eat, and subsequently suffer nutritional deficiencies. Excessive use of alcohol by pregnant women may cause birth defects. Heavy drinking can cause cirrhosis of the liver, brain damage, and increase the risk of cancer of the throat and neck.

SUMMARY

The seven Dietary Guidelines developed by the U.S. government are important tools in the maintenance of good health through good nutrition. Essentially they recommend a balanced diet. The key to a balanced diet is the use of the Basic Four food groups—vegetables and fruits, milk and milk products, meats and meat alternates, and breads and cereals. Each group has a required number of servings. Other foods may be added as desired if the requirements of the Basic Four are not omitted and if the other foods do not raise the total caloric value of the diet above that recommended.

Discussion Topics

1. List the Dietary Guidelines and state the reasons for them.
2. What groups of nutrients are provided in the vegetable and fruit group? The milk group? The meat group? The bread and cereal group?
3. How does the careful use of the Basic Four food groups eliminate the need to check menus with a chart of the recommended daily dietary allowances?
5. Discuss the sale of hollow calorie foods in school cafeterias. Is it a good policy? If so, why? If not, why not? What would your position be on this subject if you were principal of an elementary school? Of a junior or senior high school?
6. What are meat alternates? Discuss their uses.
7. Ask if anyone in class has used soybeans in cooking. If someone has, ask for an evaluation of them in terms of use, flavor, cost. What is their nutrient value?
8. Discuss the difference between nutrient content and caloric value.
9. Why should "crash" or "fad" diets be avoided? What is a better alternative? Why?
10. What would you advise your best friend if she or he was about to begin an 800-calorie reducing diet? Why would you give such advice?
11. Of what use is fiber in the diet?
12. Alcohol is not considered a food so why is there a Dietary Guideline devoted to it?
13. Discuss how the following family dinner menu might be adapted to the needs of a family member on a reducing diet:

Fried Hamburgers
Boiled Potatoes with Butter
Steamed Broccoli
Lettuce with Mayonnaise

Rolls
Angel Cake with Whipped Cream
Whole Milk

14. How might the foregoing menu be adapted to the needs of someone who must limit intake of saturated fats?

Suggested Activities

1. Visit a meat market and identify the various meat group sources (sweetbreads, muscle meats, shellfish, etc.). What essential nutrients does each of these foods provide? Price these foods at the store. Look up a recipe for each and explain its preparation to the class. If possible, prepare it for the class.

2. Organize a campaign to educate your fellow students in regard to the Basic Four food groups. Consider using classroom and lunchroom bulletin boards, flyers, assembly programs with speakers, or a short play and lunchroom demonstrations of foods and their preparation.

3. Buy some fruits and vegetables that are new to you. Bring these to class and prepare and sample them. Share ideas as to their potential uses. Perhaps these might be added to your home menus occasionally.

4. Using a restaurant menu, choose a breakfast, lunch, and dinner. Check the selection of foods used with the Basic Four food groups. Are they balanced meals? Discuss the problems that people who eat all their meals in restaurants might have in maintaining a well-balanced diet.

5. Using the following table, fill in the "Menus" column with the foods eaten in the past two days. In the "Food Groups Used" column list the groups to which each food belongs. To evaluate personal dietary habits, fill in the "Food Groups Not Used" column. Compare the table with those of the rest of the class and discuss how eating habits may be improved.

	MENUS	FOOD GROUPS USED	FOOD GROUPS NOT USED
Breakfast			
Lunch			

Dinner _____

Snacks _____

Review

Multiple Choice. Select the *letter* that precedes the best answer.

1. A balanced diet is one that includes
   a. equal amounts of carbohydrates and fats
   b. no animal products
   c. all of the essential nutrients
   d. more vegetables than fruits

2. The Basic Four food groups include
   a. vegetables and fruits   c. breads and cereals
   b. milk and meats   d. all of these

3. The size of a serving from the meat group should be approximately
   a. 1/4 pound   c. 3 ounces
   b. 1 ounce   d. 1/2 pound

4. Foods included in the normal diet should
   a. provide enough calories to satisfy energy requirements
   b. contain an adequate amount of the essential nutrients
   c. be based on the Basic Four food groups
   d. all of the above

5. When a food lends satiety to meals, it
   a. is always fattening
   b. provides enormous amounts of bulk
   c. gives satisfaction
   d. is very chewy

6. When planning meals
   a. the nutrient content of meals is the main consideration
   b. both nutrient content and caloric value must be considered
   c. only the caloric value need be considered
   d. none of the above is true

7. The minimum number of servings of fruits and vegetables that should be included in the diet each day is
   a. 2   c. 4
   b. 3   d. 6

8. Fruits and vegetables are rich sources of
   a. vitamins
   b. fats
   c. proteins
   d. all of these

9. Teenagers should have a serving of milk (or its substitute)
   a. not more than twice a day
   b. at least four times a day
   c. not more than four times a week
   d. not at all if they are overweight

10. Milk products are made from milk and include
    a. butter and margarine
    b. yogurt and cottage cheese
    c. bean curd and coconut milk
    d. all of the above

11. Milk and its products provide rich sources of
    a. proteins and fats
    b. carbohydrates
    c. minerals and vitamins
    d. all of the above

12. The minimum number of servings of breads and cereals that should be included in the diet each day is
    a. 1
    b. 2
    c. 3
    d. 4

13. Breads and cereals are rich sources of
    a. vitamin D
    b. fats
    c. carbohydrates
    d. all of these

14. Foods from the meat group should be served at least
    a. once a day
    b. twice a day
    c. three times a day
    d. four times a day

15. Foods from the meat group are rich sources of
    a. proteins
    b. carbohydrates
    c. vitamin C
    d. all of these

References

Bodinski, Lois H. 1982. *The Nurse's Guide to Diet Therapy*. New York: John Wiley & Sons.

Iowa Dietetic Association, 1984. *Simplified Diet Manual with Meal Patterns*, 5th ed. Ames: Iowa State University Press.

Krause, Marie V., and L. Kathleen Mahan. 1979. *Food, Nutrition and Diet Therapy*, 6th ed. Philadelphia: W. B. Saunders Co.

Robinson, Corinne H. 1978. *Fundamentals of Normal Nutrition*, 3rd ed. New York: Macmillan Publishing Company.

Robinson, Corinne H., and Marilyn R. Lawler. 1982. *Normal and Therapeutic Nutrition*, 16th ed. New York: Macmillan Publishing Company.

U. S. Department of Agriculture. *Composition of Food*. 1963, 1975.

Whitney, Eleanor Noss, and Eva May Nunnelley Hamilton. 1984. *Understanding Nutrition*, 3rd ed. St. Paul: West Publishing Co.

Chapter 8

PLANNING APPETIZING MEALS

VOCABULARY

aroma	croquette	jellied fruit
bland	custom	meringue
casserole	flavor	patties
consistency	fondue	souffle
convenience food	fruit whip	texture
cottage pudding	hash	

OBJECTIVES

After studying this chapter, you should be able to

- State and define criteria for planning appetizing meals

- Identify the purpose of a menu pattern

- Adapt a menu pattern to suit individual requirements or preferences

To build and maintain healthy bodies, the knowledge of basic nutrition must be combined with imagination when planning meals. Appetite appeal is as important as nutritive value in meal planning because the best food is nutritious only when it is eaten. Although the Basic Four food groups serve as the elementary guide in meal planning, the following criteria must also be considered: variety, appearance, flavor and aroma, texture, satiety, and individual likes and dislikes.

Variety

Even favorite foods become less interesting when they are prepared day after day without variation. The finest cut of steak is no longer appetizing if it is served seven days a week. It is important to consider variety within each of the Basic Four food groups each day.

Appearance

Because the initial reaction to food is based on its appearance, it is essential to consider the colors and shapes of food when planning meals. Colors and shapes should vary and blend in a harmonious way. Although a meal of tomato soup, corned beef, red cabbage, beets, and raspberry sherbet is nutritious, it lacks variety in color. Melon balls, fish balls, small boiled potatoes, brussels sprouts, and cherries lack variety in shape.

Flavor and Aroma

Flavor and aroma are so closely related that they should be considered together.

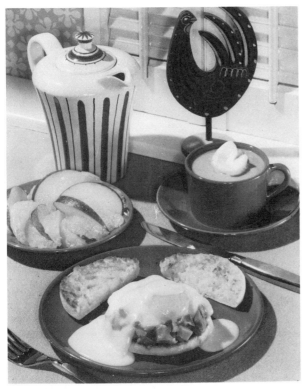

Figure 8-1 Breakfast can stimulate the appetite by a pleasing variety of shape and color of food. *(Courtesy of the National Dairy Council)*

Imagine eating a meal of onion soup, spiced sausage, mustard, sauerkraut, and hot peppers. Compare it, in terms of flavor and aroma, with a meal of chicken consomme, unspiced veal, mashed potatoes, and custard. Both menus are unappetizing. The first has too many foods with strong flavor and aroma, and the second has an excess of bland foods. *Bland* foods have mild flavors.

Texture

The *texture* (consistency or feel) of foods must also vary. For example, cream soup, baked fish, mashed potatoes, squash, and rice pudding would make a dull meal. On the other hand, jaws would tire while eating a meal in which all of the foods required considerable chewing.

Satiety

A feeling of satiety, or satisfying fullness in the stomach, should linger after a meal, but the individual should not feel as if he or she has overeaten. One reason meals should include some protein and fat is that these nutrients stay in the stomach longer than carbohydrates, thus giving satiety value to the meal. Carbohydrate is necessary, however, to satisfy taste and provide quick energy.

Individual Likes and Dislikes

It is especially important to consider the individual likes and dislikes of various family members. If a particular food is disliked by everyone, it may be possible to substitute its nutritional equal. When a particular food is disliked by only one member of the family, it is advisable to serve it during that person's absence. Naturally, family and religious customs are respected when planning meals.

THE MENU PATTERN

A pattern must be used in planning a meal just as in sewing a garment. Figure 8-2 shows basic menu patterns for a day, based on the Basic Four food groups. Evaluate them in terms of nutritional adequacy. Most people add to the basic patterns.

The menus in figure 8-3 are based on the menu patterns in figure 8-2. Evaluate them in terms of nutritional adequacy, attractiveness, economy, and efficiency of preparation.

Breakfast	Lunch	Dinner
Fruit	Meat or Substitute	Meat or Substitute
Cereal	Fruit or Vegetable	2 or 3 Vegetables
Bread	Bread	Bread
Milk	Milk	Milk

Figure 8-2 A day's menu pattern is formed from the Basic Four food groups.

Adapting the Menu Pattern

Sometimes there are family members such as young children, elderly people, or the ill, who are unable to conform to the family meal plan. In such circumstances, the menu should be adapted to suit the person with the particular needs. This means minor changes are made in the basic plan.

Individual variations in the menu should require little or no extra preparation. Suppose the sample menu were planned for a family that included a young couple, a 3-year-old boy, and an 80-year-old grandmother. The foods served should appeal to everyone and be easy for the elderly woman and the child to chew and digest.

In figure 8-3, breakfast is especially adaptable because a variety of ready-to-eat cereals can be served. The remaining foods on the menu should be suitable for everyone. The coleslaw on the sample dinner menu might present a problem, but a substitution of a cooked vegetable for the grandmother and the little boy could solve it. For lunch or supper, the cheese sandwiches might be made with enriched white bread instead of whole wheat, and a cooked vegetable could be substituted for the celery sticks. If a fresh fruit is served for dessert, it should be something easily chewed and digested, such as a banana.

If a member of the family is ill, that person may require a special diet prescribed by the doctor. Even in such cases, the family

Breakfast	Dinner	Lunch or Supper
Orange Juice	Meat Loaf	Cheese Sandwich on Whole Wheat Bread
Cereal	Baked Potato	
Milk-Sugar	Corn Pudding	Celery Sticks
Toast	Coleslaw	Fruit
Butter-Jelly	Bread-Butter	Milk
Milk	Ice Cream	
(Coffee for adults)	Milk	
	(Coffee, Tea for adults)	

Figure 8-3 These three meals demonstrate how foods are selected from menu patterns.

VEGETABLES AND FRUITS

COOKED SNAP BEANS, LIMA BEANS, CORN, PEAS and CARROTS: casseroles, croquettes, meat and vegetable pie, salads, sauces, souffles, soup, stew, stuffed peppers, stuffed tomatoes, vegetables in cheese sauce

COOKED LEAFY VEGETABLES (CHOPPED): creamed vegetables, soup, meat loaf, meat patties, omelet, souffle

COOKED POTATOES: croquettes, fried or creamed potatoes, meat-pie topping, potatoes in cheese sauce, stew or chowder

COOKED or CANNED FRUITS: fruit cup, fruit sauces, jellied fruit, quick breads, salads, shortcake, upsidedown cake, yeast breads

---

MILK & MILK PRODUCTS

SOUR MILK: cakes, cookies, quick breads

SOUR CREAM: cakes, cookies, dessert sauces, meat stews, pie or cake fillings, salad dressing, sauce for vegetables

---

BREADS & CEREALS

COOKED WHEAT, OAT and CORN CEREALS: fried cereal, meat loaf or patties, souffles, sweet puddings

COOKED RICE, NOODLES, MACARONI and SPAGHETTI: casseroles, meat or cheese loaf, timbales

STALE BREAD: slices for French toast, dry crumbs for apple betty, croquettes, fondues, coating for fried chops, soft crumbs for bread pudding, meat loaf, stuffings

CAKE and COOKIES: apple betty, cake balls with fruit or chocolate sauce, cottage pudding, crumb crust pies, refrigerator cake, trifle (cake strips with custard sauce)

MEAT

EGG YOLKS: cakes, cookies, cornstarch pudding, custard and custard sauce, eggnog, pie and cake fillings, salad dressing, sauce for vegetables

EGG WHITES: cakes, frostings, fruit whip, meringue, souffles

HARD-COOKED EGG or YOLK: casserole dishes, garnish, salads, sandwiches

COOKED MEATS, POULTRY and FISH: casserole dishes, hash, meat patties, meat pies, salads, sandwiches, stuffed vegetables

Figure 8-4 Using leftovers from the Basic Four food groups

menu should be adapted whenever possible to save time and expense in preparation and to make the patient feel that he or she is not causing extra work.

Weekly Planning

Efficiency in planning is increased by planning meals for several days or a week at one time. It is also economical to plan several meals at one time to allow for adequate use of leftovers, figure 8-4. The nurse as well as the homemaker soon learns that practical short-cuts are invaluable. Modern convenience foods may be used as often as the budget and family desires will allow. *Convenience foods* are partially prepared foods such as frozen foods, baking mixes, TV dinners, etc. Meals that can be prepared in the oven are efficient and economical.

SUMMARY

The Basic Four food groups serve as a guide for planning nutritionally sound menus. To stimulate appetites, meals should provide satiety value and variety in color, flavor, aroma, texture, and shape. Menus should be flexible so they can be easily adapted to the special needs of individual family members. This flexibility helps save time and money. Planning several meals at one time is efficient and economical. The use of leftovers, convenience foods, and oven meals should be considered in weekly planning.

Discussion Topics

1. What criteria, in addition to the Basic Four food groups, should be considered when planning family meals? Why?
2. Evaluate the menu in figure 8-3 in terms of its appetite appeal.
3. How may leftover meats be used?
4. How may leftover vegetables be used?
5. Why is it advisable to adapt the family meal to suit the special needs of the patient rather than prepare a separate meal for the patient?
6. Discuss the advantages and disadvantages of convenience foods.
7. How does one "fry" cereal?

Suggested Activities

1. Visit a local supermarket and make a list of the various convenience foods available. Compare their prices to the same foods that have not been partially prepared.
2. Look up recipes that use leftover roast beef. Present them to the class.
3. Look up definitions of any terms in Fig. 8-4 that are unfamiliar to you.

4. Plan a week's menu for a family of four who have no special dietary needs. Use the sample menus as a guide for listing the foods in proper order. Consider each of the following criteria in planning the menu:

nutritive quality   attractiveness
economy   efficiency of preparation

5. Select a menu for one day from the planned menu in activity 4. Adapt it for a visiting grandmother who has difficulty chewing.

Review

A. Multiple Choice. Select the *letter* that precedes the best answer.

1. An example of a meal plan that lacks variety is preparing
   a. two vegetables for dinner every day
   b. various dishes using meat each day
   c. a fried egg with cinnamon toast each morning
   d. fruit for lunch and dinner on the same day

2. Food products that are partially prepared commercially are called
   a. hollow calorie foods   c. bland foods
   b. convenience foods   d. brand name foods

3. The appearance of food refers to the way it
   a. tastes   c. looks
   b. smells   d. all of these

4. The flavor of food refers to its
   a. taste   c. satiety value
   b. smell   d. cost

5. The aroma of food refers to its
   a. appearance   c. taste
   b. smell   d. satiety value

6. The texture or consistency of food refers to its
   a. appearance   c. aroma
   b. feel   d. satiety value

7. Menus should be evaluated in terms of
   a. nutritional adequacy
   b. attractiveness and economy
   c. efficiency of preparation
   d. all of the above

8. Changing a menu to meet the special needs of a family member is called
   a. planning the menu
   b. adapting the menu
   c. the pattern of the menu
   d. varying the menu

9. Two examples of bland foods are
   a. grapefruit and oranges
   b. mashed potatoes and custard
   c. Italian sausage and salami
   d. all of the above
10. Foods that provide satiety value
   a. also provide large amounts of vitamin C
   b. give a lasting feeling of satisfying fullness in the stomach
   c. are those that all family members like
   d. are sugars and starches

B. Plan two dinners, selecting menus from the foods listed below. Consider variety in color, texture, and flavor. Adapt the steak menu to suit an 80-year-old woman who finds it difficult to chew.

Baked halibut, broiled steak, creamed corn, stewed tomatoes, jellied vegetable salad, tossed green salad, mashed potatoes, baked potatoes, cherry upside-down cake, rice pudding with pineapple.

C. Briefly answer the following questions.

1. In addition to the Basic Four food groups, name seven other criteria that should be considered when planning meals.

2. Why should several meals be planned at one time?

efficiency
economical

3. Why is it important for a meal to be attractive?

Because the best food is
nutrious only when it is eaten
stimulate appetite

References

Anderson, Jean. 1979. *Jean Anderson's Processor Cooking.* New York: William Morrow & Company, Inc.

Anderson, Jean, and Elaine Hanna. 1975. *The Doubleday Cookbook.* Garden City, N.Y.: Doubleday and Company, Inc.

Charley, Helen. 1982. *Food Science*, 2nd ed. New York: John Wiley & Sons.

Kinder, Faye, Nancy Green, and Natholyn Harris. 1984. *Meal Management*, 6th ed. New York: Macmillan Publishing Company.

Poleman, Charlotte M., and Christine Locastro Capra. 1984. *Shackelton's Nutrition Essentials and Diet Therapy*, 5th ed. Philadelphia: W. B. Saunders Co.

Chapter 9
FOOD CUSTOMS

VOCABULARY

anorexia	lacto-vegetarians	social status
crash reducing diets	leavened bread	staple food
cuisine	legumes	tamales
cultural	meat analogs	tempura
dietary laws	ovo-lacto-	tortillas
economic status	vegetarians	vegans
environment	peers	wok
food customs	physical disability	
homous	rate of growth	
	shoyu	

OBJECTIVES

After studying this chapter, you should be able to

- Describe the development of food customs
- List some food customs of various cultural groups
- Identify at least three nutritionally poor food habits
- Adapt menus to suit a cultural or religious group with strict dietary laws

---

The rules of good nutrition as discussed in Chapter 7 are more easily recited than practiced. It is important not only to know these rules, but to follow them daily. It is much easier to help other people correct their eating habits after evaluating and correcting one's own eating habits.

Some of the more common bad eating habits include eating an excess of foods containing fats and carbohydrates, attempting to control weight gain by crash reducing diets, and skipping meals. Obesity and malnutrition may be caused by an excess of carbohydrates or fats in the diet. Such malnutrition can develop if foods containing primarily these two nutrients are substituted for foods containing the other essential nutrients. *Crash reducing*

diets typically consist of only a narrow selection of foods, thus limiting the types of nutrients obtained. Skipping meals may also limit the variety of nutrients eaten. Ironically, this may also cause an increase in the total daily caloric intake since one is subsequently apt to overeat after being without food for a long period of time.

Habits are not easily changed. However, the key to change rests on understanding the reasons eating habits develop.

DEVELOPMENT OF FOOD CUSTOMS

People from each country have favorite foods. Frequently, there are distinctive food customs originating in just a small section of a particular country. People of a particular area favor the foods that are produced in that area. They are available and economical. Some religions have dietary laws that require particular food practices. Because most people prefer the foods they were accustomed to while growing up, food habits are often based on nationality and religion. One's economic and social status also contributes to food habits. For example, the poor do not grow up with a taste for caviar, while the wealthy may at least be accustomed to it—whether or not they like it. Those in a certain social class will be apt to use the same foods as others in their class. And the foods they choose will probably depend on the work they do. For example, people doing hard, physical labor will require higher calorie foods than those in sedentary jobs.

When people move from one country to another, or from one area to another, their economic circumstances sometimes change. They may be introduced to new foods and new food customs. Although their original food customs may have been nutritionally adequate, their new environment may cause them to change their eating habits. For example, if milk was a staple in their diet before moving and is unusually expensive in the new environment, milk may be replaced by a cheaper, nutritionally inferior beverage such as soda, coffee, or tea. Candy, a luxury in their former environment, may be inexpensive and popular in their new environment. As a result, a family might increase consumption of soda or candy, and reduce purchases of more nutritious foods. Someone who is not familiar with the nutritive values of foods can easily make such mistakes in their food selection.

The meal patterns of nationalities and religious groups different from one's own may seem strange. However, the foods used often fall into the Basic Four food groups, making the diet nutritionally adequate. When a patient's eating habits need to be corrected, such corrections are easier if the food customs of the patient are known. To gain this knowledge, it is advisable to talk with the patient and learn about her or his background. This knowledge can be used to plan nourishing menus consisting of foods that are appetizing to the patient. The necessary adjustments in the diet can then be made gradually and effectively.

FOOD PATTERNS BASED ON CULTURE

American cuisine is a marvelous composite of countless national, regional, cultural, and religious food customs. Consequently, it can be difficult to categorize a patient's food habits. Nevertheless, it is sometimes helpful to be able to do so to a certain extent. When people are ill, it is not uncommon for them to have little interest in food, and sometimes foods that were familiar to them during their childhood and youth are more apt to tempt them than other types. The following section briefly discusses some of the food patterns that are typical of various cultures, regions, religions, and philosophies. It is important to remember that there can be and usually are enormous variations within any one classification.

American Indian

It is thought that approximately half of the edible plants commonly eaten in the United States today originated with the Native Americans. Examples are corn, potatoes, squash, cranberries, pumpkins, peppers, beans, wild rice, and cocoa beans. In addition, they used wild fruits, game, and fish. Foods were commonly prepared as soups and stews, and dried. The original Native American diets were probably more nutritionally adequate than their current diets, which frequently consist of too high a proportion of sweet and salty, snack-type, hollow calorie foods. American Indian diets today may be deficient in calcium, vitamins A, C, and riboflavin.

U.S. South

Hotbreads such as corn bread and baking powder biscuits are very common in the U.S. South because the wheat grown in the area does not make good quality yeast breads. Grits and rice are also popular carbohydrate foods. Favorite vegetables include sweet potatoes, squash, green beans, and lima beans. Green beans cooked with pork are commonly served. Watermelon, oranges, and peaches are popular fruits. Fried fish is served often, as are barbecued and stewed meats. There is a great deal of carbohydrate and fat in these diets and limited amounts of protein in some cases. Iron, calcium, vitamins A and C may sometimes be deficient.

Mexican

Mexican food is a combination of Spanish and American Indian foods. Beans, rice, chili peppers, tomatoes, and corn meal are favorites. Meat is often cooked with the vegetable as in chili con carne. Corn meal is used in a variety of ways to make tortillas and tamales, which serve as bread. The combination of beans and corn makes a complete protein. While tortillas filled with cheese (called enchiladas) provide some calcium, the use of milk should be encouraged. Vitamin A

deficiency is thought to be the most common nutritional deficiency among Mexican-American children.

Puerto Rican

Rice is the basic carbohydrate food in Puerto Rican diets. Vegetables commonly used include beans, plantains, tomatoes, and peppers. Bananas, pineapple, mangoes, and papayas are popular fruits. Favorite meats are chicken, beef, and pork. Milk is not used as much as would be desirable from the nutritional point of view.

Italian

Pastas with various tomato or fish sauces, and cheese are popular Italian foods. Fish and highly seasoned foods are common to Southern Italian cuisine while meat and root vegetables are common to northern Italy. The eggs, cheese, tomatoes, green vegetables, and fruits common to Italian diets provide excellent sources of many nutrients, but additional milk and meat would improve the diet.

Northern and Western Europe

Northern and Western European diets are similar to those of the U.S. Midwest, but with a greater use of dark breads, potatoes, and fish, and fewer green vegetable salads. Beef and pork are popular as are various cooked vegetables, breads, cakes, and dairy products.

Central Europe

Citizens of Central Europe obtain the greatest portion of their calories from potatoes and grains, especially rye and buckwheat.

Pork is a popular meat. Cabbage cooked in many ways is a popular vegetable as are carrots, onions, and turnips. Eggs and dairy products are used abundantly.

Middle East

Grains, wheat, and rice provide energy in these diets. Chickpeas in the form of *homous* are popular. Lamb and yogurt are commonly used as are cabbage, grape leaves, eggplant, tomatoes, dates, olives, and figs. Black, very sweet coffee is a popular beverage.

Chinese

The Chinese diet is varied. Rice is the primary energy food and is used in place of bread. Foods are generally cut into small pieces because of an ancient law of Confucius. Vegetables are lightly cooked and the cooking water is saved for future use. Soybeans are used in many ways and eggs and pork are commonly served. Soy sauce is extensively used, but it is very salty and could present a problem with patients on low-salt diets. Tea is a common beverage. This diet may be low in fat.

Japanese

Japanese diets include rice, soybean paste and curd, vegetables, fruits, and fish. Food is frequently served *tempura* style, which means fried. Soy sauce (*shoyu*) and tea are commonly used. Current Japanese diets have been greatly influenced by Western culture.

Southeast Asian

Many Indians are vegetarians who use eggs and dairy products. Rice, peas, and beans are frequently served. Spices, especially curry, are popular. Indian meals are not typically served in courses as Western meals are. They generally consist of one course with many dishes. Eating with one's fingers is considered quite acceptable.

Thailand, Viet Nam, Laos and Cambodia

Rice, curries, vegetables, and fruits are popular in Thailand, Viet Nam, Laos and Cambodia. Meat, chicken, and fish are used in small amounts. The *wok* (a deep, round fry pan) is used for sautéing many foods. A salty sauce made from fermented fish is commonly used.

FOOD PATTERNS BASED ON RELIGION OR PHILOSOPHY

Jewish

Interpretations of the Jewish dietary laws vary. Those who adhere to the Orthodox view consider tradition very important and always observe the dietary laws. Conservative Jews are inclined to observe the rules only at home. Reform Jews consider their dietary laws to be essentially ceremonial and so minimize their significance. Essentially the laws require the following:

- Slaughtering must be done by a qualified person, in a prescribed manner. The meat or poultry must be drained of blood, first by severing the jugular vein and carotid artery, then by soaking in brine before cooking.
- Meat or meat products may not be prepared or eaten with milk or milk products.

- The dishes used in the preparation and serving of meat dishes must be kept separate from those used in the serving of dairy foods.
- A specified time, 6 hours, must elapse between consumption of meat and milk.
- The mouth must be rinsed after eating fish and before eating meat.
- There are prescribed fast days—Passover Week, Yom Kippur, and Feast of Purim.
- No cooking is done on the Sabbath—from sundown Friday to sundown Saturday.
- Food is not used from a Kosher market that remains open on the Sabbath.

These laws forbid the eating of the following:

- the flesh of animals without cloven (split) hoof or that do not chew their cud
- hind quarters of any animals
- shellfish or fish without scales or fins
- fowl that are birds of prey
- creeping things and insects
- leavened bread during Passover

Generally, the food served is rich. Fresh smoked, and salted fish, and chicken are very popular as are noodles, egg, and flour dishes. These diets may be deficient in fresh vegetables and milk.

Roman Catholic

Although the dietary restrictions of the Roman Catholic religion have been liberalized, meat is not allowed its adherents on Ash Wednesday and Fridays during Lent.

Eastern Orthodox

Followers of this religion may include Christians from the Middle East, Russia, and Greece. Although interpretations of the dietary laws may vary, meat, poultry, fish, and dairy products are restricted on Wednesdays and Fridays and during Lent and Advent.

Seventh Day Adventists

Generally, Seventh Day Adventists are *ovo-lacto-vegetarians*, which means they use milk products and eggs, but no meat, fish, or poultry. They may also use nuts, legumes, and meat *analogs* (substitutes) made from soybeans. They consider coffee, tea, and alcohol to be harmful.

Mormons (Latter Day Saints)

The only dietary restriction observed by the Mormons is the prohibition of coffee, tea, and alcoholic beverages.

Islam

Adherents of Islam are called Moslems. Their dietary laws prohibit the use of pork and alcohol, and other meats must be slaughtered according to specific laws. During the month of Ramadan, Moslems do not eat or drink during daylight hours.

Hindu

To the Hindus, all life is sacred because small animals may contain the souls of ancestors. Consequently, Hindus are usually vegetarians. They do not use eggs as they represent life.

Vegans

Vegans avoid all animal foods. They do use soybeans, chick peas, and meat analogs made from soybeans. It is important that their meals be carefully planned to include appropriate combinations of the nonessential amino acids in order to provide the nine essential amino acids. For example, beans served with corn or rice, or peanuts eaten with wheat, are better in such combinations than any of them would be if eaten alone. Vegans may show deficiencies of calcium, zinc, vitamins A, D, and B_{12}.

Lacto-vegetarians

Lacto-vegetarians are vegetarians that use dairy products.

Ovo-lacto-vegetarians

Ovo-lacto-vegetarians are vegetarians who use both eggs and dairy products.

F Macrobiotic Diets

The macrobiotic diet is a system of ten diet plans, developed from Zen Buddhism. Adherents progress from the lower number diet to the higher, gradually giving up foods in the following order: desserts, salads, fruits, animal foods, soups, and ultimately, vegetables, until only cereals—usually brown rice—are consumed. Beverages are to be kept to a minimum and only "organic" foods (see Chapter 10) are used. Foods are grouped as "Yang" (male) or "Yin" (female). A ratio of 5:1 Yang to Yin is considered important. Most of the macrobiotic diets are deficient in vitamin C. As the adherents give up foods according to plans, their diets can become increasingly inadequate. These diets can be especially dangerous because avid adherents promise medical cures from the diets that cannot be attained and so medical treatment may be delayed when needed.

SUMMARY

Food habits have many, diverse origins. One's nationality, religion, economic, and social status all affect their development. When such customs result in inadequate diets, corrections should be made gradually. Corrections are easier and more effectively made when the reasons for the food habits are understood.

Discussion Topics

1. Discuss the reasons why nurses and homemakers should practice the rules of good nutrition themselves.
2. How do food habits originate?
3. What effects does environment have on particular food habits? When do the effects of a new environment improve diets and when do they impair them?
4. From personal experience, explain why certain foods are enjoyed more than others that are commonly available in the local area.
5. Discuss the dangers of skipping meals and explain how this habit can result in an *increased* caloric intake.
6. Ask if anyone in class has been on a crash reducing diet. Ask that

person to describe the diet and its ultimate result. Would that person recommend this diet? Why?

7. Why are hot breads more popular with people from the U.S. South than yeast breads?

(8.) Would a banker or a bricklayer be more apt to choose a chef's salad for lunch? Explain.

Suggested Activities

1. Give a series of short reports on food customs. Each student should select a different country or area within a country for study. After the reports have been presented, hold a class discussion on whether climate, availability of food, and economic factors determine the food customs of the country studied. Include the following points in the reports. What is the climate of the country? What crops are grown? Are modern methods of agriculture used? Does the country depend on imports for a large part of its food supply? If so, what foods are imported? Is a large part of the population poor? What foods are most popular? Are they produced in the country itself? Are they expensive or cheap?

2. Plan a Good Friday menu for a patient of the Roman Catholic faith.

3. Investigate the lunch program of a local school. Have a panel discussion on its purpose, limitations, favorable characteristics, and suggested improvements.

4. Make attractive posters for the school lunchroom or cafeteria in which the improvement of eating habits is stressed.

Review

A. Multiple Choice. Select the *letter* preceding the best answer.

1. Food customs means one's
   - a. food nutrients
   - b. food habits
   - c. food requirements
   - d. all of the above

2. Some bad eating habits that are common include
   - a. skipping meals
   - b. eating an excess of carbohydrates and fats
   - c. using crash reducing diets
   - d. all of the above

3. The basis for food customs may be
   - a. religion
   - b. nationality
   - c. foods available locally
   - d. all of these

4. Moving to a new environment or experiencing a change in salary
   a. rarely changes established food habits
   b. usually influences established food habits
   c. always reduces the amount of food eaten
   d. never reduces the quality of food eaten

5. Crash reducing diets
   a. may limit the types of nutrients obtained
   b. are an acceptable way to control weight gain
   c. contain a wide selection of foods
   d. all of the above

6. Hotbreads are common to diets of people from
   a. Mexico   c. China
   b. the Midwest   d. the U.S. South

7. Rice is a popular carbohydrate food in
   a. Puerto Rico   c. Northern Europe
   b. Central Europe   d. all of the above

8. Sedentary jobs include those of
   a. physical education teachers   c. dancers
   b. bricklayers   d. secretaries

9. Generally, the diets of U.S. Southerners, Mexicans, Puerto Ricans, and Italians would be improved by the addition of more
   a. rice   c. milk
   b. corn   d. pasta

10. A diet of dried beans, corn, and chili peppers would most likely be used by a (an)
    a. Mexican family   c. Armenian family
    b. Italian family   d. Orthodox Jewish family

B. Adapt the following menu for a person of the Orthodox Jewish faith, using figure 9-1.

Baked Ham
Scalloped Potatoes
Buttered Peas
Bread and Butter
Fresh Fruit
Milk or Coffee

C. Matching.
Write "B" for Breads and Cereals, "M" for Meats and Meat Substitutes, "V" for Vegetables and Fruits, and "D" for Dairy Foods. Some foods may fit into more than one group.

D 1. Yogurt
B 2. Cornbread

B	3.	Grits
V	4.	Collard greens
V	5.	Yams
D	6.	Buttermilk
M V B	7.	Pizza
N	8.	Tofu made from Soybeans
M	9.	Caviar
B	10.	Tortillas

References

Hui, Y.H. 1983. *Human Nutrition and Diet Therapy.* Monterey, Calif: Wadsworth Health Sciences Division of Wadsworth Inc.

Luke, Barbara. 1984. *Principles of Nutrition and Diet Therapy.* Boston: Little Brown & Co.

Robinson, Corinne H. 1978. *Fundamentals of Normal Nutrition*, 3rd ed. New York: Macmillan Publishing Company.

Suitor, Carol W., and Merrily F. Crowley. 1984. *Nutrition Principles and Application in Health Promotion.* Philadelphia: J. B. Lippincott Company.

Williams, Sue Rodwell. 1982. *Essentials of Nutrition and Diet Therapy.* 3rd ed. St. Louis: C. V. Mosby Co.

Chapter 10

EVALUATING AND PRESERVING FOOD QUALITY

VOCABULARY

accompaniment dish
bacteria
beverage
blemish
buttermilk
caffeine
certified milk
coagulate
consumer

decaffeinated
dried milk
evaporated milk
fillet
food additives
hare
homogenized milk
milling
nutritional value
opaque

pasteurization
process cheese
raw milk
skim milk
steak
stimulant
sweetened condensed milk
venison
whole milk

OBJECTIVES

After studying this chapter, you should be able to

* State criteria for evaluating the quality of meat, poultry, fish, eggs, vegetables, and fruit

* Describe methods of storing and cooking various kinds of food to preserve nutrient content

* Identify the different types of milk and explain how milk is pasteurized

* Explain why food additives are sometimes used

Today's supermarkets provide such a variety of foods that it is essential for the *consumer* (one who buys and uses marketed items) to be able to determine the *nutritional value* (nutrient content) of foods. In addition, the consumer should have a basic knowledge of quality, appropriate uses, preparation, and storage of foods. There is no point in purchasing a food because it is rich in a specific nutrient if the food cannot be properly stored or prepared.

BEVERAGES

Beverages are fluids that relieve thirst, and provide nourishment. Water is the base of all beverages, and is necessary to regulate body processes.

Milk is an important beverage because of its high nutritive value. Chocolate flavored syrup, eggs, or sweeteners may be added to increase its nutritive and caloric values or change its flavor.

Vegetables and fruit juices are refreshing, provide vitamins, especially vitamin C, and stimulate appetites. Fruit juices should be kept cold, covered, and in *opaque* (blocks out light) containers to preserve their flavor and vitamin content. Fruit drinks (not juices), and carbonated beverages usually provide only calories in the form of sugar, and sometimes additives.

Coffee and tea have no food value without cream or sugar. Both contain the stimulant caffeine, which makes them inappropriate for children. Boiling makes coffee and tea bitter, and increases their strength. *Decaffeinated* coffee products have had 95 percent or more of the caffeine removed. To preserve flavor, both coffee and tea should be kept tightly covered, and coffee should be stored in a cool place.

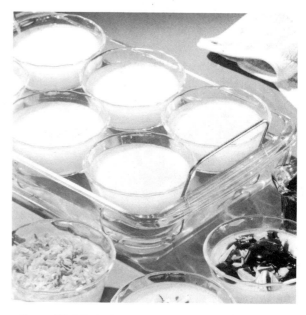

Figure 10-1 Baked custard is one of the many ways in which milk can be added to the diet. *(Courtesy of the National Dairy Council)*

MILK AND MILK PRODUCTS

Milk is considered the most nearly perfect food. It is easily digested, and contains complete protein, carbohydrate, fat, calcium, phosphorus, and vitamins A and B. Milk is low in vitamin C and iron. Most milk sold in the United States has been irradiated with 400 IU of vitamin D per quart, which otherwise is present only in small amounts.

Since *bacteria* (microorganisms) thrive on milk, there are health regulations that must be scrupulously observed by people handling it. Milk that has been handled according to these regulations is *certified*. To assure its safety, most milk is pasteurized. *Pasteurization* is a process named for Louis Pasteur, its originator. In one method of pasteurization, the milk is heated to at least 62.8°C (145°F) for at least 30 minutes and then immediately cooled to 10°C (50°F). Another method is to heat milk very quickly to 71.7°C (161°F) for at least 15 seconds and then cool it immedi-

ately. The pasteurization process kills all harmful bacteria and checks the growth of some harmless bacteria that can cause milk to sour. Milk that has not been pasteurized is called *raw milk*.

Fresh milk is available in quart, half gallon, three quart, and gallon containers. Usually the larger containers provide the lowest cost, ounce per ounce. These containers will undoubtedly be replaced by liter-sized containers.

Frequently there is a date on the milk container. Milk should not be purchased after the date indicated because it will not remain fresh for more than a day or two. Milk and milk products should be refrigerated in clean, covered containers to preserve nutrient content and inhibit the growth of bacteria. Low temperatures must be used during cooking because milk and its products scorch easily.

Although milk is most often used as a beverage, it is frequently combined with other foods such as soups, gravies, casseroles, baked products, cereals, and desserts. Milk is available in several forms, some of which are listed here.

- *Whole milk*—milk with all its natural nutrients.
- *Low-fat Milk*—milk with fat removed to no more than .5 percent, 1 percent, 1.5 percent, or 2 percent, as indicated on the label.
- *Skim milk*—milk with all or nearly all of its fat removed.
- *Chocolate milk*—milk with chocolate added; may be whole or low fat.
- *Dried milk*—milk with all of its water removed.
- *Buttermilk*—skim milk that is a by-product of making butter. Commercial buttermilk is made by adding harmless bacteria to skim milk. The bacteria change some of the lactose (milk sugar) to lactic acid. The resulting product is called *cultured buttermilk*.
- *Homogenized milk*—whole milk that has been processed to break the fat into small drops and distribute it evenly throughout the liquid so that it does not separate.
- *Evaporated milk*—whole milk with approximately 60 percent of its water removed.
- *Sweetened condensed milk*—milk that has been evaporated after the addition of sugar.

Cream

Cream is the fat in milk that rises to the surface. It may also be separated from milk by mechanical means. Cream is classified as light or heavy, depending upon its fat content. The higher the percentage of fat, the heavier the cream. "Half and half" is equal parts milk and cream. Cream is available in one-half pint, pint, and quart containers and should be kept covered and refrigerated.

Cheese

When milk coagulates, the curd that results is cheese. The hundreds of types available vary according to the kind of milk used, the amount of moisture, types of seasonings, and the method of ripening. Some cheddar cheese is graded according to quality with Grade AA the best, Grade A nearly as good, and Grade B being the lowest in flavor and cost. Natural cheese is commonly classified according to moisture content: hard, semisoft and soft, table 10-1. Another popular

Table 10-1 Natural Cheese Classification According to Moisture Content

Hard	Semisoft	Soft
Parmesan	Mozzarella	Brie
Cheddar	Roquefort	Camembert
Swiss	Blue	Cream
Edam	Gorgonzola	Cottage
Gouda	Muenster	Ricotta

cheese in the United States is *process cheese.* This is natural cheese that has been blended with additional moisture and sometimes, seasonings, to make cheese spreads.

Cheese is rich in protein, minerals, and vitamins. It is generally easy to digest. The mild-flavored cheeses can usually be served to the patient during convalescence. It is an acceptable meat alternate and is used in sandwiches, casseroles, sauces, salads, and desserts.

Because cheese toughens easily in cooking, low temperatures are recommended. To store cheese, keep it tightly wrapped in a cool place. Since the flavor of cheese is most pronounced at room temperature, it should be removed from the refrigerator an hour before serving.

Butter

Butter might be called a by-product of milk since it is made from the fat in milk. It is an excellent source of fat and contains some vitamin A. It is available as sweet butter, which means it has had no salt added, or as salt or regular butter that has had salt added. The choice depends on taste or specific diet requirements. It is available as Grade AA, A, and B. The best flavored and most expensive is AA. It must be kept refrigerated and covered because it picks up other food odors readily.

EGGS

Eggs are a rich source of protein, minerals, and vitamins that may be used as a meat alternate. They are inexpensive and easily digested. Because of their high cholesterol content, it is advisable to limit eggs to four each week.

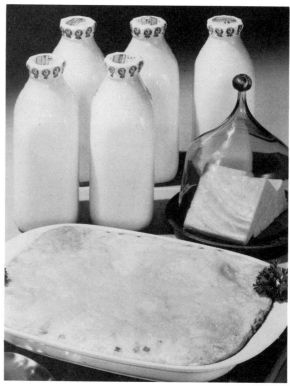

Figure 10-2 Cheese, milk, and eggs can be combined with other foods to make attractive dishes. *(Courtesy of the National Dairy Council)*

Eggs are graded according to size and quality. Large eggs usually cost more per dozen than small, but the size has nothing to do with the quality. When an egg is fresh, it sinks in water; an old egg floats because air has seeped into the shell. The freshest, highest quality eggs have a thick white that stays together. The white of eggs that are old or of poor quality is thin and runny. Grade AA and A eggs are excellent, and recommended when eggs are to be fried, poached, or presented whole in some manner. Grade B eggs are seldom available at retail level because they are typically dried or frozen. If available, they are quite acceptable for combining with other foods. Because the yolks break quite easily, Grade B eggs are not recommended for use when the whites and yolks must be separated.

Eggs should be stored in their cartons with the small end down, since this keeps the air cell at the rounded end and prevents the yolk from slipping out of place. They should be refrigerated until used unless they are to be used in cakes. Because they blend better with other cake ingredients if they are at room temperature, they should be removed from the refrigerator about an hour before the cake is made.

Eggs are a favorite breakfast, lunch, or supper dish and can be prepared in many different ways. They are used in sandwiches, salads, desserts, and baked products. Eggs, like most protein foods, become tough when cooked at high temperatures. They should never be boiled—only simmered.

MEATS, POULTRY, AND FISH

Meats, poultry, and fish provide the greatest source of protein in the adult diet. They are also rich in minerals and vitamins. Lean meats are easily digested. Some form of these foods should be served daily. Usually they are the foundation of meals. The purple stamp (vegetable dye) on meat is a government seal indicating that the meat is free from disease and has been handled under sanitary conditions.

Meat

The types of meat generally available are beef, veal, lamb, pork, and variety meats (organs). In some places, *venison* (deer meat), *hare* (rabbit meat), and other wild game are available during certain seasons. Meat is graded as prime, choice, good, standard, and commercial. Choice and good are usually the highest grades available in supermarkets. Meat markets usually carry prime, and some restaurants use prime grades.

Because the grade of quality is not always marked on packaged meats, one should know how to distinguish good quality meats. Usually, a higher grade meat is more economical than a lower grade because there is less bone, gristle, and fat in the higher grade.

In addition to a pleasant odor, good quality meat should be firm, yet resilient to the touch. Beef should be bright red and marbled with white or creamy fat. Veal should be light pink with some white, brittle fat. Lamb should be reddish pink with creamy white fat. Pork may vary from a grey pink to a deeper rose color with white fat.

Organ meats include liver, kidney, tripe, tongue, sweetbreads, and brains. These are especially good sources of minerals and vitamins as well as protein, but their cholesterol content is high. They are quite inexpensive because they contain little or no waste.

Meats are available in various cuts, figures 10-3 through 10-7. The muscles that the animal uses most are the least tender. Although the less tender cuts are usually less expensive, the choice of cut should depend on the method of cooking to be used. Tender cuts may be cooked by *dry heat* methods such as roasting, broiling, or frying. Less tender cuts should be cooked covered by *moist heat* methods such as braising or stewing. The nutrient value of meat is not related to its tenderness.

Poultry

The common types of poultry available are chicken, turkey, duck, goose, and game

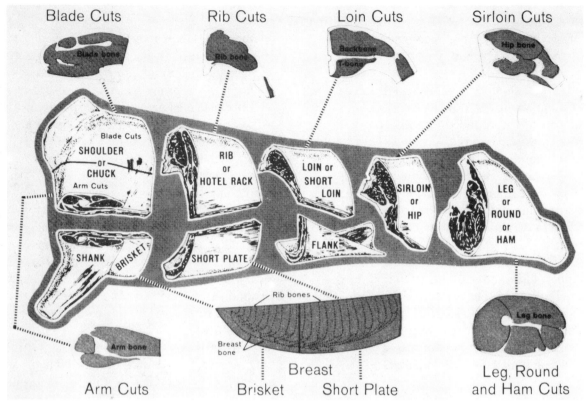

Figure 10-3 Seven basic retail cuts are used to prepare veal, lamb, beef, or pork. *(Courtesy of the National Live Stock and Meat Board)*

hen. Although the modern methods of raising poultry have resulted in a relatively standardized degree of tenderness, young birds are generally more tender and flavorful than old birds. Poultry may be graded *A* (highest quality) or *B* (less attractive, thinner birds) or *C* by government inspectors, but only when the seller pays for the inspection. If the label on the package includes the words "young," "broiler," or "fryer," the birds should be tender. If the label does not specify or says "stewing hen," or "mature turkey," the poultry will probably require moist heat methods of cooking.

Fish

Seafood may be divided into two groups: fish and shellfish. It may be purchased fresh, canned, frozen, and cured, or smoked. Seafood is graded according to size and quality, but standards of enforcing the grading are not uniform.

Some of the common fish available are cod, flounder, haddock, trout, salmon, and tuna. When purchased fresh, they should be firm with little slime, have red gills and clear, unsunken eyes. They are packaged as *round* (with head, bones, and scales), *fillets* (long,

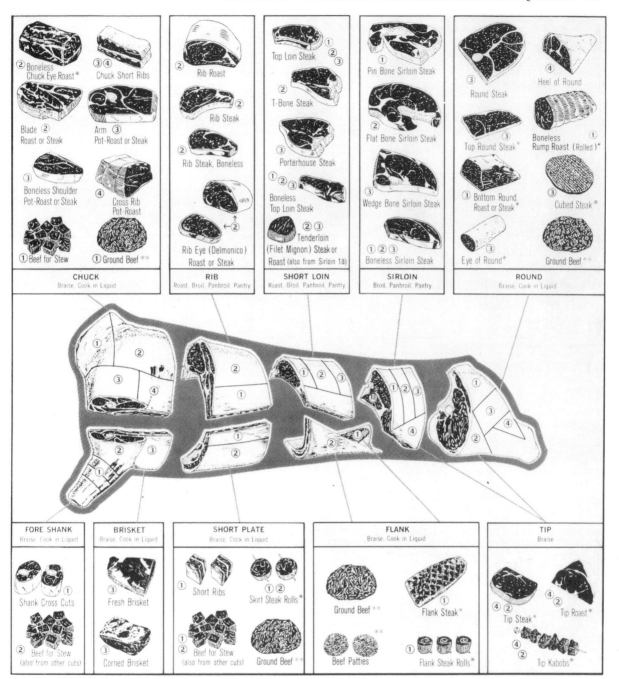

Figure 10-4 Beef cuts and cooking suggestions *(Courtesy of the Live Stock and Meat Board)*

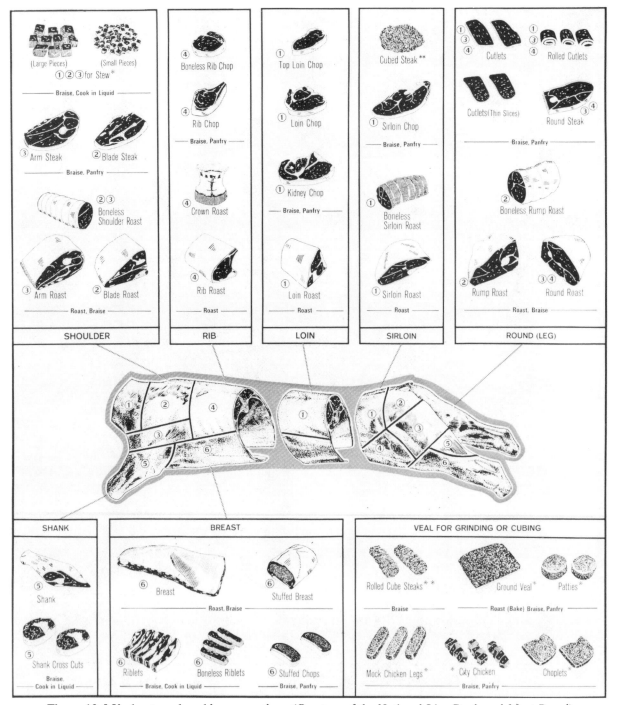

Figure 10-5 Veal cuts and cooking suggestions *(Courtesy of the National Live Stock and Meat Board)*

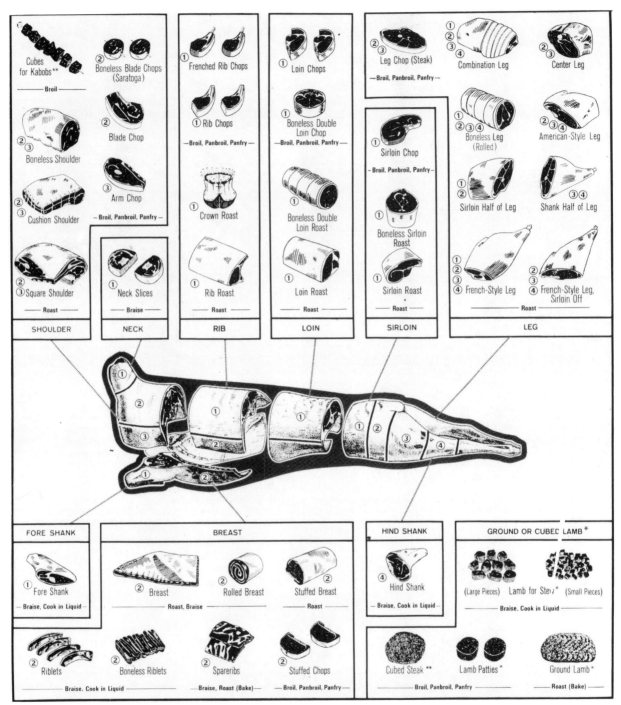

Figure 10-6 Cuts of lamb and cooking suggestions *(Courtesy of the National Live Stock and Meat Board)*

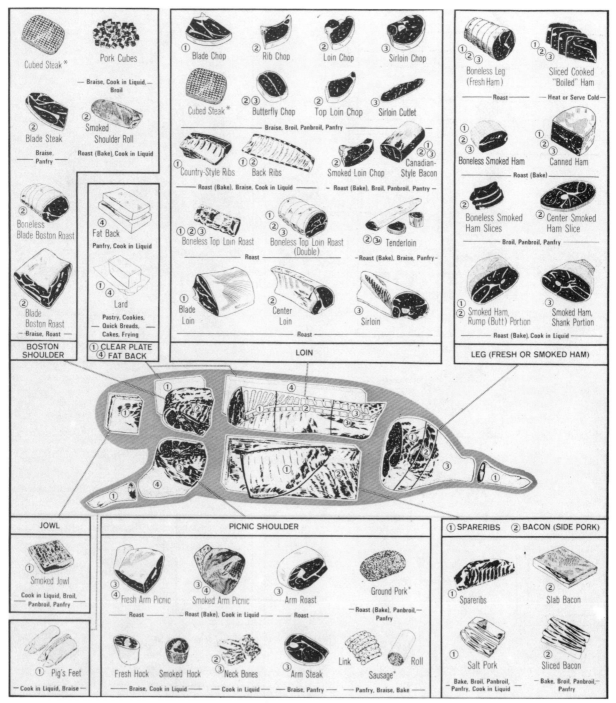

Figure 10-7 Cuts of pork and cooking suggestions (*Courtesy of the National Live Stock and Meat Board*)

thin strips of flesh, free of bone, which are cut from the sides of the fish), *steaks* (even, crosswise slices), and various fish sticks and fish balls.

The shellfish usually available include shrimp, oysters, crab, clams, lobsters, scallops, and mussels. They may be purchased raw in the shell, raw without the shell, and cooked, canned, or frozen.

Storage and Cooking of Meats, Poultry, and Fish

Because of the additional elements that make up protein, it decomposes more readily than carbohydrate and fat. Therefore, meat, poultry, and fish must be kept in the refrigerator to prevent or delay decomposition. When purchased fresh, poultry and meat should be unwrapped, lightly covered with wax paper or plastic wrap, and stored in the refrigerator. Fish should be covered well and stored in the refrigerator. Frozen foods should be well wrapped, stored in the freezer, and defrosted for use according to package directions. They should never be refrozen before cooking.

Proteins coagulate during cooking. Therefore, most foods containing large amounts of protein should be cooked at low temperatures to prevent them from becoming tough, and to prevent shrinkage. Exceptions are tender cuts of meat such as steaks and chops, which, if cooked to a rare or medium state of doneness, may be cooked at a high temperature for a short time in the broiler or on top of the stove. Roasting for a longer period of time at a low temperature is also advisable for tender cuts.

Roasting, broiling, and frying are called dry heat methods of cooking. Less tender cuts must be cooked for a longer time by a moist heat method such as stewing or braising. Older

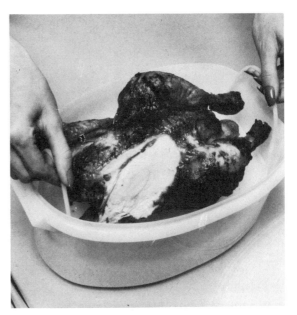

Figure 10-8 Leftover poultry should be stored in the refrigerator in a container with a tight fitting cover. *(Courtesy of Tupperware)*

fowl should also be cooked by moist heat to ensure flavor and tenderness. Larger fowl such as turkey, goose, and roasting chickens must be roasted slowly at a medium-low temperature. Fish is tender and is usually baked in liquid or sauteed to prevent it from drying out.

These foods, when left over, should be refrigerated and, when cold, tightly covered. They may be used advantageously in sandwiches, creamed dishes, salads, and soups.

VEGETABLES

Vegetables are edible plants that provide vitamins, minerals, carbohydrates, and sometimes proteins. Fresh vegetables may be

Table 10-2 Yield of Cooked Meat Per Pound of Raw Meat

Meat as purchased	Meat after Cooking (less drippings)	
	Parts weighed	Approximate weight of cooked parts per pound of raw meat purchased
Chops or steaks for broiling or frying:		ounces
With bone and relatively large amount of fat, such as pork or lamb chops; beef rib, sirloin, or porterhouse steaks	Lean, bone, fat	10-12
	Lean and fat	7-10
	Lean only	5-7
Without bone and with very little fat, such as round of beef	Lean and fat	12-13
veal steaks	Lean only	9-12
Ground meat for broiling or frying, such as beef, lamb, or pork patties	Patties	9-13
Roasts for oven cooking (no liquid added):		
With bone and relatively large amount of fat, such as beef rib, loin, chuck; lamb shoulder, leg; pork, fresh or cured	Lean, bone, fat	10-12
	Lean and fat	8-10
	Lean only	6-9
Without bone	Lean and fat	10-12
	Lean only	7-10
Cuts for pot-roasting, simmering, braising, stewing:		
With bone and relatively large amount of fat, such as beef chuck, pork shoulder	Lean, bone, fat	10-11
	Lean and fat	8-9
	Lean only	6-8
Without bone and with relatively small amount of fat, such as trimmed beef, veal	Lean with adhering fat	9-11

Source: Home and Garden Bulletin no. 72, U.S.D.A., 1971

graded U.S. Fancy, U.S. No. 1, and U.S. No. 2. However, some products may have grades above and below these. If a fresh vegetable has a grade mark, it means that the packing of the item was supervised by a U.S. Government grader. Most fresh vegetables are sold according to grades at wholesale markets, but few are marked according to grade in retail stores. Consequently, it is helpful to be able to recognize good quality fresh vegetables. They should be ripe, firm, without *blemishes* (spots) and a good, bright color. Wilted vegetables are old and have lost some of their nutritive value.

Commercially canned, frozen, and dried vegetables are convenient and retain most of their original nutrients. While their cost may be higher than the same product fresh, it must be remembered that these products contain no waste except for the package(s) in which they are packed. They usually contain additives, but their package labels should list them.

These foods are graded as U.S. Grade A (Fancy), U.S. Grade B (Choice or Extra Standard) and U.S. Grade C (Standard). The U.S. grade mark is found on very few of these items. If the label does carry a grade even without the "U.S." preceding it, it must be of the quality marked.

These items are packed and priced according to quality. Grade A is the most attractive, most tender, and most expensive. Grades B and C are less perfect in appearance and less expensive. They may be less tender and have some blemishes. The A grade is preferred when appearance is important, but all are equally nutritious.

Fresh vegetables should be stored in a cool, dry place. They should be served raw whenever possible. When cooked, they retain most nutrients by being cooked in their skins as short a time, and in as little boiling water, as possible. They should be served immediately after cooking. The liquid used in cooking should be added to soups and gravies since this liquid contains minerals and vitamins. Vegetables are commonly baked, boiled, and steamed. Some vegetables, such as potatoes, eggplant, and squash, may be fried for variety. Vegetables may be used as *accompaniment dishes* (food that is served along with the *entree*, or main dish), or in salads and soups. Leftovers should be stored in the refrigerator and covered when cold. They can be added to soups and salads.

FRUITS

Fruits are the fleshy parts surrounding the seeds of plants. They contribute valuable

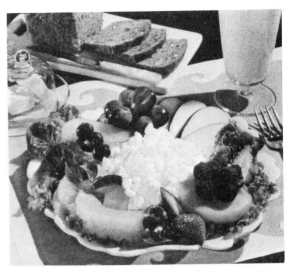

Figure 10-9 When appropriate accompaniment dishes are chosen from the Basic Four food groups, a fruit salad may be served as the main course for lunch. *(Courtesy of the National Dairy Council)*

vitamins and minerals, carbohydrates in the forms of sugar and fiber, and water. Because they contain fiber, water, and fruit acids, they have a laxative effect and are useful in overcoming constipation.

There are fresh, canned, frozen, and dried fruits available. When purchased fresh, fruit should be firm, ripe, and unblemished. Both fresh and prepared fruits are graded in the same manner as vegetables. *except bananas*

Fruit keeps best and is often tastiest when stored in the refrigerator. Frozen fruits should be kept frozen until ready for use. Some fruits, such as apples and plums, are more easily digested after cooking. They must be cooked very gently and just until tender. Sugar added at the beginning of the cooking period preserves their shape while sugar added later improves their flavor.

BREADS AND CEREALS

Cereals are the seeds of grains. As stated previously, these seeds consist of three main parts. The bran contains vitamins, minerals, proteins, and fiber. The endosperm is largely starch, which is ground and used for flour in various baked products. The germ contains the B vitamins and protein. During *milling* (grinding into flour) some of these vitamins and minerals are lost. Manufacturers restore them to their original nutrient value by adding these same nutrients in synthetic form. After this process, they are known as restored cereals. When these nutrients are added in amounts greater than the grain originally contained, the cereal is called enriched or fortified.

Because cereals are easy to grow, transport, and store, they are inexpensive and very popular. Although cereals are easily digested, cooking increases their digestibility. Breakfast cereals, rice, macaroni products, cornmeal, and various flours are the most familiar forms of cereals. Airtight containers preserve their freshness. Soybean flour, because of its fat content, should be stored airtight in a cool, dry place to prevent it from becoming rancid.

Essentially, bread is made from flour, water, and yeast with sugar, fat, and flavorings added at the discretion of the baker. It is available in countless shapes and flavors. It must be kept airtight to preserve its freshness, and may be frozen for long storage.

FOOD ADDITIVES

Today's consumers are also interested in food additives. These are chemical substances added to food during its growth, processing, or packaging. All additives are chemicals. Some are produced in nature and some are produced in laboratories.

There are two basic types of additives—the intentional additives, which are added to perform specific functions in the food; and the incidental additives, which are not intentionally added, but which may be found in the foods as a result of some stage of production or packaging.

The intentional additives serve four basic purposes.

1. *Enrich nutrient content* by adding vitamins, minerals, or protein. Examples include the addition of vitamin D to milk, which is considered the major reason for the near elimination of rickets in the United States; the addition of the vitamins thiamin, niacin, and riboflavin to cereals and breads (it is the addition of niacin that is thought to have virtually eliminated pellagra from the U.S.); and the addition of iodine to salt, which has greatly reduced the incidence of goiter in the U.S.

2. *Preserve freshness and retard spoilage.* Examples include the addition of humectants to promote the retention of moisture; antioxidants to preserve color in fruit and prevent fats from becoming rancid; and nitrites which prevent the development of botulism in packaged meats.

3. *Enhance appearance and texture.* Examples are coloring agents, flavorings, and bleaching agents used in wheat flour.

4. *Facilitate food processing.* Examples include stabilizers, emulsifiers, buffers, and thickeners that aid in the maintenance of the foods' integrity.

The incidental additives that may remain on foods are the result of the farmers' use of fertilizers, pesticides, or growth hormones during production; or from the food packaging, from which certain chemicals may be absorbed by the foods.

There is controversy regarding the addition of additives to foods. Some people want additives eliminated altogether on grounds that they may cause disease. The food industry maintains that without some additives, foods would not grow or keep as well as they now do and there would be an increase in food spoilage, which could increase food costs. The Federal Food and Drug Administration (FDA) requires that the manufacturer provide proof of the safety of food additives before they may be used. When such proof has been accepted by the FDA, the substance is added to its GRAS list. This is a list of substances *generally regarded as safe*. Even after a substance has been accepted on the GRAS list, its use is still limited. It cannot be used in amounts greater than 1 percent of the amount of the product that was shown to be safe.

ORGANIC, NATURAL, AND HEALTH FOODS

The terms *organic, natural*, and *health food* are of great interest today. In evaluating foods, it is advisable that the consumer understand what these terms mean. Actually, organic materials are chemical compounds of various sorts that contain the element carbon, in addition to other elements. Nearly all food is organic. Carbohydrates, fats, and proteins all contain carbon; vitamins and minerals are found in association with these nutrients.

Organic foods by current definition are plants that have been grown without the addition of artificial fertilizers or pesticides,

and animal foods from animals raised without treatments of antibiotics or hormones and prepared for market without the use of chemicals.

Natural foods are foods that have not been treated or processed in any way. They may or may not have been organically grown.

Health food is a general term used to describe foods that some food faddists claim have large quantities of nutrients that prevent, treat, or cure certain diseases. Honey, blackstrap molasses, granola, and wheat germ are often claimed to be health foods. Honey is considered to be a health food by some because it contains B vitamins, iron, and calcium. It does contain these nutrients but only in traces. Blackstrap molasses is an excellent source of calcium and iron, if used in large amounts. However, because molasses is strong-flavored and sweet, the amounts used in the everyday diet would not provide any significant proportion of these nutrients. Some granola cereals provide fewer vitamins and minerals than well-known varieties of the restored or enriched cereals. Among cereals, wheat germ is a good source of protein. It is also a good source of vitamin E, but again the amounts used are relatively small. Consequently, the nutrient intake from it is also small.

Health foods are sometimes overrated in their ability to prevent or cure disease. Many of these so-called health foods are good sources of certain nutrients, but most are nutritionally overrated. Many foods grown or prepared traditionally are equally rich in nutrients. Product labels and prices should be compared before one product is deemed better than another. Most of these organic, natural, and health foods are no more nutritious but are far more expensive than traditional foods.

SUMMARY

Beverages are fluids necessary to regulate body processes. Their various forms include water, milk, coffee, tea, fruit juices, and soft drinks. Milk, which is available in many forms, is one of the most valuable foods. Cheese is the curd that results from milk coagulation. Natural cheese has three basic forms—soft, semisoft, and hard. Eggs, like cheese, are a suitable meat alternate. Meats are graded and cut to aid the consumer in selecting the level of quality desired. The choice of cut depends on the method of cooking to be used. Meat, poultry, fish, or a high-quality meat substitute should be eaten at least once a day. Fruits and vegetables are usually most nutritious when eaten raw. If cooking is necessary, using only small amounts of water helps preserve nutritional quality. Breads and cereals are usually restored or enriched and are relatively inexpensive because they are easy to grow, transport, and store. Organic, natural, and health foods are usually nutritionally comparable to traditional food products. Many of these foods are expensive and overrated in their overall nutritional value.

Discussion Topics

1. Discuss the reasons for cooking vegetables and fruits and the reasons for serving them raw.
2. Discuss the nutritional values of various beverages, especially fruit drinks and sodas. As a parent, could you advise your children to drink these beverages? Why?
3. Discuss various means of including milk in the diet. Why is milk a wise purchase? Why must it be refrigerated?
4. How does the grade of eggs relate to their use in the menu? Describe 5 ways of using eggs in the diet.
5. Using the meat charts in this chapter, discuss which cuts of meat are tender and which are less tender.
6. Which methods of cooking are advised for the less tender cuts of meat? Why?
7. How does the storage of fruits and vegetables affect their nutrient content?
8. Discuss various organic, natural, and health foods. What are their advantages? Disadvantages?
9. Discuss food additives. Are there some that may be unnecessary in terms of nutrition and storage? If so, why are they used?
10. At what general temperature should meat, milk, eggs, and cheese usually be cooked? Why?
11. What is a meat alternate? Name some and explain how they might be used in a menu.

Suggested Activities

1. Organize the class into groups and visit a local supermarket. Each group should make a survey of the various forms and prices of one of the groups of foods discussed in this chapter. Reports should be exchanged and filed for future use in meal preparation.
2. Visit a health food store. Compare the prices of their products with the same products in the supermarket. Are there differences? If so, why?
3. Make a chart of the various forms of milk available and include a description of each, including cost.
4. Using other sources, prepare a report to the class on the diseases caused by bacteria that may be present in raw milk. Find out what precautions are taken by dairy farmers in the local area to prevent the contamination of milk.
5. Make an appointment and visit a meat market to observe meatcutters at work. Take notes and discuss the visit when you return to class.

Review

A. Multiple-multiple Choice. Select the *letter* that precedes the best answer.

1. Milk is an important beverage because it
   1. contains complete protein and calcium
   2. has been pasteurized to increase the amount of vitamin D
   3. contains phosphorus, vitamin A, and riboflavin
   4. contains a stimulant
   5. contains vitamin C and iron
      a) all   b) 1, 3, 4   c) 1, 2, 5   d) 1, 3
2. The following forms of milk have had some of their natural nutrients removed:
   1. homogenized milk   4. buttermilk
   2. pasteurized milk   5. raw milk
   3. skim milk
      a) 1, 2, 3, 4   b) 3, 4   c) 2, 3, 5   d) all
3. Good quality beef should have the following characteristics:
   1. a pleasant odor
   2. firm, yet resilient
   3. light pink color with brittle fat
   4. a U.S. Government grade stamp
   5. marbled with white or creamy fat
      a) all   b) 1, 3, 5   c) 1, 2, 4   d) 1, 2, 5

4. To be stored properly, fresh meats should be
   1. unwrapped and uncovered
   2. unwrapped and covered with wax paper
   3. always refrigerated or frozen
   4. refrozen after thawing
   5. never frozen
      a) 2, 3   b) 1, 3, 4   c) 1, 4, 5   d) 1, 2, 4

5. Vegetables are essential to a well-balanced diet because they
   1. contain both fat-soluble and water-soluble vitamins
   2. contain only water-soluble vitamins
   3. contain carbohydrates
   4. are good sources of fiber
   5. are good sources of complete protein
      a) 1, 3, 4   b) 2, 3, 4   c) 3, 4, 5   d) all

6. Coffee should be
   1. stored in a cool place
   2. tightly covered for storage
   3. diluted by boiling for 2 minutes
   4. given to children only after the caffeine is removed
   5. added to meals for its food value
      a) 1, 2, 5   b) 1, 2, 4   c) 2, 4, 5   d) 1, 2

7. Food additives can
   1. enrich nutrient content
   2. retard spoilage
   3. enhance flavor
   4. maintain appearance
   5. maintain texture
      a) all   b) 1, 4   c) 2, 3   d) 1, 4, 5

8. Beverages
   1. regulate body processes
   2. provide nourishment
   3. relieve thirst
   4. provide the best source of fat
      a) all   b) 1, 2, 3   c) 2, 3, 4   d) 1, 3, 4

9. A specific cut of beef may be chosen according to its
   1. intended use
   2. protein content
   3. water content
   4. total carbohydrate content
      a) 1, 2, 4   b) 1   c) 1, 4   d) 3, 4

10. Organic foods are
    1. the same as natural foods
    2. only animal foods
    3. those food produced without the use of any chemicals
    4. generally nutritious if chosen from the Basic Four food groups
    5. generally more expensive than foods from the supermarket
        a) all   b)1, 2   c) 3, 4, 5   d) 1, 2, 3

B. Match the items in column I to the correct statement in column II.

Column I	Column II
H 1. additives	a. milk with fat removed
E 2. caffeine	b. one who buys and uses products
J 3. pasteurization	c. microorganisms
A 4. skim milk	d. milk with 60% of water removed
B 5. consumer	e. stimulant
C 6. bacteria	f. grinding into flour
D 7. evaporated milk	g. natural cheese with additional moisture
F 8. milling	h. may be intentional or incidental
G 9. process cheese	i. roquefort cheese
K 10. dried milk	j. process of killing harmful bacteria in milk
	k. milk with all water removed
	l. process of breaking up fat in milk

C. Briefly answer the following questions.
1. Why are coffee and tea not advisable for children?

2. How is milk pasteurized?

References

Bennion, Marion. 1980. *Introductory Foods*, 7th ed. New York: Macmillan Publishing Company.

Charley, Helen. 1982. *Food Science*, 2nd ed. New York: John Wiley & Sons.

Green, Marilyn L., and Joann Harry. 1981. *Nutrition in Contemporary Nursing Practice*. New York: John Wiley & Sons.

Hui, Y. H. *Human Nutrition and Diet Therapy*. 1983. Monterey, Calif: Wadsworth Health Sciences Division of Wadsworth Inc.

Kerschner, Velma L. 1983. *Nutrition and Diet Therapy*. Philadelphia: F. A. Davis Co.

Kinder, Faye, Nancy Green, and Natholyn Harris. 1984. *Meal Management*, 6th ed. New York: Macmillan Publishing Company.

Peckham, Gladys, and Jeanne Freeland-Graves. 1979. *Foundations of Food Preparation*, 4th ed. New York: Macmillan Publishing Company.

Chapter 11

PURCHASING FOOD

VOCABULARY

convenience food   freeze-dried   nutrition labeling
dehydrated   grade stamps   seasonal
Food, Drug and   impulsive shopper
   Cosmetic Act

OBJECTIVES

After studying this chapter, you should be able to

- Estimate correct amounts of foods to purchase for a given number of people

- Identify information commonly given on food labels

- List guidelines for selecting size and style of food packages

- Name five considerations that help the consumer maintain a balanced diet on a low food budget

The appropriate selection of food can be quite challenging. There are countless varieties of foods available in many different styles of preparation and packaging at many different prices. The wise buyer knows that the value of food is measured by its nutritional quality and not by its price. Achieving a well-balanced diet does not depend on a large food budget. A sound knowledge of nutrition is essential for the consumer.

The Basic Four food groups are the foundation upon which all food purchasing plans should be made. It is also extremely useful to have a basic understanding of how foods are prepared and packaged for consumer use.

LABELING

Reading the label on a food package is the best method of determining the value of the food. Food labeling is somewhat regulated in the United States to protect the consumer. The Federal Food, Drug and Cosmetic Act is a law that requires that food shipped from one state to another be pure, safe to eat, and prepared under sanitary conditions. It also requires that containers of food shipped from one state to another have their ingredients and weight printed on the label. Ingredients are listed according to their proportions in the product. The ingredient found in greatest proportion is listed first, the ingredient found in second greatest proportion is listed second and so on. Foods processed and sold within one state are governed by state law.

Labels may also include the number of servings, approximate quantity, size, and maturity of the product, recipes and serving suggestions, and other products available from the manufacturer. This information on food labels is particularly important to the consumer who must select foods to be used for special diets.

In an effort to aid the consumer, the United States Food and Drug Administration has issued regulations regarding nutrition labeling. *Nutrition labeling* is the listing of specific nutrition information on packages of foods that are enriched or fortified and on foods for which a nutritional claim is made. The information required on such foods must follow a standard format. The label must include serving size, total number of servings, and calories per serving. The following ingredients must also be listed per serving: grams of protein, carbohydrate, and fat, and the percentage of the United States Recommended Daily Allowances (RDA) for protein, vitamins A and C, thiamin, riboflavin and niacin, and the minerals calcium and iron, figure 11-1. The listing of cholesterol, fatty acid, sodium content, and additional vitamins and minerals may also be included. Addi-

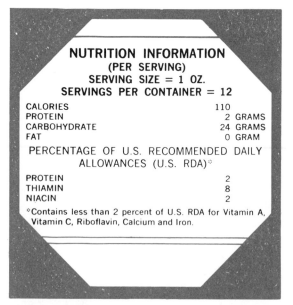

A. Certain labels include only the minimum information required.

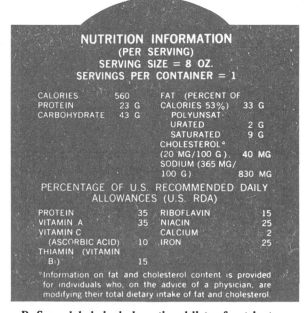

B. Some labels include optional lists of nutrients.

Figure 11-1 Nutritional labeling helps the consumer determine the nutrient value of a product. *(Courtesy of the Food and Drug Administration)*

tionally, many food manufacturers will, upon request, mail the consumer detailed nutritional information regarding their products.

GRADES

Several foods have United States Department of Agriculture (USDA) grade stamps on them, figure 11-2. The grade varies, depending upon the quality of the product. A grade stamp is not mandatory. When food is stamped, the food processor has requested and paid for the service. Foods most commonly graded are beef, lamb, chicken, turkey, butter, and eggs. When a grade stamp is found on a food product, it means that the food has been inspected by a U.S. Government expert and found to conform to specific government standards of quality. The lack of such a stamp does not mean the food is inferior in any way.

PACKAGING

The sizes and styles of food packages purchased depend on several factors. The size of the family and its members' appetites are

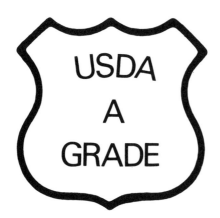

Figure 11-2 A U.S. Government grade stamp shows that the quality of a food item has been evaluated by a federal inspector.

important considerations, as are the cooking methods to be used, and the time allowed for cooking. The storage space available also determines the size of the package to be purchased. If there is sufficient storage space and the food keeps well, large packages may be economical even for small families. When there is inadequate storage space, small packages may be more practical. The consumer should select the size of the package needed according to its actual weight or volume. The consumer cannot depend on manufacturers' descriptions such as *jumbo, giant*, or *economy* size. All food containers should be checked for breaks or leaks in the packaging and, when appropriate, washed before storing.

CONVENIENCE FOODS

An extremely popular form of food today is the convenience food that requires little or no preparation. The term is used to describe cake, bread, and dessert mixes; instant puddings; brown-and-serve breads, and pastries; frozen TV dinners; and frozen or canned fruits, vegetables, meats, fish, and desserts. Most of them are high in quality and save kitchen work. These foods can be expensive for large families but economical for single or elderly people. Convenience foods reduce waste that often occurs with leftovers. When the cook spends a day away from home, convenience foods are economical in terms of time. With the addition of a fresh vegetable and milk, the frozen dinner provides a nutritionally balanced meal. It is wise to keep some of these foods on hand for unexpected situations.

Frozen Foods

It is advisable to buy frozen foods in packages that can be used at one time or in a type of package, usually a plastic bag, that allows the cook to remove only as much food as is needed for a meal. Frozen foods are sold according to weight. The labels usually indicate the number of servings per package. While frozen foods may be more expensive than fresh foods, they are sometimes more economical because they contain no waste and are always in season. Also, when they are fully-cooked foods that require only reheating, they are economical in terms of the cook's time. They do not spoil if stored properly and usually take little time to prepare.

Canned Foods

Because canned foods keep so well, they are popular and especially useful to someone with limited refrigerator space. There are few foods that are not available in cans. Except for

Table 11-1 Common Container Sizes for Canned Foods

CONTAINER			PRINCIPAL PRODUCTS
INDUSTRY TERM	CONSUMER DESCRIPTION APPROX. NET WEIGHT OR FLUID MEASURE (CHECK LABEL)	APPROX. CUPS	
8 oz.	8 oz.	1	Fruits, vegetables, specialties for small families. 2 servings.
Picnic	10 1/2 to 12 oz.	1 1/4	Mainly condensed soups. Some fruits, vegetables, meat, fish, specialties. 2 to 3 servings.
12 oz. (vac.)	12 oz.	1 1/2	Principally for vacuum pack corn. 3 to 4 servings.
No. 300	14 to 16 oz. (14 oz. to 1 lb.)	1 3/4	Pork and beans, baked beans, meat products, cranberry sauce, blueberries, specialties. 3 to 4 servings.
No. 303	16 to 17 oz. (1 lb. to 1 lb. 1 oz.)	2	Principal size for fruits and vegetables. Some meat products, ready-to-serve soups, specialties. 4 servings.
No. 2	20 oz. (1 lb. 4 oz.) 18 fl. oz. (1 pt. 2 fl. oz.)	2 1/2	Juices, ready-to-serve soups, some specialties, pineapple, apple slices. No longer in popular use for most fruits and vegetables. 5 servings.
No. 2 1/2	27 to 29 oz. (1 lb. 11 oz. to 1 lb. 13 oz.)	3 1/2	Fruits, some vegetables (pumpkin, sauerkraut, spinach and other greens, tomatoes). 5 to 7 servings.
No. 3 cyl. or 46 fl. oz.	51 oz. (3 lb. 3 oz.) 46 fl. oz. (1 qt. 14 fl. oz.)	5 3/4	Fruit and vegetable juices, pork and beans. Institutional size for condensed soups, some vegetables. 10 to 12 servings.
No. 10	6 1/2 lb to 7 lb. 5 oz.	12-13	Institutional size for fruits, vegetables and some other foods. 25 servings.

Source: National Canners Association

certain meats, canned foods are relatively inexpensive. They are sold according to the can sizes shown in table 11-1. Sometimes the weights of two different products in identical cans vary because of the different densities of the foods.

Freeze-Dried Foods

In this process, foods are frozen so rapidly that their flavors and textures are not noticeably changed. They are then *dehydrated* (have water removed). The consumer purchases them in small packages that may be kept for long periods of time without refrigeration. Directions for preparing freeze-dried foods usually include a specified period of time for soaking in a specified amount of liquid. By soaking they regain their original moisture content and appearance. After soaking they are cooked as if they were fresh foods.

ECONOMY IN PURCHASING

Economy is a major goal of the concerned shopper. Careful planning is the key to economical food purchasing. Consideration of the following factors should aid the consumer in planning economical food purchases.

Menu Planning

Careful menu planning is essential if one is to make economical food purchases. In addition, such planning saves time. Meals for the week should be planned at one time around the weekly specials advertised in local newspapers. Planning should also include the appropriate use of leftovers. The food marketing list should be made according to the weekly menu and based on the Basic Four food groups.

Intended Use

Foods should be selected according to their intended use. For example, less-expensive, small fruit is satisfactory for making peach jam, but if peaches are to be served whole or as halves, the larger, more attractive fruit should be purchased. Less tender cuts of meat are as nutritious and, when prepared appropriately, as appealing as tender cuts. However, it must be remembered that the less tender cuts of meat require longer cooking times than the tender cuts. Large cuts of meat are often less expensive per pound than small cuts. Therefore, it is economical to buy large quantities if subsequent meals are planned around leftovers. Leftovers should be properly wrapped and frozen for future use. Sometimes a few portions can be separated from the whole before cooking. The extra portions can then be wrapped and frozen for future use.

Substitutions

Cheaper foods can often be substituted for expensive foods without any loss in nutrition. Some examples include fortified margarine in place of butter, and dried milk instead of fresh milk. Such substitutions can substantially lower food costs. Recipes should be carefully checked and substitutions made whenever appropriate. Table 11-2 shows some common cooking substitutions.

Seasonal Foods

Shipping foods from distant locations is expensive and can increase the amount of food bills. For this reason it is most economical to

Table 11-2 Common Cooking Substitutions

1 square chocolate (ounce)
3 tablespoons cocoa plus 1 to 3 teaspoons fat

1 cup cake flour
1 cup all-purpose flour less 2 tablespoons

1 tablespoon cornstarch
2 tablespoons flour (for thickening)

2/3 teaspoon double-action type baking powder
1/4 teaspoon baking soda plus 1/2 teaspoon cream of tartar

1 cup fresh milk
1/2 cup evaporated milk plus 1/2 cup water
or
1/2 cup condensed milk plus 1/2 cup water with reduction of sugar used
or
1/4 cup powdered whole milk plus 1 cup water
or
1/4 cup powdered skim milk plus 2 tablespoons butter plus 1 cup water

use foods that are in season. A food's *season* is the period it is normally ripe or ready, and hence available in quantity at its lowest price. Fruits, vegetables, and certain fish are seasonal. This should be considered when planning menus. When a desired food is not locally in season, canned and frozen foods may be more economical than the fresh.

Generic Brands

Most large supermarkets now have generic brands sections carrying many products. These items do not carry a manufacturer's name or quality grade—only their generic names as, for example, "Peas," or "Peaches," or "Napkins". These items are less expensive than name brands, but qualities vary. Where quality is not a concern, they are economical purchases and should not be overlooked.

Quantities Needed

It is wise to purchase only as much food as can be used or properly stored. Because fresh fruits, vegetables, meat, fish, poultry, fats, sugar, and many cereal products are sold according to weight, it is advisable to know the number of servings per pound that each of these foods will yield. Table 11-3 can be used as a guide when first preparing market orders.

Selection of the Store or Market

The type of store or market can greatly affect the total cost of the food purchased. Typically, the large cash-and-carry supermarkets have lower prices and offer a wider selection of foods than the small neighborhood markets. Small stores sometimes charge higher prices because they are convenient, allow charge accounts, or because they make home deliveries. Large stores use a great deal of commercial advertising that can ruin the budget of the *impulsive shopper* (one who buys because of a momentary desire). The prices of the "super-specials" displayed at prominent places in the markets should be carefully checked against the regular prices of the same article. The actual value of the special should be carefully evaluated by the consumer before the purchase.

SUMMARY

Nutritious meals can be prepared on a small budget as well as on a large budget.

Table 11-3 Servings per Package or per Pound

Meat, poultry, and fish

The amount of meat, poultry, and fish to buy varies with the amount of bone, fat, and breading.

	Servings per pound[1]
MEAT	
Much bone or gristle	1 or 2
Medium amounts of bone	2 or 3
Little or no bone	3 or 4
POULTRY (READY-TO-COOK)	
Chicken	2 or 3
Turkey	2 or 3
Duck and goose	2
FISH	
Whole	1 or 2
Dressed or pan-dressed	2 or 3
Portions or steaks	3
Fillets	3 or 4

[1] Three ounces of cooked lean meat, poultry, or fish per serving.

CEREAL PRODUCTS

One serving of a cereal may vary from 1/2 cup to 1 1/4 cup. Check package labels.

	Servings per lb.
Flaked corn cereals	18-24
Other flaked cereals	21
Puffed cereals	32-38
Wheat cereals:	
Coarse	12
Fine	16-22
Oatmeal	13
Hominy grits	20
Macaroni, noodles	12
Rice	16
Spaghetti	13

Vegetables and fruits

For this table, a serving of vegetable is 1/2 cup cooked vegetable unless otherwise noted. A serving of fruit is 1/2 cup fruit; 1 medium apple banana, peach, or pear; or 2 apricots or plums. A serving of cooked fresh or dried fruit is 1/2 cup fruit and liquid.

	Servings per pound[1]
FRESH VEGETABLES	
Asparagus	2 or 3
Beans, lima[2]	2
Beans, snap	5 or 6
Beets, diced[3]	3 or 4
Broccoli	3 or 4
Brussels sprouts	4
Cabbage:	
Raw, shredded	9 or 10
Cooked	4 or 5
Carrots:	
Raw, diced or shredded[3]	5 or 6
Cooked[3]	4
Cauliflower	3
Celery:	
Raw, chopped or diced	5 or 6
Cooked	4
Kale[4]	5 or 6
Okra	4 or 5
Onions, cooked	3 or 4
Parsnips[3]	4
Peas[2]	2
Potatoes	4
Spinach[5]	4
Squash, summer	3 or 4
Squash, winter	2 or 3
Sweetpotatoes	3 or 4
Tomatoes, raw, diced or sliced	4

[1] As purchased.
[2] Bought in pod.
[3] Bought without tops.
[4] Bought untrimmed.
[5] Bought prepackaged.

	Servings per package (9 or 10 oz.)
FROZEN VEGETABLES	
Asparagus	2 or 3
Beans, lima	3 or 4
Beans, snap	3 or 4
Broccoli	2 or 3
Brussels sprouts	3
Cauliflower	3
Corn, whole kernel	3
Kale	2 or 3
Peas	3
Spinach	2 or 3

	Servings per can (16 oz.)
CANNED VEGETABLES	
Most vegetables	3 or 4
Greens, such as kale or spinach	2 or 3

	Servings per pound
DRY VEGETABLES	
Dry beans	11
Dry peas, lentils	10 or 11

	Servings per market unit[1]
FRESH FRUIT	
Apples, Bananas, Peaches, Pears, Plums	3 or 4 per pound
Apricots, Cherries, sweet, Grapes, seedless	5 or 6 per pound
Blueberries, Raspberries	4 or 5 per pint
Strawberries	5 or 6 per unit

[1] As purchased.

	Servings per package (10 or 12 oz.)
FROZEN FRUIT	
Blueberries	3 or 4
Peaches	2 or 3
Raspberries	2 or 3
Strawberries	2 or 3

	Servings per can (16 oz.)
CANNED FRUIT	
Served with liquid	4
Drained	2 or 3

	Servings per package (8 oz.)
DRIED FRUIT	
Apples	8
Apricots	6
Mixed fruits	5
Peaches	6
Pears	4
Prunes unpitted	4 or 5

Source: USDA Home and Garden Bulletin No. 1, 1975

Labels on packaged foods give contents and weight. Consumers who know how a food item will be used can select the appropriate type and size of the package as well as the level of quality needed. Planning menus around weekly specials, buying fresh foods in season, and making nutritionally equal substitutions can reduce food costs. Usually, the large supermarkets offer foods at lower prices than the small stores.

Discussion Topics

1. Bring grocery advertisements from the newspaper to class.
   a. Compare the prices of the week's specials. Remember to consider the varying qualities of food.
   b. Discuss any new foods that are listed. Ask if anyone in the class has used them.
   c. Discuss the various ways in which one of the meats "on special" can be prepared.
   d. Discuss which foods, if any, are seasonal.
2. What are convenience foods? Name six. Discuss their advantages and disadvantages.
3. Discuss the information found on food packages and how it may or may not affect the purchase and use of some foods. Why is this particularly important to a diabetic patient? To a heart patient? What is nutrition labeling?
4. Discuss quality grade stamps. Has anyone noticed them? What do they indicate?

Suggested Activities

1. Plan a week's menu for a family of four who have no special dietary needs. Assume the cost of the week's menu is $100.
   a. List some possible changes that would lower the cost, without lowering the nutritional value.
   b. Determine the amounts of food required for the menu. Refer to table 11-3.
   c. Make a market list for this menu, organized according to the Basic Four food groups.
   d. Adapt this menu to suit a single person; to suit a middle-aged couple who have no children.
2. List the fresh fruits and vegetables available at a local supermarket this week. Have the instructor explain the unfamiliar ones. Compare their

costs with the identical frozen products and with canned products. Remember to consider edible portions and waste.

3. List the information printed on the label of a canned food.

4. Check the local supermarkets to see what freeze-dried foods are available. Buy one and prepare it according to package instructions. Compare it with the same frozen food in regard to flavor, appearance, preparation, and cost.

5. Visit a supermarket and determine the number of different preparations that are available in each of the following foods (frozen, fresh, canned, etc.): green peas, potatoes, corn, orange juice, bananas, rice, milk, shrimp. Evaluate ease of home preparation and cost of each.

A. Multiple Choice. Select the *letter* that precedes the best answer.

1. The value of food is determined by its
   a. cost
   b. nutritional quality
   c. ease in preparation
   d. all of these

2. The foundation of all good food purchasing plans is
   a. the Basic Four food groups
   b. nutritional labeling
   c. the federal Food, Drug and Cosmetic Act
   d. quality grading

3. A substitute for one cup of fresh milk is
   a. 1/4 cup dried milk plus 1 cup water
   b. 1/2 cup evaporated milk plus 1/2 cup water
   c. both a and b
   d. none of the above

4. The quality of a food
   a. may be shown by a USDA grade stamp
   b. is always indicated on food labels
   c. is never determined by the federal government
   d. is always determined by the food manufacturer

5. The size of the food package purchased depends on
   a. family size
   b. size of appetites
   c. available storage space
   d. all of these

6. It is advisable to plan meals for a period of
   a. one day
   b. one week
   c. two weeks
   d. one month

7. A fresh fruit or vegetable that is in season is usually
   a. tastiest
   b. available in quantity
   c. available at its lowest cost
   d. all of these
8. An example of a convenience food is
   a. frozen dinners
   b. fresh picked vegetables
   c. bagged coffee beans
   d. Grade AA eggs
9. Under the nutrition labeling regulation, specific nutrition information must be listed on packages for
   a. all foods
   b. enriched and fortified foods
   c. foods making a nutritional claim
   d. both b and c
10. The nutrition labeling regulation was issued by the
    a. Food and Drug Administration
    b. United States Department of Agriculture
    c. National Research Council
    d. Food and Nutrition Board

B. Complete the following sentences.
1. The law requiring that food shipped from one state to another be uncontaminated, safe to eat, and prepared under sanitary conditions, is the _____.
2. This same law requires that labels on food containers list ingredients and _____.
3. An RDA is a nutrient's _____.
4. Foods that are very easy to serve because they are partially prepared are called _____.
5. Freeze-dried foods have the nutrient _____ removed.
6. USDA grade stamps on foods indicate the food's _____ , not its nutritional value.
7. A food's _____ is the period during which it is usually ripe and at its best.
8. Large cuts of meat usually cost _____ (less, more) per pound than small cuts.
9. A person who buys foods because of a momentary desire is a (an) _____ shopper.
10. A satisfactory substitute for butter is margarine which is _____ .

C. Briefly answer the following questions.
1. Name at least five considerations that help the consumer maintain a well-balanced diet on a low food budget.

2. What factors determine the size and style of food package to be purchased?

3. Why are frozen or canned foods sometimes more economical than fresh foods?

References

Howe, Phyllis Sullivan. 1981. *Basic Nutrition in Health and Disease*. Philadelphia: W. B. Saunders Co.

Hui, Y. H. 1983. *Human Nutrition and Diet Therapy*. Monterey, Calif: Wadsworth Health Sciences Division of Wadsworth Inc.

Kinder, Faye, Nancy Green, and Natholyn Harris. 1984. *Meal Management*, 6th ed. New York: Macmillan Publishing Company.

Luke, Barbara. 1984. *Principles of Nutrition and Diet Therapy*. Boston: Little Brown & Co.

Peckham, Gladys, and Jeanne Freeland-Graves. 1979. *Foundations of Food Preparation*, 4th ed. New York: Macmillan Publishing Company Inc.

Robinson, Corinne H. 1979. *Fundamentals of Normal Nutrition*, 3rd ed. New York: Macmillan Publishing Company.

Section 3
Meal
Preparation

Chapter 12

USING KITCHEN EQUIPMENT EFFICIENTLY

VOCABULARY

abrasive	durability	meat thermometer
appliance	efficiency	pastry blender
culinary	equipment	
deodorize	flatware	

OBJECTIVES

After studying this chapter, you should be able to

- State the criteria for selecting kitchen equipment

- Name three practices that can reduce accidents in the kitchen

- Explain how to smother a grease fire

Kitchen work is complicated because it involves so many different processes. Efficiency is attained when the cook learns to perform the necessary tasks quickly and well. To do this, a good deal of practice is necessary and laborsaving methods must be employed.

Before beginning any *culinary* (relating to the kitchen or cookery) task, one should collect the necessary equipment and ingredients and arrange them conveniently. Clean-up should be considered during the preparation of food. Equipment that has been used should be set apart from ingredients that have been used. To save dishwashing after meals, the equipment used during the preparation of a meal should be washed and stored before the meal

whenever possible. It is especially important to keep the school and hospital kitchens clean and orderly. Order helps prevent accidents and mistakes in the preparation of food, and increases efficiency. Cleanliness reduces the spread of disease.

DISHWASHING

Scrape off food scraps and rinse the dishes as soon as possible after meals. Those dishes or cooking pans containing sticky starch or protein foods may require soaking in cold water. When a cooking pan is very sticky, it is usually helpful to add a small amount of

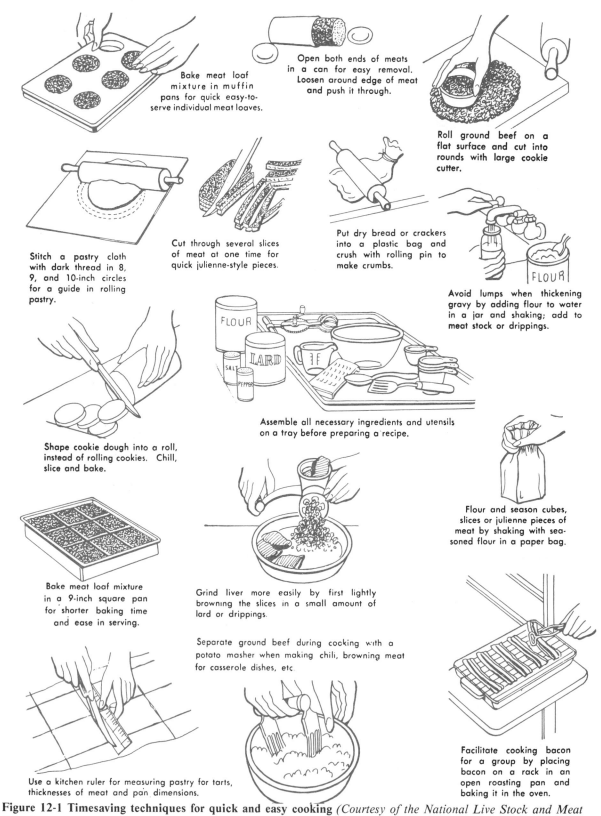

Bake meat loaf mixture in muffin pans for quick easy-to-serve individual meat loaves.

Open both ends of meats in a can for easy removal. Loosen around edge of meat and push it through.

Roll ground beef on a flat surface and cut into rounds with large cookie cutter.

Stitch a pastry cloth with dark thread in 8, 9, and 10-inch circles for a guide in rolling pastry.

Cut through several slices of meat at one time for quick julienne-style pieces.

Put dry bread or crackers into a plastic bag and crush with rolling pin to make crumbs.

Avoid lumps when thickening gravy by adding flour to water in a jar and shaking; add to meat stock or drippings.

Shape cookie dough into a roll, instead of rolling cookies. Chill, slice and bake.

Assemble all necessary ingredients and utensils on a tray before preparing a recipe.

Flour and season cubes, slices or julienne pieces of meat by shaking with seasoned flour in a paper bag.

Bake meat loaf mixture in a 9-inch square pan for shorter baking time and ease in serving.

Grind liver more easily by first lightly browning the slices in a small amount of lard or drippings.

Separate ground beef during cooking with a potato masher when making chili, browning meat for casserole dishes, etc.

Use a kitchen ruler for measuring pastry for tarts, thicknesses of meat and pan dimensions.

Facilitate cooking bacon for a group by placing bacon on a rack in an open roasting pan and baking it in the oven.

Figure 12-1 Timesaving techniques for quick and easy cooking (*Courtesy of the National Live Stock and Meat Board*)

water, cover the pan and place over direct heat just until the liquid comes to a boil. Remove it from the heat and allow to cool enough so that it may be handled. Then drain, rinse, and wash with hot, soapy water.

To prepare for washing, sort dishes according to type after they have been rinsed. Wash glassware first, then *flatware* (knives, forks, and spoons), dishes, and finally the pots and pans. Rinse in hot water and let the dishes and glassware drain and air-dry, covered with a clean towel. Air-drying is a sanitary method of drying dishes. The use of a dish towel can sometimes spread germs. A towel may be needed to dry some metal equipment to prevent water spots and rust. Store them in their proper places when they are thoroughly dry.

SELECTION OF EQUIPMENT

Equipment is chosen for its durability, efficiency, ease with which it can be maintained, and price in relation to these considerations. The student is probably familiar with small equipment or utensils such as skillets, saucepans, double boilers, and various spatulas, spoons, and hand blenders.

The use of larger equipment and appliances such as pressure pans, mixers, electric blenders, food processors, steamers, and dishwashers should be carefully explained and demonstrated. Gas, electric, and microwave cooking equipment have varying types of controls and will require special instructions before use. Observe the demonstration and care of all equipment carefully to use it efficiently and safely. When purchasing kitchen equipment, ask the salesperson to demonstrate the use of it. Read the manufacturer's instructions carefully before using any piece of equipment.

CLEANING EQUIPMENT AND KITCHEN SURFACES

The stove should be cleaned after each use. When a spot is too sticky to be removed easily with soap and water, let a small amount of soapy water stand on the sticky area for a few minutes. Then wash again and, if necessary, use a plastic cleaning pad or soap pad to remove the residue. Some cleaning pads are abrasive and should be used cautiously to prevent scratching the surface of equipment. Some surfaces such as stainless steel and enamel are dried and polished to prevent water spots. The oven and broiler should be cleaned regularly, and always after food has been spilled in them. There are commercial cleaners available for this purpose. Package directions must be followed carefully because these cleaners can be dangerous when misused.

Only food in clean, covered containers should be placed in the refrigerator. Any spills inside or outside should be removed. The refrigerator should be cleaned regularly and deodorized by washing with a baking soda solution.

The sink should be scoured and washed with hot soapy water after each use. Grease should not be poured in the sink because it increases the difficulty of cleaning and may clog the drain. If the drain should clog, there are commercial products available to clear it. However, they should be used with caution and should never come in contact with the hands or the porcelain of the sink.

Tables and countertops should be washed and dried after each use. Cupboards and storage spaces should be kept orderly and clean.

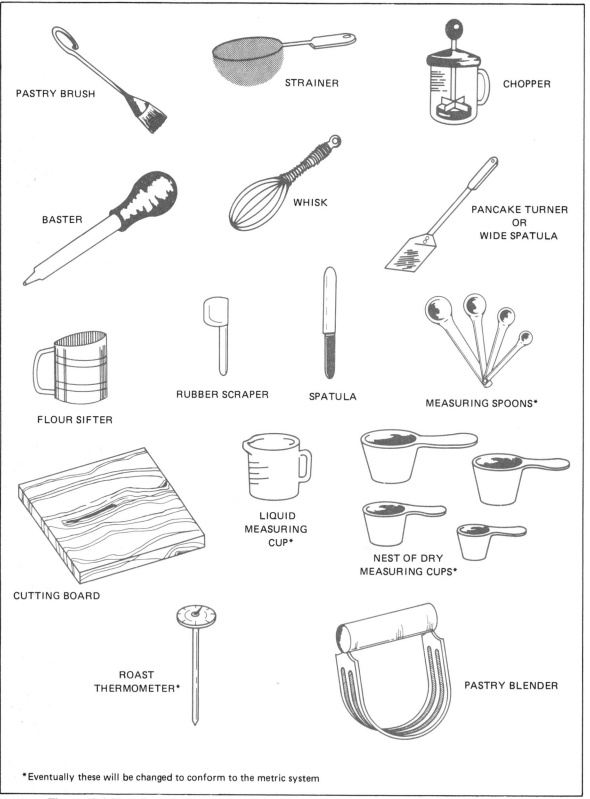

PASTRY BRUSH

STRAINER

CHOPPER

BASTER

WHISK

PANCAKE TURNER
OR
WIDE SPATULA

FLOUR SIFTER

RUBBER SCRAPER

SPATULA

MEASURING SPOONS*

CUTTING BOARD

LIQUID
MEASURING
CUP*

NEST OF DRY
MEASURING CUPS*

ROAST
THERMOMETER*

PASTRY BLENDER

*Eventually these will be changed to conform to the metric system

Figure 12-2 Use of small kitchen utensils greatly increases efficiency in food preparation.

KITCHEN SAFETY

Each year people are injured or killed as a result of careless habits in the kitchen. All of these incidents are labeled *accidents*, which means they might have been avoided.

Grease and water spilled on the floor should be wiped up immediately to prevent slips and falls. A stepladder should be used to reach articles stored on high shelves or cabinets. Knives should be washed separately and stored apart from other utensils and out of the reach of small children. Pot holders should be used for handling hot utensils but stored a safe distance from the stove burners. The handles of cooking pans should be turned inward on the stove to prevent burns. Ovens should be kept clean to prevent grease fires. Gas stoves should be turned on only after the match box is closed and one match has been lit. Matches and poisons should be kept out of reach of children. Should a grease fire develop, it must be smothered with salt, baking soda, a tight lid, or a fire blanket. **CAUTION:** Do not throw water on a stove fire since water spreads grease fires.

SUMMARY

Good planning is important in working efficiently in the kitchen. Kitchen equipment is chosen for durability, efficiency, and ease in cleaning. Equipment can only be used effectively when it is used and cleaned properly. All equipment should be washed, dried, and properly stored after use.

Discussion Topics

1. Why is it important to keep the kitchen clean?
2. Why is it especially important to keep the school and hospital kitchens clean?
3. Describe how to efficiently clean the kitchen after preparing a meal.
4. Discuss the uses of the various pieces of kitchen appliances and equipment.
5. Ask if students are familiar with the following types of cookware: cast iron, Pyrex, Teflon-coated, copper-bottom, stainless steel, and enamel. Discuss the advantages and disadvantages of this equipment. Discuss their proper care.

Suggested Activities

1. Observe a demonstration of the use and care of kitchen equipment.
2. Visit the school cafeteria kitchen. Observe the equipment and ask for demonstrations.
3. Visit a hospital kitchen and observe the use of the equipment.
4. Visit a hotel dining room kitchen and observe the use of the equipment.

5. Make a list of the special cleaning products available at the local supermarket for specific surfaces such as stainless steel, copper, silver, porcelain, enamel, and wood.
6. Visit a store that sells cooking equipment such as food processors, crockpots, electric fry pans, and so on. List the types available. Discuss the actual value of these items in terms of everyday home use.
7. Give demonstrations of proper dishwashing, oven cleaning, refrigerator cleaning, stove cleaning.

Review

A. Briefly answer the following questions.
1. What factors should be considered when purchasing kitchen equipment?

2. How can sticky substances be removed from the stove?

3. Why is it unwise to pour grease in the sink?

4. Why is it especially important to keep the storage spaces in excellent order at all times in the school or hospital kitchen?

5. List three ways the cook can increase the efficiency of food preparation?

6. If a protein food such as milk or egg is stuck to a pan, what is the best method of removal?

7. In what order should dishes be washed?

8. Name three practices that can reduce accidents in the kitchen.

9. Explain how to smother a grease fire.

B. Identify the kitchen utensils sketched below.

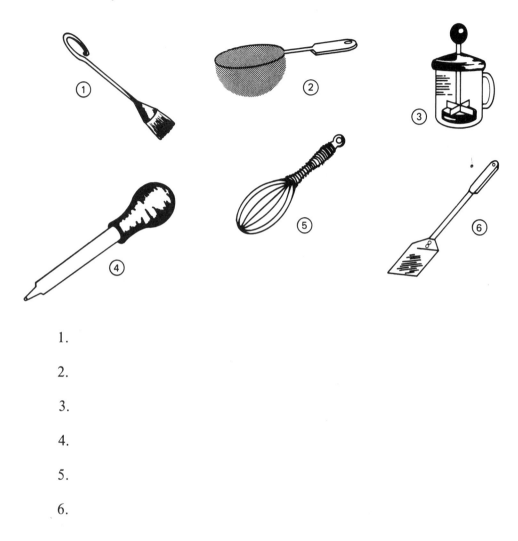

1.

2.

3.

4.

5.

6.

References

Anderson, Jean, and Elaine Hanna. 1975. *The Doubleday Cookbook*. Garden City, N.Y.: Doubleday & Company Inc.

Kinder, Faye, Nancy Green and Natholyn Harris. 1984. *Meal Management*, 6th ed. New York: Macmillan Publishing Company.

The Fannie Farmer Cookbook, 12th ed. 1979. New York: Alfred A. Knopf.

Chapter 13

PREVENTING FOOD-RELATED ILLNESS

VOCABULARY

botulism	insecticide	protozoa
carrier	microorganisms	Salmonella
diarrhea	nausea	sanitation
dysentery	parasite	Staphylococcus
environment	Perfringens	toxin
infectious	polluted water	trichinosis

OBJECTIVES

After studying this chapter, you should be able to

- Identify diseases caused by contaminated food, their symptoms, and the means by which they are spread

- List signs of food contamination

- State precautions for protecting food from contamination

The most nutritious food can cause illness if it is contaminated with harmful *microorganisms* (microscopic plants and animals such as bacteria, viruses, worms, and molds), or chemical poisons. Fortunately, in the United States there are strict federal, state, and local laws regulating the commercial production of food. Dairies, canneries, bakeries, and meat-packing houses are all subject to government inspection. The commercial processing of foods is regularly checked so that these foods are wholesome and safe to eat. Nevertheless, people do sometimes become sick because of something they ate. With few exceptions, such illnesses occur because of the ignorance or carelessness of people who handle food in the kitchen.

There are always microorganisms in the *environment* (surroundings). Sometimes they are present in the food because its animal-source contained them. When foods are undercooked these microbes may be carried to consumers and make them sick. Microorganisms may be introduced to food by a carrier. A *carrier* is a person (or animal) capable of transmitting an *infectious* (disease-causing) organism. Very often the carrier suffers no effects from the organism and therefore is unaware of the danger. A food handler may have a cut on the hand, a cold, or a skin infection, and microorganisms from this person may very easily spread to the food. Insects, dust, and animals may contaminate the food if it is improperly stored. Foods are generally moist and soft, and provide an excellent place for microorganisms to grow. When foods are not stored at proper temperatures, these microorganisms multiply very rapidly. Foods should be handled and stored in such ways as to best control the growth of these organisms.

ILLNESSES CAUSED BY MICROORGANISMS IN FOOD

Salmonellosis (commonly called Salmonella) is an infection caused by the Salmonella bacteria. Salmonella may be found in raw meats, poultry, fish, milk, and eggs. It is transmitted by eating contaminated food or by contact with a carrier. Salmonellosis is characterized by headache, vomiting, diarrhea, abdominal cramps, and fever. In very severe cases it may even result in death. Those who suffer the most severe cases are typically the very young, the very old, and the weak or incapacitated.

Refrigeration at 7.2°C (45°F) or below inhibits the growth of these bacteria. However, bacteria can remain alive in the freezer and in dried foods. Salmonella bacteria are destroyed by heating to at least 60°C (140°F) for a minimum of ten minutes. One species of Salmonella causes typhoid fever.

Perfringens poisoning is caused by the *Clostridium perfringens* bacteria. It is commonly found in soil, on food, and in the intestinal tracts of warm-blooded animals. It is transmitted by eating heavily contaminated food. It is characterized by nausea, diarrhea, and inflammation of the stomach and intestines. These are spore-forming bacteria that grow without oxygen and are very difficult to destroy. The spores can survive most cooking temperatures. The best method of controlling them is to refrigerate meats quickly at 4.4°C (40°F) or below.

Staphylococcal poisoning, commonly called *Staph*, is caused by the *Staphylococcus aureus* bacteria. These bacteria are found on the skin and in the respiratory passages. They grow in meats, poultry, fish and egg dishes, and in salads such as potato, egg, macaroni and tuna, and in cream-filled pastries. This poisoning is transmitted by carriers and by eating food that contains the toxin. It is characterized by vomiting, diarrhea, and abdominal cramps. It is considered a relatively mild illness. The growth of these bacteria is inhibited if foods are kept at temperatures above 60°C (140°F) or below 4.4°C (40°F). The toxin can be destroyed by boiling the food for several hours, or by heating it in a pressure cooker at 115.6°C (240°F) for 30 minutes. In most cases, long periods of high temperature cooking would reduce the appeal and nutritional value of food. Practically speaking, it would be better to discard foods suspected of being contaminated.

Botulism is caused by the toxin produced by the *Clostridium botulinum* bacteria. This is perhaps the rarest but most deadly of all the food poisonings. It is characterized by double vision, speech difficulties, inability to swallow, respiratory paralysis and sometimes death. The fatality rate in the United States is about 65 percent. The spores of this bacteria can divide and produce toxin without oxygen. This means that toxin can be produced in sealed containers such as cans and jars. The spores are extremely heat resistant. They must be boiled for six hours before they will be destroyed. The toxin, however, may be destroyed by boiling for twenty minutes.

Great care must be taken to prevent botulism when canning foods at home. The

Table 13-1 Bacterial Foodborne Illnesses: Causes, Symptoms, and Prevention

Name of Illness	What Causes It	Symptoms	Characteristics of Illness	Preventive Measures
Salmonellosis Examples of foods involved: Poultry, red meats, eggs, dried foods, dairy products.	**Salmonellae.** Bacteria widespread in nature, live and grow in intestinal tracts of human beings and animals.	Severe headache, followed by vomiting, diarrhea, abdominal cramps, and fever. Infants, elderly, and persons with low resistance are most susceptible. Severe infections cause high fever and may even cause death.	Transmitted by eating contaminated food, or by contact with infected persons or carriers of the infection. Also transmitted by insects, rodents, and pets. Onset: Usually within 12 to 36 hours. Duration: 2 to 7 days	Salmonellae in food are destroyed by heating the food to 140°F and holding for 10 minutes or to higher temperatures for less time, for instance, 155°F for a few seconds. Refrigeration at 40°F inhibits the increase of Salmonellae, but they remain alive in foods in the refrigerator or freezer, and even in dried foods.
Perfringens poisoning Examples of foods involved: Stews, soups or gravies made from poultry or red meat.	**Clostridium perfringens.** Spore-forming bacteria that grow in the absence of oxygen. Temperatures reached in thorough cooking of most foods are sufficient to destroy vegetative cells, but heat-resistant spores can survive.	Nausea (without vomiting), diarrhea, acute inflammation of the stomach and intestines.	Transmitted by eating food contaminated with abnormally large numbers of the bacteria. Onset: Usually within 8 to 20 hours. Duration: May persist for 24 hours.	To prevent growth of surviving bacteria in cooked meats, gravies, and meat casseroles that are to be eaten later, cool foods rapidly and refrigerate promptly at 40°F or below or hold them above 140°F.
Staphylococcal poisoning (frequently called staph) Examples of foods involved: Custards, egg salad, potato salad, chicken salad, macaroni salad, ham, salami, cheese	**Staphylococcus aureus.** Bacteria fairly resistant to heat. Bacteria growing in food produce a toxin that is extremely resistant to heat.	Vomiting, diarrhea, prostration, abdominal cramps. Generally mild and often attributed to other causes.	Transmitted by food handlers who carry the bacteria and by eating food containing the toxin. Onset: Usually within 3 to 8 hours. Duration: 1 or 2 days.	Growth of bacteria that produce toxin is inhibited by keeping hot foods above 140°F and cold foods at or below 40°F. Toxin is destroyed by boiling for several hours or heating the food in a pressure cooker at 240°F for 30 minutes.
Botulism Examples of foods involved: Canned low-acid foods, smoked fish	**Clostridium botulinum.** Spore-forming organisms that grow and produce toxin in the absence of oxygen, such as in a sealed container.	Double vision, inability to swallow, speech difficulty, progressive respiratory paralysis. Fatality rate is high, in the United States about 65 percent.	Transmitted by eating food containing the toxin. Onset: Usually within 12 to 36 hours or longer. Duration: 3 to 6 days.	Bacterial spores in food are destroyed by high temperatures obtained only in the pressure canner. More than 6 hours is needed to kill the spores at boiling temperature (212°F). The toxin is destroyed by boiling for 10 to 20 minutes; time required depends on kind of food.

Source: USDA Home and Garden Bulletin No. 162, 1975

FDA and USDA report five deaths from botulism traced to commercially canned foods in the United States between 1925 and 1974, and 700 deaths from home-canned foods during that same time period.

Trichinosis is a disease caused by the parasite *Trichinella spiralis*. A *parasite* is a life form that depends completely on another life form without making any contribution towards the needs of the host. Trichinosis is transmitted by eating inadequately cooked pork from pigs that are infected with the *Trichinella spiralis* parasite. Symptoms include vomiting, fever, chills, and muscle pain. Cooking all pork to an internal temperature of at least 58.3°C (137°F) kills the organism and prevents this disease. The parasite may also be destroyed by freezing.

Dysentery is a disease caused by a *protozoa* (a tiny, one-celled animal). The protozoa is transmitted through food by carriers or by contaminated water. It causes severe diarrhea that may occur intermittently until the patient is properly treated.

PREVENTION OF FOOD CONTAMINATION

All of the foregoing illnesses are caused by contaminated food or water. Food becomes contaminated because of poor sanitation on the part of the food handler or from improper storage.

To prevent contamination, persons preparing food must have clean hands that are not cut or infected in any way, clean clothes, and clean cooking equipment. They should touch the food as little as possible. After handling uncooked food, people should wash their hands and any knives or cutting boards used. Tests should be made regularly of people working as professional food handlers to ascertain that they are not carriers of infectious organisms.

Food poisons cannot be seen, but sometimes there are telltale signs of their existence. If a can bulges, if its contents appear different than usual, or if the food has an unusual odor, it should be discarded in a place where animals and children cannot reach it. **CAUTION:** The food should never be tasted in these circumstances because Clostridium botulinum may be present, and can be fatal. A good rule of thumb is: "If in doubt, throw it out."

Food Storage

Proper food storage is very important in inhibiting the growth of bacteria. Because bacteria grow best at temperatures between 15.6° and 51.7°C (60° and 125°F), it is important to keep food refrigerated, that is, below 15.6°C (60°F); or to keep it hot, above 51.7°C (125°F). Leftover food should always be refrigerated as soon as the meal is finished, and covered after it is cold. It should not be allowed to cool at room temperature before being refrigerated. Frozen foods should either be cooked from the frozen state or thawed in the refrigerator. (When cooked from the frozen state, cooking time will be increased by at least 50 percent.) Frozen foods should not be thawed at room temperature. Food must always be protected from dust, insects, and animals since all of these can spread contamination.

Miscellaneous Food Poisonings

Occasionally food poisoning is termed natural. This means it is caused by ingesting certain plants or animals that contain poison.

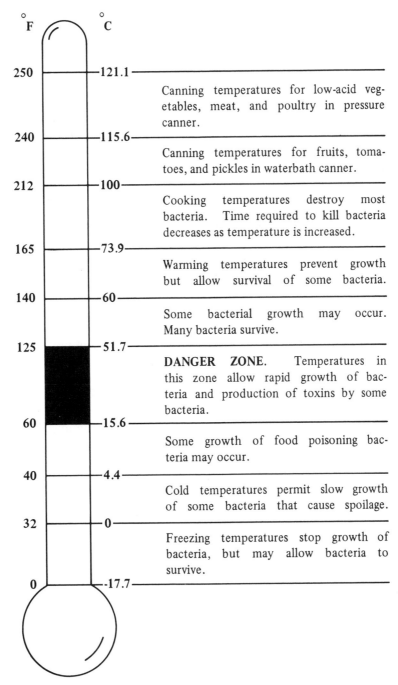

Figure 13-1 Temperatures of food for control of bacteria *(Reprinted from U.S.D.A. Home and Garden Bulletin No. 162, 1983)*

Examples are plants such as poisonous mushrooms, rhubarb leaves, and fish from polluted water.

Individuals may develop *allergies* (hypersensitivities) to certain foods. If these foods are eaten, they may cause temporary reactions. Symptoms may include nausea, diarrhea, dizziness, and sometimes serious breathing difficulties.

Poisoning also may result from ingesting cleaning agents, insecticides or excessive amounts of a drug. Children may swallow cleaning agents or medicines. The cook may mistakenly use a poison instead of a cooking ingredient. Sometimes insecticides cling to fresh fruits and vegetables. It is essential that all potential poisons be kept out of the reach of young children and kept separate from all food supplies. Fresh fruits and vegetables should be thoroughly washed before being stored.

SUMMARY

Infection or poisoning traced to food is usually caused by human ignorance or carelessness. The serving of safe meals is essentially the responsibility of the cook. Food should not be prepared by anyone who has or carries a contagious disease. All fresh fruits and vegetables should be washed before being eaten. Meats, poultry, fish, eggs, and dairy products should be refrigerated. Pork should always be cooked to the well-done stage. Food should be covered to prevent contamination by dust, insects, or animals. Garbage should also be covered so that it does not attract insects. Hands that prepare foods should be clean and free of cuts or wounds. Kitchen equipment should be spotless. Finally, the food itself should be safe. People should avoid foods containing natural poisons.

Discussion Topics

1. Name four types of food poisoning. If any class member has suffered from food poisoning, ask the person to describe the symptoms.
2. How may food become contaminated?
3. How can insects contaminate food?
4. How may food be kept free of insect and animal contamination?
5. Why should foods be refrigerated?
6. Discuss appropriate storage of cleaning agents in a home with young children.

Suggested Activities

1. Using outside sources, present a committee report on diseases that can be carried in food. Include the agent of transmission, mode of transmission, symptoms, and treatment.
2. Visit a restaurant kitchen. Look for practices that may lead to potential food poisoning. Note the practices and uses of equipment designed to prevent food poisoning.

Review

A. Multiple Choice. Select the *letter* that precedes the best answer.

1. A microorganism is a (an)
   a. unit of measurement
   b. tiny animal or plant
   c. component of a microscope
   d. individual human cell

2. Salmonella bacteria are destroyed by heating foods to 60°C (140°F) for a minimum of
   a. 2 minutes
   b. 10 minutes
   c. 30 minutes
   d. 2 hours

3. Someone who is capable of spreading an infectious organism but is not sick is called a
   a. food handler
   b. carrier
   c. transport
   d. fomite

4. When an organism is infectious, it is
   a. disease-causing
   b. prone to infections
   c. not contagious
   d. always fatal

5. Most cases of food poisoning in the United States are caused by
   a. careless processing in commercial factories
   b. lack of government inspection
   c. careless handling of food in the kitchen
   d. house pets

6. Generally, food poisoning symptoms include
   a. headache
   b. nausea
   c. abdominal upset
   d. all of these

7. Salmonella infection and staphylococcal poisoning are caused by
   a. virus
   b. bacteria
   c. protozoa
   d. worms

8. The deadliest of the bacterial food poisonings is
   a. Staphylococcus
   b. Salmonella
   c. botulism
   d. perfringens poisoning

9. The disease caused by a parasite sometimes found in pork is
   a. tularemia
   b. dysentery
   c. avitaminosis
   d. trichinosis

10. The disease caused by a protozoa and characterized by severe diarrhea is
    a. Salmonella
    b. botulism
    c. dysentery
    d. infectious hepatitis

11. Foods may be contaminated by
    a. people
    b. insects
    c. animals
    d. all of these

12. The temperatures in the danger zone that encourage bacterial growth are between
    a. 0 to 32°F (−18 to 0°C)
    b. 32 to 60°F (0 to 16°C)
    c. 60 to 125°F (16 to 52°C)
    d. 125 to 212°F (52 to 100°C)

13. A telltale sign of spoiled food may be
    a. a bulging can
    b. a peculiar odor
    c. an unusual appearance
    d. all of these

14. Leftover foods should be
    a. put in the refrigerator immediately after meals
    b. cooled to room temperature before refrigerating
    c. cooled in the refrigerator for at least an hour before freezing
    d. stored unwrapped in the refrigerator

15. Frozen foods should be
    a. thawed at room temperature
    b. refrozen if not used immediately after thawing
    c. thawed in the refrigerator
    d. any of the above

References

Luke, Barbara. 1984. *Principles of Nutrition and Diet Therapy*. Boston: Little Brown & Co.

Robinson, Corinne H. 1978. *Fundamentals of Normal Nutrition*, 3rd ed. New York: Macmillan Publishing Company.

Robinson, Corinne H. and Marilyn R. Lawler. 1982. *Normal and Therapeutic Nutrition*, 16th ed. New York: Macmillan Publishing Company.

Suitor, Carol W., and Merrily F. Crowley. 1984. *Nutrition Principles and Application in Health Promotion*. Philadelphia: J. B. Lippincott Company.

Williams, Sue Rodwell. 1984. *Mowry's Basic Nutrition and Diet Therapy*, 7th ed. St. Louis: C. V. Mosby Co.

Chapter 14
READING RECIPES

OBJECTIVES

After studying this chapter, you should be able to

- Define cookery terms commonly used in recipes
- Demonstrate the processes involved in various cookery terms

Tested recipes list specific amounts of ingredients and include directions for combining them to produce satisfactory and predictable food products. Since the preparation of meals involves the use of recipes, it is important to understand the terms used in them.

To use cookery terms and follow recipes correctly, the student should learn the definitions of these terms, observe demonstrations of the techniques defined, and practice the techniques when following recipes. It is always wise to use tested recipes to avoid disappointing results and waste. A knowledge of the following terms should prove useful.

a la king: served in a white sauce with bits of green pepper and pimiento. A common example is chicken a la king.

aspic: highly seasoned jelly made from broth, stock, or tomato juice. An example is tomato aspic.

au gratin: prepared in white sauce with cheese added. Potatoes au gratin are an example.

bake: cook in the oven as is done with cakes and cookies.

barbecue: to bake or to roast over coals or on a spit, basting with spicy sauce, as is done with chicken and pork ribs.

baste: to brush or pour hot fat on cooking foods, as is done with roasting poultry.

beat: to combine with air by mixing vigorously; this is often done with eggs.

blanch: to plunge into boiling water and then

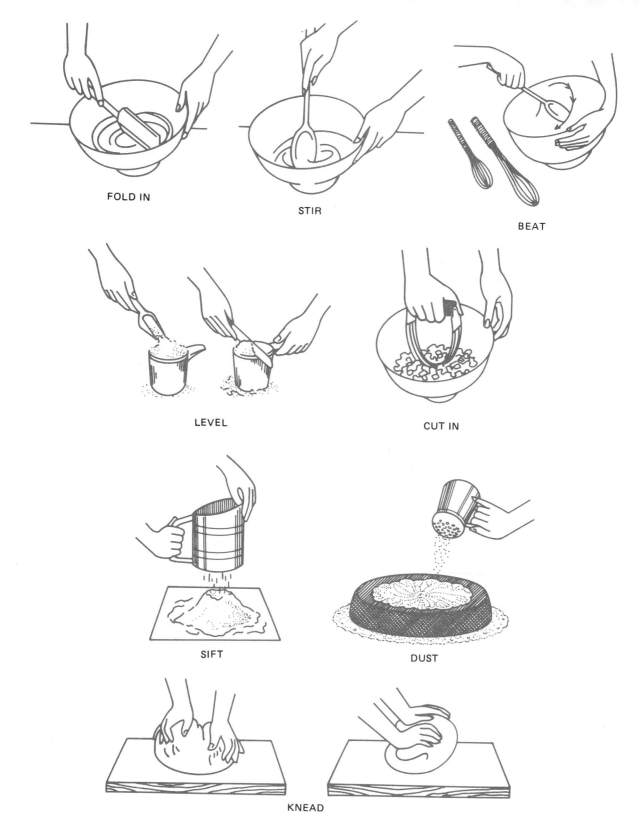

Figure 14-1 Baking instructions must be carefully followed.

into cold water. This may be done with almonds to remove their brown skins.

blend: to mix thoroughly, as is done when combining ingredients for cakes and cookies.

boil: to cook in liquid at 100°C (212°F) as is indicated when bubbles break on the surface of the liquid.

braise: to cook in a covered container with a small amount of liquid, as is done with less tender cuts of meat.

broil: to cook under or over direct heat. Tender meats can be broiled.

brush: to spread a thin amount of sauce, oil, or egg over food as is commonly done with yeast breads.

casserole: a combination of foods providing a meal in one dish; sometimes the dish itself is called a casserole.

chop: to cut into small, irregular pieces, as is done with onions, celery, hard-cooked eggs, and nuts.

combine: to mix together.

compote: fruit in syrup; also, the long-stemmed dish in which it may be served.

cream: to mix with beaters or the back of a spoon until food is smooth and creamy in consistency; done to mix shortening and sugar for cakes and cookies.

croquette: combination of finely chopped food and white sauce shaped in a ball or cone, rolled in egg and crumbs, and fried in deep fat. An example might be chicken croquettes.

cube: to dice or cut into small, regular squares, as may be done with cheese.

cut in: to blend shortening with flour using two knives or a pastry blender.

deviled: highly seasoned. An example might be deviled eggs.

dice: to cube or cut into very small, regular squares.

dredge: to coat heavily with flour, as is sometimes done before browning meat; or to coat with sugar, as may be done with some cookie dough just before baking.

dust: to sprinkle lightly with flour or sugar, as may be done to the top of baked products.

flake: to separate gently with a fork, as may be done to fish.

fold: to blend very gently with a down, across, up and over motion to retain air in a mixture, as is done when combining heavy mixtures with light, whipped ingredients.

fry: to cook in hot fat, as may be done with potatoes or chicken.

garnish: to trim or decorate food; the trimmings. Such trimmings should harmonize in color, flavor, and shape with the dish it decorates. Examples are parsley, egg slices, pickles, carrot curls.

grate: to rub on a rough surface, producing small particles, as is done with onions, lemons, and oranges.

grill: to broil.

julienne: to cut into thin strips, as may be done with meat used in salads.

knead: to mix by folding and squeezing, as in mixing yeast bread doughs.

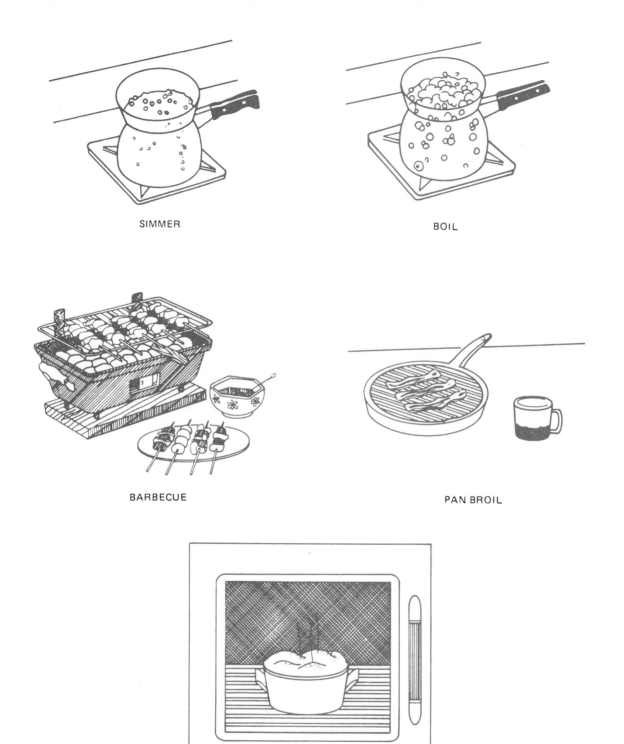

SIMMER

BOIL

BARBECUE

PAN BROIL

BAKE

Figure 14-2 Different cooking methods are used according to type and quality of food.

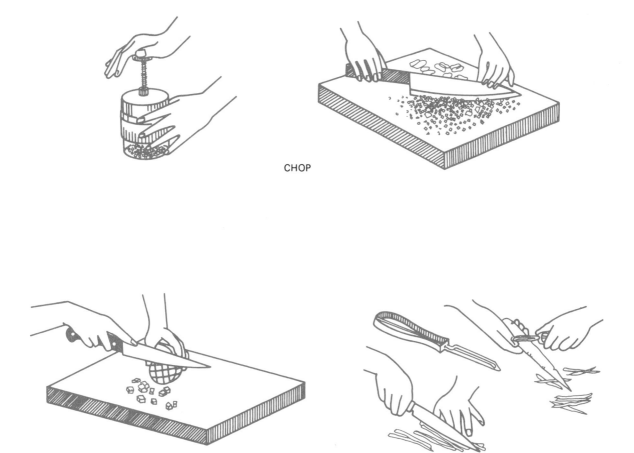

CHOP

DICE (CUBE)

JULIENNE

Figure 14-3 Cutting foods into smaller pieces is a process used in many types of cookery.

marinade: distinctive liquid or sauce in which some foods are kept for a specified time to alter their original flavors.

marinate: to let stand in a marinade.

mince: to chop as finely as possible, as may be done with celery, onions, or parsley.

mocha: combination of coffee and chocolate flavors. An example is mocha icing.

pan-broil: to fry, pouring off fat as it accumulates, as may be done when cooking bacon.

parboil: to partially cook by boiling or simmering, as may be done to julienne potatoes before frying.

poach: to cook in liquid just below the boiling point, as may be done with eggs, fish, or chicken.

puree: to press through a strainer to remove fiber; the food that has been pressed through the strainer. An example is puree of spinach.

saute: to fry slowly in a small amount of fat, as may be done with onions, peppers, or eggs.

scald: to bring a liquid just to the boiling point and immediately remove it from the heat, as may be done with milk.

score: to make shallow, even cuts on the surface; often done with ham that is to be baked.

sear: to brown quickly at a high temperature, as is sometimes done with meat.

shred: to tear or rub or cut into thin pieces, as is done with lettuce and cabbage.

sift: to put dry ingredients through a sieve to remove lumps, as is done with flour.

simmer: to cook in liquid just below the boiling point; indicated by tiny bubbles breaking just beneath the surface of the liquid.

skewer: a metal or wooden pick for fastening foods, or to fasten foods with such a pick.

souffle: light, fluffly dish having eggs as the main ingredient. Examples are cheese and chocolate souffles.

steam: to cook in covered container over, but not touching, boiling water as is done with vegetables, shellfish, and some quick breads.

steep: to let stand in hot liquid for a specified time, as is done with tea.

stew: to cook slowly in liquid or a mixture of meat and vegetables cooked by this method. An example is beef and vegetable stew.

stock: liquid in which foods have been cooked. Examples are meat or vegetable stocks.

timbale: finely chopped foods combined with eggs and baked in a mold. Examples are chicken timbales.

whip: to beat rapidly, introducing air, as may be done to egg whites or heavy cream.

SUMMARY

A thorough knowledge of the meanings of cookery terms and the ability to use them correctly is essential for efficient meal preparation. Using appropriate equipment is also necessary in applying the techniques described.

Discussion Topics

1. Why is it important for a cook to know the meaning of cooking terms?
2. Why is it wise to use tested recipes rather than untried recipes?
3. Discuss how casseroles can be prepared from leftover foods.
4. How can a chocolate frosting be changed into a mocha frosting?
5. Of what use are the words "serves two" in a recipe?
6. What is beef stock? Chicken stock?
7. Name five foods frequently used as garnishes. What are some attractive garnishes suitable for egg salad?
8. Why are purees frequently included in hospital menus?
9. Name two ingredients that are frequently folded into other ingredients.

10. What is the difference between:
    - fry and pan-broil
    - a la king and au gratin
    - dice and julienne
    - marinate and steep
    - mince and grate
    - whip and fold

Suggested Activities

1. Identify the cookery terms in the following recipe and explain them.

    Egg Salad

3 eggs	Simmer the eggs 15 minutes.
1 tbsp. grated onion	Cool and shell them. Chop the
1/2 tsp. salt	celery and grate the onion. Cube
1/4 tsp. paprika	the eggs and add the celery,
1/4 c. chopped celery	mayonnaise, salt, paprika, and
1/4 c. mayonnaise	onion. Combine gently. Serve on
	greens and garnish with tomato
	wedges. Serves two.

2. Organize two teams and have a "spell-down" on the cookery terms and their definitions.
3. Plan a menu that includes an aspic, a dish a la king, and a compote. Use cookbooks for reference.
4. Plan a menu that includes a casserole, a puree, and a souffle.
5. Divide the class into groups and have each group demonstrate one or more of the cooking terms discussed in this chapter.
6. Browse through a cookbook and look for directions that include some of the following terms. Name the recipe in which each is found.

baste	cream	fold	sear
beat	cut in	marinate	sift
blend	deviled	simmer	steam
braise	dredge	saute	whip

7. Prepare a class cookbook composed of favorite recipes from students and teacher. Include sections on appetizers, soups, fish, poultry, meats, vegetables, breads, and desserts. Allow space for additions.

Review

A. Match the foods listed in column I with the cookery terms commonly used in preparing them, listed in column II. Some choices can be used more than once.

Column I	Column II
_____ 1. egg whites	a. sift
_____ 2. almonds	b. braise
_____ 3. pot roast	c. blanch
_____ 4. lemon rind	d. mince
_____ 5. sirloin steak	e. scald
_____ 6. cookies	f. puree
_____ 7. milk	g. grate
_____ 8. flour	h. whip
_____ 9. bread	i. poach
_____ 10. parsley	j. broil
	k. bake
	l. knead
	m. dice

B. Read the following recipe. In the space provided below the recipe, write definitions of the italicized cookery terms.

Braised Beef

5 pounds top round of beef
3 cups red wine
1/2 cup chopped onion
1/2 cup diced celery
1 tablespoon minced parsley
1/2 cup flour
3 tablespoons margarine
1 cup beef stock

Put the meat in a large bowl. (1) *Chop* the onions, (2) *dice* the celery, (3) *mince* the parsley, and (4) *combine* the vegetables. Place the vegetables on top of, and around the meat. Add the wine. Cover and (5) *marinate* in the refrigerator 24 hours. Discard the (6) *marinade*. Dry the meat and (7) *dredge* with the flour. Melt the margarine in a heavy skillet. Add meat and (8) *sear*, turning as the meat browns. Place the browned meat in a casserole with a tight-fitting cover. Add the (9) beef *stock*. Cover and (10) *braise* over low heat 3 hours or until tender. 1 1/4 hours before serving, add 12 medium white potatoes. Bring to a (11) *boil*. Reduce heat and (12) *simmer* 1 hour. Slice meat. Serve with the potatoes and buttered carrots (13) *julienne*. (14) *Garnish* with parsley.

1.   3.

2.   4.

5.   10.

6.   11.

7.   12.

8.   13.

9.   14.

References

Anderson, Jean, and Elaine Hanna. 1975. *The Doubleday Cookbook*. Garden City, New York: Doubleday & Company, Inc.

The Fannie Farmer Cookbook, 12th ed. 1979. New York: Alfred A. Knopf.

Peckham, Gladys, and Jeanne Freeland-Graves. 1979. *Foundations of Food Preparation*, 4th ed. New York: Macmillan Publishing Company

Chapter 15

MEASURING AND WEIGHING INGREDIENTS

VOCABULARY

density	grams	metric system
centi- (a prefix)	kilo	micro- (a prefix)
English system of	liter	milli- (a prefix)
weights and	meter	volume
measures		
equivalent		

OBJECTIVES

After studying this chapter, you should be able to

- State metric equivalents of common household measures

- Compare weight and volume of cooking ingredients

- Convert measurements from the English to the metric system and from the metric to the English system

- Measure and weigh foods accurately

Accuracy in weighing and measuring ingredients is essential to prepare dishes that are consistent in quality and that fulfill the physician's orders when therapeutic diets are prescribed. One must be familiar with the systems of weights and measures and know how to use the measuring devices and scales.

SYSTEMS OF WEIGHTS AND MEASURES

The two systems of weights and measures commonly used are the *English* and the *metric*. The English is most commonly used in the United States. The units of measurement within it originated in various cultures. The English system includes many different measuring units such as pints, quarts, and gallons, as well as inch, foot, and yard.

The metric system is an international system of weights and measures based on the number ten. Because a power of ten is common to all measuring units, conversion within the metric system is quite simple. In this system, the basic unit of weight or mass is the *gram*. Length is measured in *meters* and volume is measured in *liters*. The metric units for weight, length, or volume all use the same *prefixes* (beginnings of words), table 15-2. Although the metric system is used in many parts of the world, the United States has been slow to accept it. However, it will soon be

Table 15-1 Metric Equivalents of Common Household Measures*

	Household	Metric
dash	less than 1/8 teaspoon	–
few grains (f. g.)	less than 1/8 teaspoon	–
drop	–	0.060 milliliter (ml)
15 drops	–	1 milliliter (same as one cubic centimeter)
1 teaspoon (tsp)	1/3 tablespoon	5 milliliters (ml)
1 tablespoon (tbsp)	3 teaspoons	15 milliliters (ml)
1 fluid ounce (oz)	2 tablespoons	30 milliliters (ml)
1 cup (c)	8 fluid ounces or 16 tablespoons	240 milliliters or 0.24 liters
1 pint (pt)	2 cups	470 milliliters or 0.47 liters
1 quart (qt)	2 pints or 4 cups	950 milliliters or 0.95 liters
1 gallon (gal)	4 quarts	3.8 liters
1 peck (pk)	2 gallons	7.6 liters
1 bushel (bu)	4 pecks	30.4 liters
1 pound (lb)	16 ounces	.454 kilograms (kg)

*The above equivalents are presented only as a guide to familiarize the user with metric measures. It is recommended that the size of rounded metric measures be learned and used.

Table 15-2 Unit Relationships Within the Metric System

Weight	Length	Volume
1000 grams = 1 *kilo*gram	1000 meters = 1 *kilo*meter	1000 liters = 1 *kilo*liter*
100 grams = 1 *hekto*gram*	100 meters = 1 *hekto*meter*	100 liters = 1 *hecto*liter*
10 grams = 1 *deka*gram*	10 meters = 1 *deka*meter*	10 liters = 1 *deka*liter*
1 gram	1 meter	1 liter
.1 gram = 1 *deci*gram*	.1 meter = 1 *deci*meter*	.1 liter = 1 *deci*liter*
.01 gram = 1 *centi*gram*	.01 meter = 1 *centi*meter	.01 liter = 1 *centi*liter*
.001 gram = 1 *milli*gram	.001 meter = 1 *milli*meter	.001 liter = 1 *milli*liter
.000001 gram = 1 *micro*gram*	.000001 meter = 1 *micro*meter*	.000001 liter = 1 *micro*liter*

* units not commonly used

widely used throughout the country and students and consumers need to know how to use it, and how to convert from one system of measurement to the other. This is not difficult but it requires practice. Quick reference and ways to convert are illustrated in tables, 15-3 and 15-4.

MEASURING DEVICES AND THEIR CORRECT USE

The measuring devices commonly available in the United States are still based on the English system. Measuring spoon sets include 1/4 teaspoon, 1/2 teaspoon, 1 teaspoon and 1 tablespoon. Measuring cups for solid and dry ingredients include 1/4 cup, 1/3 cup, 1/2 cup,

and 1 cup. To use these for dry ingredients, fill them gently, without shaking, and remove the excess with a flat spatula so they are level across the top. Shaking the measuring cup packs the dry ingredients and results in an excess of the ingredient. When a solid ingredient such as shortening must be measured or when brown sugar is packed into a cup, air pockets should be pushed out with a slender knife. The measurement is leveled by pressing down firmly and then cutting across the top of the cup with a flat spatula.

Liquids are measured in a cup that has marks indicating 1/4 cup, 1/3 cup, 1/2 cup, 2/3 cup, 3/4 cup, 1 cup, and sometimes 2 cups, figure 15-1. There is a spill area above the one-cup or two-cup mark and a pouring

Table 15-3 Converting from the English System to the Metric System

CONVERT TO METRIC	WHEN YOU KNOW	MULTIPLY BY	TO FIND
WEIGHT	ounces (oz)	28	grams (g)
	pounds (lb)	0.45	kilograms (kg)
VOLUME	teaspoons (tsp)	5	milliliters (ml)
	tablespoons (Tbsp)	15	milliliters
	fluid ounces (fl oz)	30	milliliters
	cups (c)	0.24	liters (l)
	pints (pt)	0.47	liters
	quarts (qt)	0.95	liters
	gallons (gal)	3.8	liters
	cubic feet (ft^3)	0.03	cubic meters (m^3)
	cubic yards (yd^3)	0.76	cubic meters
TEMPERATURE	Fahrenheit (°F) temperature	5/9 (after subtracting 32)	Celsius (°C) temperature

Source: Adapted from "Some References on Metric Information" by US Dept of Commerce, National Bureau of Standards, 1975

Table 15-4 Converting from the Metric System to the English System

CONVERT TO ENGLISH	WHEN YOU KNOW	MULTIPLY BY	TO FIND
WEIGHT	grams (g) kilograms (kg) metric tons (1000 kg)	0.035 2.2 1.1	ounces (oz) pounds (lb) short tons
VOLUME	milliliters (ml) liters (l) liters liters cubic meters (m^3) cubic meters	0.03 2.1 1.06 0.26 35 1.3	fluid ounces (fl oz) pints (pt) quarts (qt) gallons (gal) cubic feet (ft^3) cubic yards (yd^3)
TEMPERATURE	Celsius ($^\circ$C) temperature	9/5 (then add 32)	Fahrenheit ($^\circ$F) temperature

Source: Adapted from "Some References on Metric Information" by US Dept. of Commerce, National Bureau of Standards, 1975

Table 15-5 Equivalent Weights and Measures

Weight Equivalents

	Milligram	Gram	Kilogram	Grain	Ounce	Pound
1 microgram (μg)	.001	.000001				
1 milligram (mg)	1.	.001		.0154		
1 gram (g)	1,000.	1.	.001	15.4	.035	.0022
1 kilogram (kg)	1,000,000.	1,000.	1.	15,400.	35.2	2.2
1 grain (gr)	64.8	.065		1.		
1 ounce (oz)		28.3		437.5	1.	.063
1 pound (lb)		453.6	.454		16.	1.

Volume Equivalents

	Cubic Millimeter	Cubic Centimeter	Liter	Fluid Ounce	Pint	Quart
1 cubic millimeter (mm^3)	1.	.001				
1 cubic centimeter (cm^3)	1,000.	1.	.001			
1 liter (l)	1,000,000.	1,000.	1.	33.8	2.1	1.06
1 fluid ounce (fl oz)		30. (29.57)	.03	1.		
1 pint (pt)		473.	.473	16.	1.	
1 quart (qt)		946.	.946	32	2.	1.

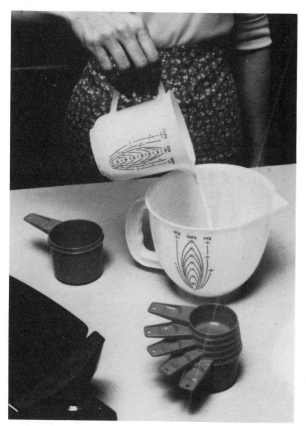

Figure 15-1 Measuring cups are useful in many sizes.
(Courtesy of Tupperware)

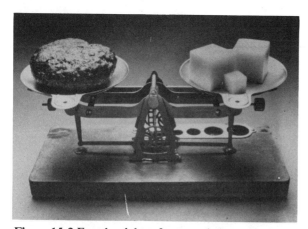

Figure 15-2 Equal weights of meat and cheese can best be determined on a scale. *(Courtesy of Tupperware)*

Table 15-6 Cooking Ingredients Compared in Weight and Volume

Breadcrumbs

4 ounces	3/4 cup less 1 tablespoon
100 grams	1/2 cup

Currants and Raisins

1 pound	2 3/8 cups
100 grams	1/2 cup plus 1 tablespoon

Nuts

4 ounces	2/3 cup, chopped
100 grams	1/2 cup plus 1 tablespoon (chopped)

Brown sugar

1 pound	2 1/4 cup
100 grams	1/2 cup plus 2 tablespoons

Granulated sugar

1 pound	2 cups
100 grams	1/2 cup less 1 tablespoon

Butter, margarine, solid fats and cheese

1 pound	2 cups
1 ounce	2 tablespoons
100 grams	7 tablespoons

Flour

1 pound	3 1/2 to 4 cups
1 ounce	3 tablespoons
100 grams	3/4 cup less 2 tablespoons

Rice, uncooked

1 pound	2 cups

Powdered sugar

1 pound	3 3/4 cups
100 grams	3/4 cup

spout. To use the cup accurately, it must be on a level surface at eye level and the liquid being measured should come exactly to the line of measurement specified. This equipment is inexpensive and is available at most supermarkets or variety stores.

Most food scales measure weight in grams or ounces. It is helpful to remember that one ounce equals approximately 30 grams. Measuring foods and weighing them with the scales should be practiced until it can be done quickly and accurately. Learning weights and measurements, their equivalents, and their abbreviations becomes easier with practice.

Weight and volume of food depends on its density. Therefore, two foods of equal weight may differ in volume. For example, one pound of butter equals 2 cups, but one pound of powdered sugar equals 3 3/4 cups. When the cook is comparing amounts of food, both weight and volume must be considered, table 15-6.

SUMMARY

Foods must be weighed and measured accurately to maintain quality in cooking and to conform to the physician's prescription when special diets are ordered. There are convenient devices for measuring and weighing foods. The common weights and measures in both the English and metric systems should be learned.

Discussion Topics

1. Why is it important to measure and weigh foods accurately at home? In the hospital kitchen?
2. Why are liquid measuring cups inappropriate for measuring dry ingredients and vice-versa?
3. Discuss the units of measurement in the English and those in the metric systems. Make comparisons of commonly used units in cooking.
4. Why are there 3 1/2 to 4 cups of flour in one pound, but only two cups of granulated sugar in one pound?
5. Which would weigh more, one cup of dry cereal or one cup of cooked cereal? Why?

Suggested Activities

1. Observe demonstrations of measuring sugar, flour, and water. Practice measuring these items. Check each other for accuracy.
2. After the use of scales has been demonstrated, practice weighing one cup each of flour, sugar, and water. Remember to subtract the weight of the measuring cup from the total weight to find out the net weight of

each item. Write a report of the experiment, listing the items from lightest to heaviest.

3. Weigh a piece of meat with bone before and after cooking. What percentage of the meat is waste? Weigh just the bone. What percentage of the meat was bone? What accounts for the remainder of the waste?

4. Prepare two ground beef patties of equal weight from the same package of ground meat. Fry one patty over medium-low heat until it is cooked through. Fry the second patty over high heat until it has a dark brown crust on the outside. Weigh each again. Is there a difference in the weights of the two patties? If so, which cooking temperature resulted in the lighter-weight patty? Compare the palatability of the two patties.

5. Convert the following recipe to metric measurements:

Meatloaf
2 1/4 pounds ground beef
2 eggs
1/2 cup bread crumbs
2 tbsp. minced onion
1 cup milk
1 tsp. pepper

6. Convert one or more of your favorite recipes to metric measurements. Test one.

7. Convert the following recipe to the English system of measurements

Pound Cake
250 g butter
750 g sugar
6 eggs
250 g flour
5 ml baking soda
250 g sour cream

Review

A. Briefly answer the following questions.

1. How many teaspoons are there in one tablespoon?

2. How many ounces are there in 1/2 cup of water?

3. How many cups are there in 1 pint?

4. How many quarts are there in 1 gallon?

5. How many cups are there in 1 pound of butter?

6. How many cups are there in 1 pound of flour?

7. How many cups are there in 5 pounds of granulated sugar?

8. How many grams are there in 2 kilograms?

9. How many grams are there in 3 ounces?

10. How many quarts are there in 1 liter?

11. How many pounds are there in 1 kilogram?

12. How many grams are there in 1 pound?

13. How many kilograms are there in 4 pounds?

14. On what number is the metric system based?

B. Make the alterations indicated in the following measurements for a brownie recipe.

1/4 c. butter   1 oz. chocolate
1 c. sugar   1/4 c. whole milk
1 tsp. vanilla   1 c. all-purpose flour
2 eggs   1 tsp. salt
1. Double the recipe.

2. Convert the measurements to the metric system.

3. How many brownie recipes can be prepared from each of the following ingredients?
   a. 1 lb. of sugar   c. 1 qt. of milk
   b. 1 lb. of butter   d. 1 doz. eggs

References

Anderson, Jean, and Elaine Hanna. 1975. *The Doubleday Cookbook*. Garden City, N.Y.: Doubleday & Company, Inc.

Charley, Helen. 1982. *Food Science*, 2nd ed. New York: John Wiley & Sons.

The Fannie Farmer Cookbook, 12th ed. 1979. New York: Alfred A. Knopf.

Peckham, Gladys, and Jeanne Freeland-Graves. 1979. *Foundations of Food Preparation*, 4th ed. New York: Macmillan Publishing Company.

Chapter 16

PREPARATION OF THE PATIENT'S MEAL

OBJECTIVES

After studying this chapter, you should be able to

- Adapt a family menu to suit the needs of the patient

- Demonstrate correct procedures for feeding a bedridden patient

- List dietary information that should be included in a patient's chart

In the home, the family menu should serve as the basis of the patient's meal whenever possible. This usually pleases the patient because it makes her or him feel a part of the family. Working from the same basic menu reduces food preparation time and avoids unnecessary food costs.

Family meals are quite easily adapted to the patient by omitting or adding certain foods or by varying the method of preparation. Suppose the patient was to limit fat intake and the family menu was the following:

Fried Hamburgers
Mashed Potatoes with Butter
Buttered Peas
Lettuce
with
French Dressing
Ice Cream
with
Fresh Strawberries
Whole Milk

Broiling the hamburgers instead of frying would help to limit the fat content. The patient's mashed potatoes might be served with little or no butter and the peas with only salt and pepper and perhaps a suitable spice or herb. The patient could be served lettuce with lemon and for dessert, strawberries without ice cream. Skim milk is a simple substitute for whole milk.

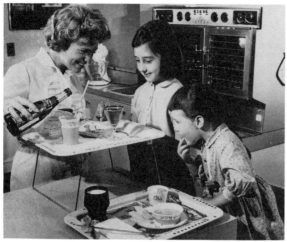

Figure 16-1 Note how attractively this tray has been prepared for a small patient. *(Courtesy of Parent's magazine)*

SERVING THE MEAL

To serve a meal at the bedside, the tray should be lined with a pretty cloth or paper liner. Attractive dishes that fit the tray conveniently without crowding it should be used. The food should be arranged attractively on the plate, with a colorful garnish such as a slice of fruit, parsley, a pickle, or vegetable stick. The garnish must fit into the patient's diet plan. Utensils must be arranged conveniently. Water should be served as well as another beverage (unless it is prohibited by the physician). Foods must be served at proper temperatures.

When the patient is on complete bedrest, special preparations are required before the meal is served. The patient should be given the opportunity to use the bedpan and to wash before the meal is served. The room can be ventilated and the bedcovers straightened. The patient should be helped to a comfortable position and any unpleasant sights removed

before the meal is served. Pleasant conversation during the preparations can improve the patient's mood considerably. Certain topics of conversation can help stimulate the patient's interest in eating. The patient might be told that the family is anticipating the same meal. Perhaps the recipes used will interest some patients. Appropriate remarks on the patient's progress, whenever possible, are helpful.

When the meal preparations are complete, the tray should be placed so it is easy for the patient to feed herself or himself, or if necessary, convenient for someone else to do the feeding. If the patient needs help, the napkin should be opened and placed, the bread spread, the meat cut, the eggs shelled and the straw offered. The patient should be encouraged to eat and be allowed sufficient time. If the meal is interrupted by the physician, the tray should be removed and the food kept at proper temperatures in the kitchen. It should be served again as soon as the physician leaves.

Some patients are unable to feed themselves. The person doing the feeding should sit near the side of the bed. Small amounts of food should be placed toward the back of the mouth with a slight pressure on the tongue with the spoon or fork. If the patient is suffering from one-sided paralysis, the food and drinking straw must be placed in the non-paralyzed side of the mouth. The patient must be allowed to help herself or himself as much as possible. If the patient begins to choke, help her or him sit up straight. Do not give food or water while the patient is choking. The patient's mouth should be wiped as is needed.

Special care must be taken in serving a meal for a blind patient. An appetizing description of the meal can help create a desire to eat. To help the blind patient feed herself or himself, arrange the food as if the plate were

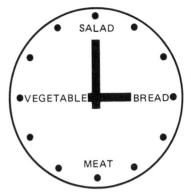

Figure 16-3 To a blind patient a plate of food can be pictured as the face of a clock.

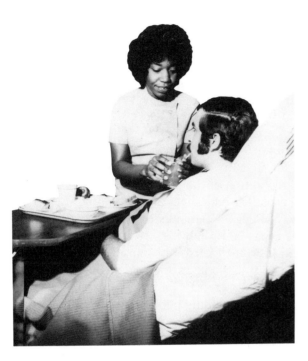

Figure 16-2 Some patients require assistance with eating.

the face of a clock. The meat might be put at 6 o'clock, vegetables at 9 o'clock, salad at 12 and bread at 3 o'clock. The person who regularly arranges the meal should remember to use the same pattern for all meals. Blind people usually feel better when they can help themselves.

The tray should be removed and the patient helped to brush her or his teeth when the meal is finished. The kinds and amounts of food refused, the time, the type of diet, and the patient's appetite should be recorded on the patient's chart after each meal. At times, the doctor requests an accurate report of the types and amounts of uneaten food.

SUMMARY

A patient's meal should be adapted from the family's meal whenever possible. This saves time and expense, and allows the patient to feel more a part of the family. A patient on bedrest should be given the bedpan and allowed to wash her or his hands before the meal. Patients should be encouraged to feed themselves. However, help should be offered if it is needed. The blind patient can eat more easily if food is arranged in a set pattern on the plate. Pleasant conversation and cheerfulness on the part of the nurse can improve the patient's appetite. The type of diet, time of meal, patient's appetite, type and amount of food eaten should all be recorded on the patient's chart.

Discussion Topics

1. Why is it wise to adapt the family menu to suit the patient's special requirements?

2. Discuss the following menu in terms of nutrient value and attractiveness. Adapt it to a patient on a low-calorie diet?

Cream of Chicken Soup

Roast Beef with Gravy

Baked Potatoes

Buttered Green Beans

Rolls and Butter

Angel Cake

with

Chocolate Ice Cream

3. Discuss the importance of proper preparation of the patient and room before the meal. What can disturb a patient and affect appetite?
4. How may the appearance of the tray affect the patient's appetite?
5. What is a garnish? Why may some types be prohibited?
6. Why should the patient be encouraged to feed herself or himself?
7. Why is it important to remove the tray as soon as the patient has finished the meal?
8. How can the behavior and attitude of the attending person affect the appetite of the patient?

Suggested Activities

1. Plan a family dinner and adapt it to the needs of a patient who should limit carbohydrate intake.
2. Arrange a tray suitable for serving this meal.
3. Have two students participate in the following role-playing situation. The class should evaluate and discuss the "nurse's" tact and skill in dealing with the "patient."
   Mrs. Jones is a young, active woman with a family. She is recovering from viral pneumonia. Although she is allowed out of bed, she is not supposed to prepare meals or do housework until her condition improves. Dr. Malcolm has told Miss Wilson, the nurse, that it is important for Mrs. Jones to regain her lost weight. One day before her dinner was served, Mrs. Jones complained to Miss Wilson. She was discouraged about her lack of energy and stated that her family needs her. Miss Wilson noted that she ate very little for breakfast and lunch. What should she say to Mrs. Jones?
4. Practice feeding each other. Ask the "nurse" to fill in the "patient's" chart.
5. Practice feeding a blindfolded "patient."

Review

A. A patient on a limited fat intake should avoid foods that are rich in fat. Indicate which foods she or he may eat on the following list by writing Y (yes). Write N (no) for the foods to be avoided.

_____ 1. fried hamburger   _____ 6. butter

_____ 2. mashed potatoes   _____ 7. ice cream

_____ 3. peas   _____ 8. fresh strawberries

_____ 4. lettuce   _____ 9. whole milk

_____ 5. French dressing

B. Briefly answer the following questions.

1. How may the following menu be adapted for a patient who must avoid foods high in cellulose?

Fresh Fruit Cup
Roast Turkey
Rice with Peas
Mashed Sweet Potatoes with Pecans
Celery and Carrot Sticks
Whole Wheat Bread
Butter
Cherry-Nut Ice Cream
Milk and Coffee

2. What should be done if the patient's meal is interrupted by a visit from the doctor?

3. What dietary information should be recorded on the patient's chart after a meal?

4. Give two examples of a colorful garnish.

References

Kinder, Faye, Nancy Green, and Natholyn Harris. 1984. *Meal Management*, 6th ed. New York: Macmillan Publishing Company.
Poleman, Charlotte M., and Christine Locastro Capra. 1984. *Shackelton's Nutrition Essentials and Diet Therapy*, 5th ed. Philadelphia: W. B. Saunders Co.

Section 4
Nutrition
During Life
Stages

Chapter 17

DIET DURING PREGNANCY AND LACTATION

VOCABULARY

adolescent	mortality rate	retardation
craving	nausea	skeletal structure
eclamptic stage	obstetrician	trimester
fetus	pica	toxemia
hemoglobin	placenta	vitamin
lactation	preeclampsia	supplement
morning sickness	proteinuria	

OBJECTIVES

After studying this chapter, you should be able to

- Identify nutritional needs during pregnancy and lactation

- Modify the normal diet to meet the needs of pregnant and lactating women

THE IMPORTANCE OF GOOD NUTRITION DURING PREGNANCY

Good nutrition during pregnancy is essential to both the mother-to-be and her child. In addition to her normal nutritional requirements, the pregnant woman must provide nutrients and kcal for increased breast and uterine tissue, blood volume, placenta (structure that forms around the human embryo to nourish and protect it inside the uterus), and the embryo. The pregnant woman who follows a nutritionally appropriate diet is more apt to feel better, to retain her health, and to bear a healthy infant than one who chooses her foods thoughtlessly.

Studies have shown a relationship between the mother's diet and the health of the baby at birth. It is also thought that the woman who consumed a nutritious diet before pregnancy is more apt to bear a healthy infant than one who did not. Malnutrition of the mother is believed to cause growth retardation in the *fetus* (infant developing in the mother's uterus). Low birth weight infants have a higher *mortality* (death) rate than those of normal birth weight. Also, a relationship is suspected between maternal nutrition and the subsequent mental development of the child.

NUTRITIONAL NEEDS DURING PREGNANCY

Although it is often said, "a pregnant woman must eat for two", this is true only in terms of nutrients and not in terms of kilocalories. The saying may have originated because the appetite is usually very good during the second and third *trimesters* (three-month periods) of pregnancy. During the first trimester, the mother may suffer from some degree of nausea and have a slightly fickle appetite.

It is true that energy needs increase during pregnancy because of the developing fetus, increasing maternal tissue, and an increased basal metabolism rate. During the first trimester, there is little tissue growth so energy needs increase only slightly. There is a substantial increase in maternal tissue during the second trimester, and the placenta and the fetus grow a great deal during the third trimester. However, the pregnant woman commonly reduces her activities as the pregnancy progresses which reduces her energy expenditure. Consequently, the additional energy need during pregnancy is low. On the average, a pregnant woman requires only an additional 300 kcal per day.

It must be stressed that 300 kcal is an *average* amount. When the mother is very young and still growing herself, or is engaged in a highly active occupation, 300 kilocalories may not be sufficient to meet her energy needs. In any event, the daily caloric intake during pregnancy should never be reduced below 36 kcal per kilogram of pregnant weight.

Some of the specific daily nutrient requirements, however, are increased dramatically. The pregnant adolescent requires more of the essential nutrients than the mature woman because the adolescent is still growing herself. These requirements are shown on Table 17-1. These figures are recommended requirements for the general U.S. population; the physician may suggest alternate figures based on specific knowledge of the patient and her activities.

The protein requirement is increased by 30g, from 44g to 74g for the mature pregnant woman, and from 46g to 76g for the pregnant adolescent. It is essential for tissue building, and the protein-rich foods are excellent sources of many other essential nutrients,

Table 17-1

	Age (years)	Weight (kg)	Weight (lb)	Height (cm)	Height (in)	Energy Needs (with range) (kcal)		Protein (g)	Vita-min A (µg RE)	Vita-min D (µg)	Vita-min E (mg α-TE)
Females	11–14	46	101	157	62	2200	(1500–3000)	46	800	10	8
	15–18	55	120	163	64	2100	(1200–3000)	46	800	10	8
	19–22	55	120	163	64	2100	(1700–2500)	44	800	7.5	8
	23–50	55	120	163	64	2000	(1600–2400)	44	800	5	8
Pregnant						+300		+30	+200	+5	+2
Lactating						+500		+20	+400	+5	+3

Reprinted from Food and Nutrition Board, National Academy of Sciences—National Research Council, 1980

especially iron, zinc, magnesium, and the B vitamins. An inexpensive way to include extra protein in the diet is to add dried milk to creamed foods.

Requirements for vitamins A and E are increased by 25 percent to allow for their storage by the fetus as well as their roles in maintaining healthy eyes, skin, bones, and blood tissue. The requirement for vitamin D is increased from 50 to 100 percent, depending on the age of the mother. It is necessary for helping calcium and phosphorus build the baby's skeletal structure, and for maintaining the mother's skeletal structure. It is important that the estimated intake of 70 to 140mcg of vitamin K is met to maintain normal clotting ability of the blood.

Requirements for the B vitamins are all substantially increased during pregnancy, with the greatest increase in folacin and B_{12} because of their roles in blood building.

The vitamin C requirement is increased by 33 percent, or more if the mother is under 15 years of age. This is necessary because the percentage of vitamin C in fetal blood is 50 percent greater than in maternal blood.

The calcium and phosphorus requirements are increased by 400 mg each. These figures represent a 50 percent increase in the adult's requirement, and a 33 percent increase in the adolescent's requirement. The adolescent's non-pregnant requirement is 1200mg for calcium and phosphorus while the non-pregnant adult's normal requirement for each is only 800mg. Calcium and phosphorus are essential for building bones and teeth. The magnesium requirement is increased by 50 percent to 150mg. Magnesium is necessary for bone, muscle, and blood tissue. The iron requirement increases from 18mg to 30—60mg because the increased maternal tissue, placenta, and especially the fetus all need iron for the hemoglobin in their blood. The fetus increases its hemoglobin level to 20g to 22g per 100ml of blood. This is nearly twice the normal human hemoglobin level of 13g to 14g per 100ml of blood. The infant's hemoglobin level is reduced to normal shortly after birth as the extra hemoglobin breaks down. The resulting iron is stored in the liver and is available when needed during the infant's first few months of life when the diet is essentially milk. Zinc, which is essential for growth and enzymatic action, must be increased by 33 percent during pregnancy. The iodine requirement during pregnancy—although increased by only

Table 17-1 (*Continued*)

Water-Soluble Vitamins							Minerals					
Vita-min C (mg)	Thia-min (mg)	Ribo-flavin (mg)	Niacin (mg NE)	Vita-min B-6 (mg)	Fola-cin (μg)	Vitamin B-12 (μg)	Cal-cium (mg)	Phos-phorus (mg)	Mag-nesium (mg)	Iron (mg)	Zinc (mg)	Iodine (μg)
50	1.1	1.3	15	1.8	400	3.0	1200	1200	300	18	15	150
60	1.1	1.3	14	2.0	400	3.0	1200	1200	300	18	15	150
60	1.1	1.3	14	2.0	400	3.0	800	800	300	18	15	150
60	1.0	1.2	13	2.0	400	3.0	800	800	300	18	15	150
+20	+0.4	+0.3	+2	+0.6	+400	+1.0	+400	+400	+150	+30	+5	+25
+40	+0.5	+0.5	+5	+0.5	+100	+1.0	+400	+400	+150	+30	+10	+50

Table 17-2 Suggested 2400 Calorie Menu for a Pregnant Woman

Breakfast	Lunch	Dinner
Orange Juice	Citrus Fruit Cup	Tomato Juice
Scrambled Egg	Roast Beef Sandwich with	Calves Liver
Toast with Peanut Butter	Mayonnaise & Lettuce	Baked Potato with Butter
	Vanilla Pudding	Baked Squash
Skim Milk	Skim Milk	Fresh Spinach Salad with Oil and Vinegar
		Ice Milk
		Skim Milk

Snack	Snack
Apple	Yogurt

about 15 percent—is, nevertheless, essential for the prevention of maternal goiter.

To meet the nutritional requirements of pregnancy, the diet should, of course, be based on the Basic Four food groups. Special care should be taken in the selection of food so that the necessary additional nutrients and not just additional kilocalories are provided.

One of the best ways of providing these nutrients is by drinking an additional pint (470ml) of milk each day, or using appropriate substitutes. This additional amount brings the total amount of milk required by the mature pregnant woman to one quart (about 1 liter or 950 milliliters). The amount required by the pregnant adolescent, then, would be slightly over one and one-half quarts (1 1/2 liters or 1,500 ml). An additional pint of milk provides 350 kcal if whole milk is used, and 190 kcal if skim milk is used. This additional pint of milk also provides 16 grams of protein—half the

additional requirement of 30 g; 580 mg of calcium and 460 mg of phosphorus—more than the additional amounts required; approximately 65 mg of magnesium, or nearly one-half of the additional requirement; 1.86 mg of zinc, or nearly half of the additional requirement; four times the additional thiamin required; nearly three times the additional riboflavin required; one-fifth of the additional niacin required and even some of the additional iron and vitamin C required.

Some obstetricians may prescribe a vitamin supplement for the mother-to-be. However, it is not advisable for the mother to take any unprescribed nutrient supplement, as an excess of vitamins or minerals can be toxic to mother and baby.

The unusual cravings for certain foods during pregnancy do no harm unless eating them interferes with the normal balanced diet or causes excessive weight gain.

CONCERNS DURING PREGNANCY

Nausea

Sometimes *nausea* (the feeling of a need to vomit) may occur during the first *trimester* (3-month period) of pregnancy. This type of nausea is commonly known as *morning sickness*. It typically passes as the pregnancy proceeds to the second trimester. Dry crackers or dry toast eaten before rising, eliminating some of the fat in the diet, and avoiding liquids at mealtimes may help to reduce it. If nausea persists it should be treated by the doctor.

Weight

Usually there is little weight gain during the first three months of pregnancy. A woman gains about .45 kg (1 pound) a week during the last six months of pregnancy. The average weight gain during pregnancy is 11 kg (24 pounds) and should not be less than 9 kilos (20 pounds).

Adolescents tend to gain more than mature women since many of them are still growing themselves. Women having their first babies are apt to gain more than women having their second or third babies; and very thin women are inclined to gain more than stout women. Excessive weight gain should be avoided because it may predispose a woman to toxemia, cause complications during delivery, and overweight after delivery.

If weight gain becomes excessive, the pregnant woman should reevaluate her diet and eliminate the foods (except for the extra pint of milk) that do not fit within the Basic Four food group plan. Examples of these include candy, cookies, rich desserts, potato chips, salad dressings, and sweet beverages. In addition, she might substitute skim milk for whole milk, which would reduce her caloric intake by 160—200 kcal per day. Except in cases where the woman cannot tolerate lactose (the sugar in milk), it is not advisable to substitute calcium pills for milk because this reduces the protein, vitamin, and total mineral content of the diet as well as the caloric content.

A bowl of clean, crisp, raw vegetables such as broccoli or cauliflower tips, carrots, celery, cucumber, zucchini sticks, and radishes can provide interesting snacks that are nutritious, filling, satisfying, and low in calories. Fruits and custards made with skim milk make nutritious satisfying desserts that are not high in calories. Broiling, baking, or boiling foods instead of frying can further reduce the caloric content of the diet.

It is important, however, that there is weight gain during pregnancy. Pregnancy is no time for the overweight woman to reduce. She should gain the same average amount during pregnancy as the woman who is not overweight. Weight loss can be undertaken after the pregnancy.

Toxemia

Toxemia or *preeclampsia* is a condition that sometimes occurs during the third trimester of pregnancy. It is characterized by high blood pressure, the presence of albumin in the urine (*proteinuria*), and edema. The edema causes a somewhat sudden increase in weight. If the condition persists and reaches the *eclamptic* (convulsive) stage, convulsions and coma may occur. The cause of toxemia is not known, but it occurs more frequently among pregnant women on inadequate diets (particularly when the diets are inadequate in protein) than among pregnant women on good diets.

Pica

Pica is the craving for nonfood substances such as starch or clay. The diets of pregnant women who indulge such cravings tend to be low in protein, calcium, and iron. Pica has been associated with iron-deficiency anemia. Obviously, this is not a healthy practice and should be discouraged.

Nutritional Anemia

Anemia is a condition caused by an insufficiency of red blood cells, hemoglobin, or blood volume. The patient suffering from it does not receive sufficient oxygen from the blood, and consequently feels weak and tired, has a poor appetite, and appears pale. Nutritional anemia is caused by a lack of specific nutrients. Iron-deficiency *anemia* is its most common form. During pregnancy, the increased volume of blood creates the need for additional iron for the hemoglobin of this blood. When this need is not met by the diet or by the iron stores in the mother's body, iron-deficiency anemia develops. Because the need for iron increases to such an extent during pregnancy, it is difficult to provide sufficient iron in the diet. Therefore, it is quite common for the obstetrician to prescribe a daily iron supplement of 30—60 mg during pregnancy. Pregnant women should be warned against self prescription of iron, however, since excess amounts can be toxic. A simple method of improving the absorption of iron is the inclusion of a vitamin C-rich food at meals. Vitamin C acts as an *iron enhancer* because it greatly improves the absorption of iron.

Folic acid deficiency anemia is also of concern during pregnancy because the body requires a great deal of folic acid when new cells are being formed. Consequently, the obstetrician may prescribe a folic acid supplement of 400mcg per day.

Alcohol, Caffeine, and Tobacco

Controversy continues regarding the use of alcohol, caffeine, and tobacco during pregnancy because research has not yet determined conclusively that their effects are permanently harmful to the fetus. However, there are indications that these substances do harm the fetus.

Alcohol appears to be associated with abnormal physical and mental development of the fetus. When the mother drinks alcohol, it enters the fetal bloodstream in the same concentration as it does the mother's. Unfortunately, the fetus does not have the capacity to metabolize it as quickly as the mother, so it stays longer in the fetal blood than it does in the maternal blood.

Caffeine is known to cross the placenta, but its longlasting effects on the human fetus have not been determined. Birth defects in newborn rats whose mothers were fed caffeine during pregnancy have been observed.

Tobacco smoking by pregnant women has for some time been associated with babies of reduced birth weight.

Obviously, because of the indications of toxicity to the fetus, it is advisable that pregnant women limit, if not avoid, the use of these substances.

LACTATION

Lactation is the period during which the mother nurses her baby. This causes her

Table 17-3 Suggested 2600 Calorie Menu for a Lactating Woman

Breakfast	Lunch	Dinner
Grapefruit Half	Orange Juice	Melon
Poached Egg	Creamed Chicken on Toast	Pot Roast of Beef
Bacon		Potato
Toast	Green Salad with Oil & Vinegar	Carrots
Peanut Butter		Coleslaw
Skim Milk	Baked Apple	Roll & Butter
	Skim Milk	Baked Custard
		Skim Milk

Snack	Snack
Fruit Juice	Milk

kilocalorie and nutrient requirements to increase because she is producing about 5.5 ounces (165 ml) of milk for every 2.2 pounds (1 kilogram) of the baby's weight each day. Each ounce (30ml) of human milk contains 20 kilocalories. To determine the baby's daily caloric requirement, one would first multiply the baby's weight in kilograms by 5.5 ounces. This number of ounces of milk would then be multiplied by 20 kcal. For example, to determine the caloric requirement for a ten-pound (4.5 kilo) infant, one would multiply its weight in kilograms (4.5) by 5.5 ounces. This answer (24.75 ounces) must then be multiplied by 20 kcal to determine the total daily caloric requirement of 495 kcal. Because the mother produces milk very efficiently, and she has presumably stored some fat during pregnancy that can be used for energy in milk production during lactation, the increase in her kcal requirements during lactation is relatively small. The estimated average additional caloric requirement during lactation is 500 kcal (2100 kilojoules) per day. See Table 17-1. This would, in fact, depend on the size of the baby and its appetite, as well as the size and activities of the mother.

Care should be taken to ensure that the extra protein, vitamins, and minerals required are provided in the foods chosen to fulfill the additional caloric requirement. The nursing mother should be advised to choose her foods from among the Basic Four food groups and to remember that potato chips, soda, and candy provide little more than calories.

It is advisable that the adult nursing mother have at least 950ml (one quart) of milk each day. The adolescent nursing mother should have one and a half quarts. Cheese may be substituted for part of the milk, and milk may be included in other foods such as white sauces, custards, and puddings. This milk will provide many of the additional nutrients required, as well as many of the additional kcal.

It is important that the nursing mother have sufficient fluids to replace those lost in the infant's milk. There is no particular beverage that is better than any other.

The mother should be made aware that she must reduce her caloric intake at the end of the nursing period to avoid adding unwanted weight.

follows a well-balanced diet. Research has shown that maternal nutrition can affect the subsequent mental and physical health of the child. Anemia and toxemia during pregnancy are two conditions that may be the result of inadequate nutrition. Both caloric and nutrient requirements increase for pregnant women (especially adolescents) and women who are breast feeding. The average weight gain during pregnancy is 9—11 kilograms (20—25 pounds).

SUMMARY

A pregnant woman is more likely to remain healthy and bear a healthy infant if she

Discussion Topics

1. Discuss the truth of the statement, "A pregnant woman must eat for two."
2. Why is it especially important for a pregnant woman to have a highly nutritious diet?
3. Discuss weight gain during pregnancy from the first month through the ninth. What types of women are apt to gain more than the average? Why is an excessive weight gain during pregnancy undesirable? Is pregnancy a good time to reduce? Why?
4. Of what value are protein-rich foods during pregnancy?
5. It is common for an iron supplement to be prescribed during pregnancy. Why? What may happen if the mother-to-be does not receive an adequate supply of iron? And how may such a condition affect her baby? Discuss the advisability of the pregnant woman's taking a self-prescribed iron or vitamin supplement in addition to that prescribed by the obstetrician.
6. Discuss why the obstetrician regularly checks the pregnant woman's blood pressure, urine, and weight during her pregnancy.
7. Discuss the effects of lactation on the mother's diet.
8. What is morning sickness and how may it be alleviated? If any class member has been pregnant, ask her questions regarding morning sickness.
9. How many servings of each of the Basic Four food groups may be found in the menus in tables 17-2 and 17-3?

Suggested Activities

1. Using table A-7 in the Appendix, plan a day's menu for a normal 20-year old pregnant woman. Adapt it to meet the needs of a pregnant 16-year old. Adapt both menus to suit women who dislike drinking milk.
2. Adapt the first menu in Activity 1 to meet the needs of a 29-year old pregnant woman.
3. Using table A-7 in the Appendix, plan a day's menu for a nursing mother who normally requires 2400 calories.
4. Using table A-7 in the Appendix, list the nutrients in one quart (500 ml) of skim milk. Do the same for 1 quart of whole milk.
5. Make a list of different ways of including milk in the diet. Compare notes and recipes with other class members.
6. List the foods that you have eaten in the past 24 hours. Adapt these menus to meet your nutritional requirements if you were pregnant.
7. Ask a physician or a nurse to speak to the class on the importance of adequate nutrition before and during pregnancy. Ask the speaker questions regarding the effects of good or poor nutrition on the health of the mother, prenatal development, infant mortality, and the growth and development of the child.

Review

A. Multiple Choice. Select the *letter* that precedes the best answer.

1. The infant developing in the mother's uterus is called the
   a. sperm   c. placenta
   b. fetus   d. ovary
2. Anemia would most likely result from
   a. pica   c. a lack of iron
   b. an excess of vitamin A   d. improper cooking of meat
3. High blood pressure, edema, and albumin in the urine are symptoms of
   a. nausea   c. pica
   b. anemia   d. toxemia
4. A common name given nausea in early pregnancy is
   a. morning sickness   c. toxemia
   b. pica   d. mortality

5. Folacin and vitamin B_{12} requirements increase during pregnancy because of their roles in
   a. building strong bones and teeth
   b. fighting infections in the placenta
   c. blood building
   d. enzyme action

6. The average additional daily energy requirement for the pregnant woman is
   a. 100 calories
   b. 300 calories
   c. 500 calories
   d. 1000 calories

7. The additional nutrients required during pregnancy are largely met by
   a. eating steak each day
   b. drinking a malted each day
   c. using an additional pint of milk each day
   d. using an iron supplement

8. Craving for nonfood substances during pregnancy is known as
   a. anemia
   b. toxemia
   c. nausea
   d. pica

9. During pregnancy, the average weight gain is
   a. 10 to 15 pounds
   b. 15 to 20 pounds
   c. 9 to 11 kilograms
   d. 11 to 15 kilograms

10. The period during which a mother nurses her baby is known as
    a. pregnancy
    b. trimester
    c. lactation
    d. obstetrics

11. A nursing mother should have at least
    a. 1 cup of milk each day
    b. 1 pint of milk each day
    c. 1 and 1/2 pints of milk each day
    d. 1 quart of milk each day

12. Some appropriate substitutes for milk include
    a. orange juice and tomato juice
    b. cheese and custard
    c. breads and cereals
    d. vegetables and fruit juices

13. The average daily additional energy requirement for a nursing mother is
    a. 100 calories
    b. 300 calories
    c. 500 calories
    d. 1000 calories

14. The daily diet during pregnancy and lactation should
    a. be based on the Basic Four food groups
    b. include at least a quart of milk
    c. be limited in hollow calorie foods
    d. all of the above

15. Appropriate snacks for pregnant and lactating women include

    a. fruits and milk   c. sodas

    b. potato chips and pretzels   d. hard candies

B. True or False

The following usually contain milk or cream:

1. Eggnog
2. Chocolate pudding
3. Meat Loaf
4. Strawberry yogurt
5. Pineapple cottage cheese
6. Creamed chicken
7. Caramel custard
8. New England clam chowder
9. Hot cocoa
10. Quiche Lorraine
11. Chicken gravy
12. Banana cream pie
13. Cream of broccoli soup
14. Sour cream pie
15. "Light" coffee
16. Cheesecake
17. Chipped beef on toast
18. Macaroni and cheese
19. Apple pie a la mode
20. Grilled cheese sandwich
21. Vanilla shake
22. Chocolate malt
23. Pizza
24. Tuna melt
25. Rice pudding

References

Diet Manual. Massachusetts General Hospital Dietary Department. Boston: Little, Brown & Co. 1976.

Eschleman, Marian M. 1984. *Introductory Nutrition and Diet Therapy.* Philadelphia: J. B. Lippincott Company.

Luke, Barbara. 1979. *Maternal Nutrition.* Boston: Little Brown & Co.

Luke, Barbara. 1984. *Principles of Nutrition and Diet Therapy.* Boston: Little Brown & Co.

Roberts, Bonnie S. Worthington, Joyce Vermeersch and Sue Rodwell Williams. 1981. *Nutrition in Pregnancy and Lactation*, 2nd ed. St. Louis: C. V. Mosby Co.

U.S. Department of Agriculture. *Composition of Food.* 1963; 1975.

University of Iowa Hospitals and Clinics. 1979. *Recent Advances in Therapeutic Diets.* Iowa City: Iowa State University Press.

Chapter 18

DIET DURING INFANCY

VOCABULARY

aseptic	pediatrician	sterilizing
bubbled	psychological	process
coordination	development	synthetic
emotional bond	regurgitation	terminal
immunity	sterile	weaning

OBJECTIVES

After studying this chapter, you should be able to

- State the effect inadequate nutrition has on an infant

- Identify the ingredients used in infant formulas

- Explain the aseptic and terminal methods of formula preparation

- Describe when and how foods are introduced into the baby's diet

Food and its presentation are extremely important during the baby's first year. Physical and mental development are dependent on the food itself and psychological development is affected by the time and manner in which the food is offered.

Infants react to their parents' emotions. If food is forced on a child, or withheld until the child is uncomfortable, or if the food is presented in a tense manner, the child reacts with tension and unhappiness. If the parent is relaxed, the infant's mealtime can be a pleasure for both parent and child.

NUTRITIONAL REQUIREMENTS OF THE INFANT

The first year of life is a period of the most rapid growth in one's life. A baby doubles its birth weight by six months of age and triples it within the first year. This explains why the infant's energy, vitamin, mineral, and protein requirements are higher per unit of body weight than those of older children or adults. During this first year, the normal child needs about 100 kcal per kilo-

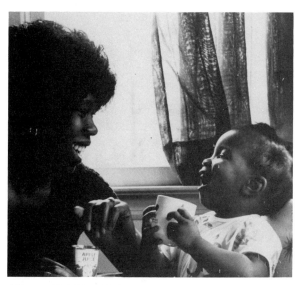

Figure 18-1 Food is better accepted and digested in a happy and relaxed atmosphere.

Table 18-1 Recommended Daily Dietary Requirements for Infants from Birth to One Year of Age

Age	0–5 mo.	5 mo.–1 yr.
Weight		
(kg)	6	9
(lb)	13	20
Height		
(cm)	60	71
(in)	24	28
Protein		
(g)	kg × 2.2	kg × 2.0
Fat-Soluble Vitamins		
Vitamin A		
(μg RE)	420	400
Vitamin D		
(μg)	10	10
Vitamin E		
(mg α-TE)	3	4
Water-Soluble Vitamins		
Vitamin C		
(mg)	35	35
Thiamin		
(mg)	0.3	0.5
Riboflavin		
(mg)	0.4	0.6
Niacin		
(mg NE)	6	8
Vitamin B-6		
(mg)	0.3	0.6
Folacin		
(μg)	30	45
Vitamin B-12		
(μg)	0.5	1.5
Minerals		
Calcium		
(mg)	360	540
Phosphorus		
(mg)	240	360
Magnesium		
(mg)	50	70
Iron		
(mg)	10	15
Zinc		
(mg)	3	5
Iodine		
(μg)	40	50

Source: Food and Nutrition Board, National Academy of Sciences—National Research Council, 1980

gram of body weight each day. This is approximately two to three times the adult requirement. A diet of less than 80 kcal per kilogram of body weight is considered inadequate, and one that contains more than 120 kcal per kilogram of body weight may lead to obesity. However, low birth weight infants and infants who have suffered from malnutrition or illness require more than the normal number of kcal per kilogram of body weight.

The basis of the infant's diet is milk. It is a highly nutritious, digestible food containing protein, fat, carbohydrate, vitamins, minerals, and water.

It is, however, a poor source of iron and vitamin C. Consequently, these nutrients are usually provided as supplements to the infant's milk diet. The baby's store of iron is typically depleted by the age of four months and the pediatrician usually prescribes an iron supplement at that time. Bottle-fed babies may receive a supplement of vitamin C by the age of 10 days because the sterilizing process for the formula frequently destroys this vitamin. Except for iron and vitamin C, the normal infant's appetite will ensure the provision of sufficient nutrients whether the child is nursed or given properly-mixed formula.

The RDA of nutrients for infants may be seen in Table 18-1.

METHODS OF FEEDING

Infants may be breast-fed or bottle-fed. Both breast milk and formula provide 20 kcal per ounce. Each is composed of approximately 10 percent protein, 50 percent fat, and 40 percent carbohydrate. Breast feeding is nature's way of providing a good diet for the baby. It is economical, nutritionally adequate, sanitary, and saves time otherwise spent in formula preparation. Mother's milk gives the baby temporary *immunity* (resistance) to some infectious diseases. Since it is sterile and so easy to digest, it usually does not cause gastrointestinal disturbances. Additionally, it helps establish an emotional *bond* between mother and child that is beneficial to both.

Many mothers prefer to bottle feed their babies. Certain women are unable to produce enough breast milk; others who are employed or involved in many activities outside the home find bottle feeding more convenient. Still others simply prefer not to breast feed. Either way is acceptable provided the infant is given love and attention during the feeding. The infant should be cuddled and kept comfortable and warm during the feeding. During and after the feeding, the infant should be *bubbled* (burped) to release gas in the stomach. Bubbling helps prevent *regurgitation* (spitting up food).

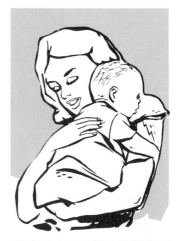

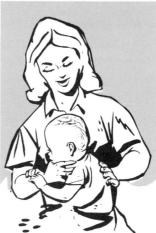

Figure 18-2 To bubble a baby, hold him in one of the two positions shown and gently stroke his back.

Although babies have been fed according to prescribed time schedules in the past, it is preferable to feed infants *on demand*, which means when they are hungry. Feeding on demand prevents the frustrations that hunger can bring, and helps the child develop trust in people. The newborn may require more frequent feedings, but normally the demand schedule averages out to approximately every four hours by the time the baby is two or three months old.

Formulas and Their Preparation

If the baby is bottle-fed, parents receive instructions for feeding from the *pediatrician* (baby and children's doctor). One of the convenient, prepared products may be prescribed. There are many ready-to-use formulas available in disposable bottles and cans. Some of these preparations require the addition of water, but many are complete and ready to serve. Some have vitamins and iron added. The cost of milk formula is directly related to convenience—the most convenient is the most expensive. If parents are more concerned with economy than convenience, the pediatrician can prescribe a homemade formula.

Normally, cow's milk is used in formulas because it is most abundant and easily modified to resemble human milk. It is modified because it has more protein and mineral salts and less milk sugar (lactose) than human milk. Water and sugar are usually added to dilute these nutrients. When an infant is extremely sensitive or allergic to cow's milk a *synthetic* (man-made) milk may be given. Synthetic milk is commonly made from soybeans. Goat's milk is sometimes used as a substitute for cow's milk in situations where the baby is allergic to cow's milk, or the baby may be breast fed.

If the infant is given a formula prepared at home, it is essential that it be carefully and accurately prepared. Typically, it is made from water, pasteurized cow's milk, and a sweetener. The milk may be fresh, evaporated, dried, whole, or skim. The usual forms of sugar used are granulated (sucrose), corn syrup (glucose and maltose), or malt sugar (maltose). The pediatrician prescribes a formula that suits the needs of the baby, and adjusts it as the child grows.

The following formula is recommended by Dr. Spock in his book, *Baby and Child Care* (Pocket Books, Inc., New York, N.Y., 1976).

evaporated milk: 13 oz.
water: 19 oz.
corn syrup: 2 Tbsp.

Two basic methods for preparing formulas are the terminal and the aseptic. The *aseptic* method includes sterilization of each item used in the formula preparation before the formula is poured into the bottles. In the *terminal* method, the bottles and formula are sterilized together. The terminal method is effective and simpler than the aseptic method. Using the terminal method, all equipment is first washed and rinsed. The formula is mixed in a pitcher and poured into the bottles. The bottles are loosely capped and then sterilized by boiling for 25 minutes. The bottles should be allowed to cool in the covered pan until they are lukewarm. The nipples are then tightened, and the bottles refrigerated.

The equipment for preparing formulas should consist of a kettle, wire rack for sterilizing, long brush for cleaning, measuring cups and spoons, saucepans, funnel, spoon, can opener, bottles, nipples, nipple caps, and tongs for removing hot bottles.

It is essential that all equipment used in preparing formulas be clean. Milk is an excellent medium for the growth of microorganisms. Bottles, caps, and nipples should be thoroughly cleaned after each feeding.

The formula may be given cold, at room temperature, or warmed, but it should be given at the same temperature consistently. To warm the formula for feeding, bottles should be placed in a saucepan of warm water or a bottlewarmer. The bottles should be shaken occasionally to warm the contents evenly. The temperature of the milk can be tested by shaking a few drops on one's wrist. The milk should feel lukewarm.

Even if the baby is breast-fed, sterile bottles will be needed for water and fruit juices. Sterilization of nipples, rings, and bottles is simple, and it is very important in preventing the growth of harmful micro-organisms. To sterilize these items, they must be boiled for the number of minutes specified by the pediatrician. The nipple and ring must be attached to the bottle with sterile tongs.

Supplementary Foods

In addition to milk, an infant may be given vitamin drops as early as ten days of age and fruit juice shortly after. However, these should be given only on the advice of the pediatrician. *The age at which new foods are introduced is highly variable.* Some pediatricians encourage early introduction of cereals and fruits while others discourage it. Pediatricians are increasingly advising that

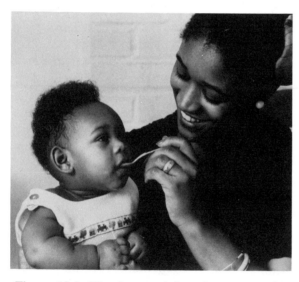

Figure 18-3 Weaning an infant from the bottle actually begins when food is given with a spoon.

semi-solid foods not be introduced into the child's diet until the child is four to six months old. By this age a child is better able to move food from the front of the mouth to the throat. A delayed introduction of solids may prevent some food allergies because as the intestines mature, they are more capable of handling a variety of foods. Delayed introduction of solids may help prevent overnutrition of the child that can lead to obesity. In any event, there is no nutritional need to introduce solids before the child is three-months old so long as the child is nursed or fed a proper formula. By the age of six months, however, mothers' milk or formula cannot supply sufficient energy to the growing child. Solid foods are introduced at this stage. These must be introduced gradually and individually. One food is introduced and then no other new food for four or five days. If there is no allergic reaction, another food may be introduced, a waiting period allowed, then another, and so on. The typical order of introduction is rice cereal; other cereals; cooked or pureed fruits, or in the case of bananas, simply mashed; cooked and pureed vegetables; and finally finely ground meats. Between 6 and 12 months, toast, zwieback, teething biscuits, custards, puddings, and ice cream may be added. By the age of one year, most babies are eating foods from all of the Basic Four food groups, and may have most any food that is easily chewed and digested. The child's few teeth and lack of coordination may limit the types of foods that can be eaten. It is important that the child be given a well-balanced diet. The Basic Four food groups are an excellent guide. Foods should be selected according to the advice of the pediatrician. Care should be taken to avoid excess sugar and salt in the baby's diet.

Weaning (teaching the infant to drink from a cup instead of the breast or bottle)

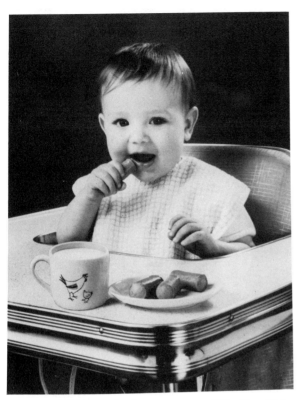

Figure 18-4 Finger foods encourage self-feeding. This baby is enjoying meat sticks specially manufactured for toddlers. *(Courtesy of Gerber Products Company)*

actually begins when the infant is first given food from a spoon. It progresses as the child shows an interest in, and ability to drink from a cup. The child will ultimately discard the bottle. If the child shows great reluctance to discard the bottle, the pediatrician's advice should be sought.

SUMMARY

It is particularly important that babies have adequate diets so their physical and mental development is not impaired. Breast feeding is nature's way of feeding an infant, although formula feeding is equally acceptable. Cow's milk is usually used in formulas because it is most available and is easily modified to resemble human milk. To modify milk, sugar and water can be added to fresh, evaporated, or dried milk. Two methods of preparing formulas are the aseptic and the terminal methods. The young child's diet is supplemented on the advice of the pediatrician. Added foods should be based on the Basic Four food groups.

Discussion Topics

1. Do any of the students know a woman who has breast-fed her baby? What were her reactions to the experience?
2. Why is breast feeding not always possible?
3. Why are some babies not allowed cow's milk? What kind of milk can these children have?
4. Discuss the possible effects of regularly propping the baby's bottle instead of holding the baby during feeding.
5. Why is a rigid time schedule for feeding a baby not advisable?
6. What foods is an 8-month baby usually allowed to eat?
7. How may weaning be accomplished?

Suggested Activities

1. Have a panel discussion on the advantages and disadvantages of breast feeding.
2. Observe demonstrations of the preparations of formula by the aseptic and the terminal methods. Practice preparing formula by both methods. Calculate the cost of the ingredients.
3. Observe a demonstration of the actual feeding and bubbling of a baby.
4. Visit a store that carries prepared infant formulas and check prices of these products. Compare the prices of these products with the cost of preparing the formulas yourself.

Review

A. Complete the following statements:

1. The mother's milk gives the infant temporary _____ to certain diseases.
2. An infant _____ (does, does not) react to the emotions of the person feeding her or him.
3. The doctor who decides what kind of formula to give the baby is the _____ .
4. Cow's milk has more _____ and _____ than human milk.
5. Cow's milk has less _____ than human milk.
6. Usually, the first solid food added to the infant's milk diet is a

   _____ .
7. Because milk contains little vitamin _____ the formula should be supplemented early.
8. Usually, an infant may have any food that is easily chewed and digested when she or he is approximately _____ months old.
9. When an infant is allergic to cow's milk, _____ may be substituted.
10. Inadequate nutrition during infancy may impair the infant's _____ and _____ development.

B. Match the items in column I to the correct statement in column II.

Column I	Column II
_____ 1. milk	a. baby doctor
_____ 2. supplement	b. teaching the child to drink from a

_____ 3. immunity

_____ 4. regurgitation

_____ 5. bubbling

_____ 6. pediatrician

_____ 7. synthetic

_____ 8. terminal method

_____ 9. aseptic method

_____ 10. weaning

    cup instead of a nipple

c. addition

d. basis of the infant's diet

e. burping

f. spitting up of food

g. sterilization of formula equipment
   before formula is mixed

h. man-made

i. sterilization of formula and equipment
   together

j. protection from disease

k. doctor who delivers the baby

C. Briefly answer the following questions.

1. Why should the mother give her baby special attention during feedings?

2. How is a bottle warmed? Is this always necessary?

3. Name two factors that determine the infant's ability to manage solid foods.

References

Green, Marilyn L. and Joann Harry. 1981. *Nutrition in Contemporary Nursing Practice.* New York: John Wiley & Sons.

Massachusetts General Hospital Dietary Departments. 1976. *Diet Manual.* Boston: Little, Brown & Co.

Pipes, Peggy L. 1981. *Nutrition in Infancy and Childhood*, 2nd ed. St. Louis: C. V. Mosby Co.

U.S Department of Agriculture. *Composition of Foods.* 1963, 1975.

Williams, Sue Rodwell. 1984. *Mowry's Basic Nutrition and Diet Therapy*, 7th ed. St. Louis: C. V. Mosby Co.

Chapter 19

DIET DURING CHILDHOOD AND ADOLESCENCE

OBJECTIVES

After studying this chapter, you should be able to

* Identify nutritional needs of children aged 1 to 10

* Identify nutritional needs of adolescents

* State the effects of inadequate nutrition during the growing years

* Adapt family menus to suit the needs of both children under 10 and adolescents

* Evaluate the nutritive value of the fast-food products available in the U.S. today

CHILDREN AGED ONE TO TEN

Although specific nutritional requirements change as children grow, nutrition always affects physical, mental, and emotional growth and development. Studies indicate that the mental ability and size of an individual are directly influenced by the diet during the early years. Children who have an inadequate supply of nutrients—especially protein—and calories during their early years may be shorter and less intellectually able than children who receive an adequate diet.

Eating habits usually develop during childhood. When people develop poor eating habits then, they are apt to continue them throughout their lives. Poor eating habits can exacerbate emotional and physical problems such as irritability, depression, anxiety, fatigue, and illness.

Because children learn partly by imitation, learning good eating habits is easier if the parents have good habits and are calm and relaxed about the child's. Nutritious foods should be available at snack time as well as at mealtime, and meals should include a wide variety of foods to ensure good nutrient intake.

Parents should be aware that it is not uncommon for children's appetites to vary. The rate of growth is not constant. As the child grows, the rate of her or his growth actually slows. In addition, children's attention is increasingly focused on their environment rather than their stomachs. Consequently, their appetites and interest in food commonly decrease during the early years. The caloric requirement for a child of four drops to approximately 80 kcal per kilo of body weight. Children's likes and dislikes may change. They also like to assert themselves to show their independence. New foods should be introduced gradually, in small amounts, and as attractively as possible. Allowing the child to assist in marketing and in the preparation of a new food are often good ways of arousing interest in the food and a desire to eat it. Children very often prefer foods in small pieces that are simply prepared. They are wary of foods covered by sauce or gravy.

Nutritional Requirements of Young Children

Although children need the same nutrients as adults, the amounts differ. However, just because the child is smaller and lighter than an adult, the child's RDA are not always less than the adult's. Compare the child's RDA with those of the adult's in Table 19-1. Children under four require more iron and vitamin D than adults do. Pediatricians often prescribe supplements of these two nutrients. Parents must be advised against prescribing

them for their children, however, since excess amounts of these nutrients can be toxic. Calcium and phosphorus requirements are the same as for adults. The caloric requirement for children under six is substantially less than the adult's, so the child's food must be chosen very carefully.

The Basic Four food groups should be used as the basis for building menus for people of all ages. Its use reduces the work of the meal planner as it ensures good nutrition for the family.

ADOLESCENCE

Adolescence is typically a period of rapid growth that is accompanied by an enormous appetite. When good eating habits have been established during childhood and there is nutritious food available, the teenager's food habits should present no problem.

Adolescents are imitators, like children, but instead of imitating adults, adolescents prefer to imitate their peers and do what is popular. Unfortunately, the foods that are popular are often hollow calorie foods such as potato chips, sodas, and candy. Hollow calorie foods provide mainly carbohydrates and fats, and very few proteins, vitamins, and minerals, except for salt, which is usually provided in excess.

When the adolescent's food habits need improvement, it is wise for the adult to tactfully inform her or him of nutritional needs and of the inferiority of the hollow calorie foods. The adolescent has a natural desire for independence and may resent being told what to do.

Before attempting to change an adolescent's food habits, her or his food choices should be carefully checked for nutrient con-

Table 19-1 Recommended Daily Dietary Allowances

	Age (years)	Weight		Height		Protein (g)	Fat-Soluble Vitamins		
		(kg)	(lb)	(cm)	(in)		Vitamin A (µg RE)	Vitamin D (µg)	Vitamin E (mg α-TE)
Children	1–3	13	29	90	35	23	400	10	5
	4–6	20	44	112	44	30	500	10	6
	7–10	28	62	132	52	34	700	10	7
Males	11–14	45	99	157	62	45	1000	10	8
	15–18	66	145	176	69	56	1000	10	10
	19–22	70	154	177	70	56	1000	7.5	10
	23–50	70	154	178	70	56	1000	5	10
	51+	70	154	178	70	56	1000	5	10
Females	11–14	46	101	157	62	46	800	10	8
	15–18	55	120	163	64	46	800	10	8
	19–22	55	120	163	64	44	800	7.5	8
	23–50	55	120	163	64	44	800	5	8
	51+	55	120	163	64	44	800	5	8

Source: Food and Nutrition Board, National Academy of Sciences—National Research Council, 1980

tent. It is too easily assumed that because the adolescent chooses the food, the food is automatically a poor choice in regard to nutrient content. This is not always the case. If the adolescent has a problem maintaining a minimum weight, she or he may need some advice regarding diet.

Nutritional Requirements of Adolescents

Because of their rapid growth, adolescents have higher kcal requirements and, in most cases, higher nutrient requirements than adults. See Table 19-1. Frequently, boys' nutritional requirements are greater than that of girls because boys are generally bigger in stature and more active physically. The exception is the nutritional need for iron. Girls' needs are the same as those of boys until the age of 19, when the boys' needs drop to almost

half of their former requirement. Girls' requirement remains high throughout the childbearing years.

PROBLEMS OF WEIGHT CONTROL DURING ADOLESCENCE

Anorexia Nervosa

Generally, adolescent boys in the United States are considered well nourished. This is not always the case with girls, whom, studies show, are sometimes found to have diets deficient in kilocalories, iron, and protein. This may be due to poor eating habits because of concern about weight. A moderate concern about weight is understandable, and possibly even beneficial, so long as it does not cause diets to be deficient in essential nutrients or

Table 19-1 (*Continued*)

		Water-Soluble Vitamins					Minerals					
Vita-min C (mg)	Thia-min (mg)	Ribo-flavin (mg)	Niacin (mg NE)	Vita-min B-6 (mg)	Fola-cin (µg)	Vitamin B-12 (µg)	Cal-cium (mg)	Phos-phorus (mg)	Mag-nesium (mg)	Iron (mg)	Zinc (mg)	Iodine (µg)
45	0.7	0.8	9	0.9	100	2.0	800	800	150	15	10	70
45	0.9	1.0	11	1.3	200	2.5	800	800	200	10	10	90
45	1.2	1.4	16	1.6	300	3.0	800	800	250	10	10	120
50	1.4	1.6	18	1.8	400	3.0	1200	1200	350	18	15	150
60	1.4	1.7	18	2.0	400	3.0	1200	1200	400	18	15	150
60	1.5	1.7	19	2.2	400	3.0	800	800	350	10	15	150
60	1.4	1.6	18	2.2	400	3.0	800	800	350	10	15	150
60	1.2	1.4	16	2.2	400	3.0	800	800	350	10	15	150
50	1.1	1.3	15	1.8	400	3.0	1200	1200	300	18	15	150
60	1.1	1.3	14	2.0	400	3.0	1200	1200	300	18	15	150
60	1.1	1.3	14	2.0	400	3.0	800	800	300	18	15	150
60	1.0	1.2	13	2.0	400	3.0	800	800	300	18	15	150
60	1.0	1.2	13	2.0	400	3.0	800	800	300	10	15	150

Table 19-2 Mean Heights and Weights and Recommended Energy Intake

Category	Age (years)	Weight (kg)	Weight (lb)	Height (cm)	Height (in.)	Energy Needs (with range) (kcal)		Energy Needs (with range) (MJ)
Infants	0.0–0.5	6	13	60	24	kg × 115	(95–145)	kg × 0.48
	0.5–1.0	9	20	71	28	kg × 105	(80–135)	kg × 0.44
Children	1–3	13	29	90	35	1300	(900–1800)	5.5
	4–6	20	44	112	44	1700	(1300–2300)	7.1
	7–10	28	62	132	52	2400	(1650–3300)	10.1
Females	11–14	46	101	157	62	2200	(1500–3000)	9.2
	15–18	55	120	163	64	2100	(1200–3000)	8.8
Males	11–14	45	99	157	62	2700	(2000–3700)	11.3
	15–18	66	145	176	69	2800	(2100–3900)	11.8

Source: Food and Nutrition Board, National Academy of Sciences—National Research Council, 1980

lead to a potentially fatal condition called *anorexia nervosa.*

Anorexia nervosa, commonly called anorexia, is a psychological disorder that is more common among girls than boys. It causes the patient to so drastically reduce her kilocalorie intake that it can upset metabolism, cause weakness, amenorrhea, and sometimes lead to death. Its causes are not clear. It appears that some anorexia patients have been overweight and have irrational fears of regaining lost weight. Others seem to have an excessive need to control their families. Some may simply want to resemble the photos of the

Table 19-3 A Family Menu with a Kcal Value That Can Range from 1300 to 2800, Depending on the Sizes of the Servings. (This would be suitable for children of 1 year, adolescents, and their parents.)

Breakfast	Lunch	Dinner
Orange Juice	Macaroni & Cheese	Meat Loaf
Cereal and Milk	Green Beans	Baked Potato
Toast	Bread	Shredded Lettuce with Tomatoes
Butter or Margarine	Butter or Margarine	and
Milk	Pineapple Chunks	Dressing
Coffee	Milk	Roll
		Butter or Margarine
		Custard
		Milk

Morning Snack	Afternoon Snack
Crackers and Cheese	Banana
Apple Juice	

very slim fashion models not realizing that fashion photography can be deceptive. Some have poor mother-daughter relationships. In any event, a great deal of psychotherapy and time, usually involving the entire family, are typically required for the patient to overcome the disorder.

Bulimia

Bulimia is a syndrome where the patient alternately *binges* (eats excessively) and fasts. *Bulimarexia* is a condition where the patient binges and then induces vomiting and sometimes uses laxatives and diuretics to get rid of

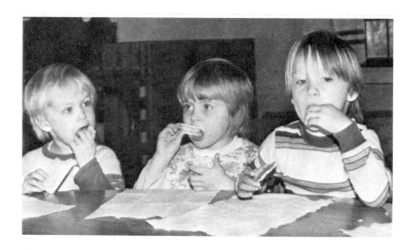

Figure 19-1 Snacks are enjoyed with friends in the playroom. *(Reprinted from Lesner,* Pediatric Nursing, *Figure 5-8)*

the food ingested during the binge. Both of these problems are due to an inordinate and frequently unexplained fear of gaining weight. In either case, it is probable that the patient will require help from a psychological counselor in order to end the syndrome.

Obesity in Adolescence

Obesity during adolescence is especially sad because it tends to diminish the individual's self-esteem and consequently excludes her or him from the normal social life of the teen years, which further diminishes self-esteem. Also, it tends to make the individual prone to obesity as an adult. Its cause is difficult to determine, but overfeeding during childhood may be a contributing factor. It is a particularly difficult problem to solve until the individual really decides to reduce. After such a decision. the individual should see a medical doctor to make certain that her or his health is good and to learn the amount of weight that should be lost, the time that this will require, and the daily kcal allotment. Meals must be carefully planned around the Basic Four so that all nutrient requirements are met, and the kcal allotment is not exceeded. Daily menus should include some snacks.

Fast Foods

Many Americans have become extremely fond of the "fast foods" that are so readily available. Many others are highly critical of their nutrient content. Examples of these foods—most of which are favorites of teenagers—include hamburgers, cheeseburgers, milkshakes, franks, pizza, sodas, hot chocolate, tacos, chili, fried chicken, and onion rings. Because of the criticism they have received, some of these fast food companies have run tests to determine the nutritional content of their products and have made their results public.

A comparative study of products from three chains showed that their hamburgers contained an average of 250 kcal, 12g protein, 30 gm carbohydrates, 10g fat, and 540 mg of sodium. In addition, these hamburgers were shown to contribute small amounts of vitamin A, vitamin C, thiamin, riboflavin, niacin, calcium, and iron.

Milkshakes contained approximately 375 kcal, 10g protein, 60 gm carbohydrates, 9 gm fat, and 300 mg of sodium, plus small amounts of vitamin A, vitamin C, thiamin, niacin, iron, and substantial amounts of riboflavin and calcium.

French fries were shown to contribute essentially carbohydrates and fat totalling 250 kcal per 2 1/2 ounce serving.

Pizza was also evaluated and one average slice was found to contain approximately 370 kcal. It contributes carbohydrates, fat, protein, substantial amounts of calcium and iron, plus fair amounts of thiamin, riboflavin, and niacin.

To sum up, the calorie count is high, as is the fat and sodium content, while the vitamin, mineral, and fiber content of fast food meals are low. These foods are, nevertheless, a great deal more nutritious than sodas, cakes, and candy. When used with discretion in a balanced diet, they cannot be considered harmful.

Alcohol and the Adolescent

The use of alcohol by adolescents is increasing. This is particularly regrettable because the health of teenagers and their unborn children may be seriously harmed by excessive use of alcohol. Heavy drinkers may not eat properly and consequently may not get the necessary nutrients at a time when they are still growing. They are also creating the potential for liver damage. Rehabilitation programs should include nutrition counseling.

Nutrition for the Athlete

Good nutrition during the period of life when one is involved in athletics can prevent unnecessary wear and tear on the body as well as maintain the athlete in top physical form. The specific nutritional needs of the athlete are not numerous, but they are important. The athlete needs additional water, kilocalories, thiamin, riboflavin, niacin, sodium, potassium, iron, and protein.

The body uses water to rid itself of excess heat through perspiration. This lost water must be regularly replaced during the activity to prevent dehydration. Plain water is the recommended liquid because the commercial "athletes'" or "electrolyte" drinks contain more sugar, salt, and potassium than is advisable. If these commercial beverages are used, they must be diluted with equal parts of plain water. Salt tablets are not recommended because despite the loss of salt and potassium through perspiration, the loss is not equal to the amount contained in the tablets. If there is an insufficient water intake, these very salt tablets can increase the risk of dehydration.

The increase in kcal will depend on the activity and the length of time it is performed. The requirement could be double the normal, up to 6,000 kcal per day. Because glucose and fatty acids are used for energy, and rot protein, the normal diet proportions of 45—55 percent carbohydrate, 35—40 percent fat, and 10—15 percent protein are advised.

There is an increased need for B vitamins because they are necessary for energy metabolism. Some extra protein is necessary, but only during training when muscle mass and blood volume are increasing. Protein needs are not increased by physical activity. In fact, excess protein can cause increased urine production, which can lead to dehydration.

The minerals sodium and potassium are needed in larger amounts because of loss through perspiration. This amount of sodium can usually be replaced just by salting food to taste. And orange juice can provide the extra potassium.

A sufficient supply of iron is important to the athlete, particulary to the female athlete. Iron-rich foods eaten with vitamin C-rich foods should provide sufficient iron. The onset of menstruation can be delayed by the heavy physical activity of the female athlete and amenorrhea may occur.

When weight is a concern of the athlete, such as with wrestlers, care should be taken that the individual does not become dehydrated by refusing liquids in an effort to "make weight" for the class.

In general, the athlete should select foods using the Basic Four food plan. The pregame meal should be eaten 3 hours before the event, and should consist primarily of carbohydrates, and small amounts of protein and fat. Concentrated sugar foods are not advisable because they may cause extra water to collect in the intestines, creating gas and possibly diarrhea.

Glycogen loading (carboloading) is sometimes used for long activities. This means that muscle stores of glycogen are increased. To accomplish this, the athlete begins six days before the event. For 3 days the athlete eats a diet consisting of only 10 percent carbohydrate and mostly protein and fat as she or he performs heavy exercise. This depletes the current store of glycogen. The last three days, the diet is 70 percent carbohydrate and the exercise is very light so that the muscles become loaded with glycogen. However, the longterm effects of glycogen loading are not known, and it should be noted that the heart is a muscle.

After the event, the athlete may prefer to drink fruit juices until relaxed, and then fulfill the appetite with sandwiches or a full meal.

There are no magic potions or diet supplements that will increase an athlete's prowess as may be touted by health food faddists. Good diet, good health habits, and practice combined with innate talent remain the essentials for athletic success.

SUMMARY

Children's nutritional needs vary as they grow and develop. Although a young child's kcal requirement is substantially less than an adult's, her or his nutrient requirements are not. Adolescents have higher nutrient and kcal requirements than adults. Anorexia nervosa and obesity are two problems of weight control that can occur during adolescence. Fast foods are acceptable when used with discretion in a balanced diet. The nutritional needs of athletes are similar to those of non-athletes except for increased needs for kcal, B vitamins, sodium, potassium, iron, and protein.

Discussion Topics

1. Discuss how parents' anxieties about children's food habits may affect those habits.
2. Discuss the manner in which depression may affect food habits.
3. In what ways does obesity affect an adolescent's self-esteem?
4. Discuss ways of arousing a six-year old's interest in new foods.
5. Why do young children require more iron and more vitamin D than adults?
6. Why can it be especially difficult for a parent to influence her or his adolescent's attitudes about food?
7. Discuss the nutrient content of some fast foods. Explain why they can be useful additions to the diet, and also why they should not be used exclusively.
8. What could be assumed to be a logical result if a 30-year old lawyer continued to eat as he did at 16? Why?
9. Describe anorexia nervosa. Ask if anyone in the class has suffered from it or knows anyone who has. Ask that individual for descriptions of the patient's attitude, physical condition, possible causes, and case results (if any).
10. Discuss how snack foods can affect one's overall nutrition.
11. Discuss the pros and cons of glycogen loading.

Suggested Activities

1. List your favorite snack foods. List nutritious snack foods. Check kcal values of these foods (see Table A-7 in the Appendix) and compare lists for nutrition and taste. Discuss possible improvements in your list of favorite snacks.

2. Role-play a situation where an over-weight, middle-aged patient has been told by her physician that she must lose 25 pounds. Try to convince her to change her food habits. (Remember to consider types of foods as well as amounts, meal hours, and reasons she is overeating.)

3. Plan a talk for fourth grade students on the importance of good food habits. Begin with an outline and develop it into a narrative that nine-year old children will understand. If possible, ask permission of a fourth-grade teacher to deliver this talk to the class.

4. Role-play a situation where your younger sister, who is considerably overweight, has just asked you how she can lose weight. Ask her why she wants to lose weight; how much weight she wants to lose; how long she is willing to be on a reducing diet; what her favorite foods are; when she eats; the amounts she eats; where she eats; and with whom she eats.

5. Plan a talk for the athletic department of the high school on "The Diet of the Athlete."

Review

A. Multiple Choice

_____ 1. Nutrition affects one's
   a. size
   b. mental ability
   c. emotional growth and development
   d. all of the above

_____ 2. Poor eating habits can exacerbate
   a. anxiety and depression
   b. fatigue
   c. illness
   d. all of the above

_____ 3. Children's appetites
   a. vary
   b. are static
   c. are irrelevant to their nutritional status
   d. are entirely dependent on the size of the child

_____ 4. Of the following foods, children are most apt to prefer
   a. carrot-zucchini casserole   c. raw carrot sticks
   b. creamed carrots with peas   d. carrot and pineapple gelatin
                                     salad
_____ 5. Young children's and adults' nutritional requirements are the
   same for
   a. protein   c. calcium
   b. vitamin D   d. kcal
_____ 6. Children's iron requirement is high because it is needed for
   a. healthy bones and teeth   c. prevention of nightblindness
   b. fighting infections   d. blood building
_____ 7. As a child grows, his or her kcal requirement per pound of body
   weight
   a. remains unchanged   c. becomes less
   b. increases   d. doubles each year
_____ 8. Meatloaf is a good source of
   a. protein   c. iron
   b. B vitamins   d. all of the above and more
_____ 9. Hollow calorie foods provide
   a. carbohydrate and fat   c. no calories
   b. proteins, minerals, and d. fiber
      vitamins
_____ 10. Although boys usually need more kcal than girls, girls usually
   need more
   a. protein   c. iron
   b. vitamin C   d. vitamin D

B. Completion
   1. A psychological disorder that causes people to drastically
      reduce their kcal intake is called _____ .
   2. An overweight adolescent who has decided to reduce should
      plan meals based on _____ .
   3. A real criticism of fast foods is their high _____ , _____ , and
      _____ content, and low _____ , _____ , and
      _____ content.
   4. Because of young children's high need for these two nutrients,
      pediatricians sometimes prescribe nutritional supplements of
      _____ and _____ for children under four years of age.
   5. Eating habits usually develop during _____ .
   6. As the child grows, its rate of growth _____ .
   7. Excessive amounts of vitamins and minerals can be _____ .

8. Although a child's need for most nutrients increases as the child grows into adulthood, the exceptions are _____ , _____ , _____ , and _____ .

9. The cessation of menstruation is called _____ and can be caused by _____ .

10. The first step in a substantial weight-loss program should be to see one's _____ .

C. Answer the following questions as they relate to this menu.

Breakfast	*Lunch*	*Dinner*
Orange Juice	Macaroni & Cheese	Meat Loaf
Cereal & Milk	Green Beans	Baked Potato
Toast	Bread	Shredded Lettuce
Butter or Margarine	Butter or Margarine	with Tomatoes
Milk	Pineapple Chunks	and Dressing
Coffee	Milk	Roll
		Butter or Margarine
		Custard
		Milk

Morning Snack	*Afternoon Snack*
Crackers & Cheese	Banana
Apple Juice	

1. Vitamin C is considered an iron enhancer and should be eaten at each meal. Where is the vitamin C in this menu?

2. Protein should be included in every meal. Where is the protein in this menu?

3. List 8 sources of iron in this menu.

4. A teenager should have 4 cups of milk each day. List the sources of milk in this menu and estimate the approximate amounts included.

5. List each of the following groups separately, as found in this menu:

   breads and cereals

   fruits and vegetables

   meats and meat substitutes

6. Does this menu fulfill the requirements of the Basic Four food groups for an adult; for an adolescent; for a child under ten; for the athlete?

References

Green, Marilyn L., and Joann Harry. 1981. *Nutrition in Contemporary Nursing Practice.* New York: John Wiley & Sons.

Howard, Roseanne B., and Nancie H. Herbold. 1982. *Nutrition in Clinical Care*, 2nd ed. New York: McGraw Hill Book Company.

Hui, Y. H. 1983. *Human Nutrition and Diet Therapy.* Monterey Calif: Wadsworth Health Sciences Division of Wadsworth Inc.

Mahan, L. K., and J. M. Rees. 1984. *Nutrition in Adolescence.* St. Louis: Times Mirror/ Mosby College Publishing.

White, Marlene Boskind, and William C. White, Jr. 1983. *Bulimarexia.* New York: W. W. Norton & Co.

Whitney, Eleanor Noss, and Eva May Nunnelley Hamilton. 1984. *Understanding Nutrition*, 3rd ed. St. Paul: West Publishing Co.

Winick, Myron. 1980. *Nutrition in Health and Disease.* New York: John Wiley & Sons.

Chapter 20
DIET DURING YOUNG ADULTHOOD AND MIDDLE-AGE

VOCABULARY

adipose tissue
caloric
  requirement
diabetes mellitus
energy imbalance

hypertension
kcal intake
nutrient
  requirement

nutritional
  requirement
obesity

OBJECTIVES

After studying this chapter, you should be able to

- Identify the nutritional needs of young adults and the middle-aged
- Explain sensible, long-range weight control for these people
- Adapt menus to meet their nutritional requirements

Adulthood can be broadly divided into three periods: young adulthood, middle age, and old age. The first two periods will be discussed in this chapter.

Young adulthood is a time of excitement and exploration. Individuals are alive with plans, desires, and energy as they begin searching for and finding their places in the mainstream of adult life. They appear to have boundless energy for both social and professional activities. They are usually interested in exercise for its own sake, and often participate in athletic events as well.

Middle age is a period when the physical activities of young adulthood typically begin to decrease, resulting in a lowered caloric requirement for most individuals. At this age

people seldom have young children to supervise, and the strenuous physical labor of some occupations may be delegated to younger people. Middle-aged people may tire more easily than they did when they were younger. Therefore, they may not get as much exercise during their leisure hours as they did in earlier years. Because appetite and food intake may not decrease, there is a common tendency toward overweight during this period.

NUTRIENT REQUIREMENTS

Except during pregnancy and lactation, nutrient requirements remain unchanged between the ages of 23 and 50. And they drop very slightly for only four of the listed nutrients between the age groupings of 19—22 and 23—50. See Table 20-1. Nutrient needs do not diminish during adult life because the body continues replacing worn out cells and producing heat and energy until death.

The kcal requirement, however, does diminish with age. Adults usually reach their peak kcal requirement between the ages of 19 and 22. From 23 years on, kcal requirements diminish. See Table 20-2. The average kcal requirement for males between the ages of 19 and 22 is 2900 while the average kcal requirement for males between the ages of 23 and 50 is 2700. This does not seem to be a large number, but it must be remembered that it takes only 3500 kcal to add one pound of weight to the body. An individual who over-eats by only 200 kcal a day can gain 20 pounds in one year. Obviously, when nutrient requirements remain static, but kcal requirements decrease, people must choose their foods carefully to fulfill their nutrient requirements without adding unwanted kcal.

Despite men's generally larger size, less than half the nutrient requirements for men are larger than for women. Women's iron requirement remains higher throughout the child-bearing years, after which it is the same as that for men.

During pregnancy and lactation, women's requirements outpace men's except for kcal. See Table 20-1. A woman who settles for a piece of pie at lunchtime while her husband eats a hamburger and salad is being very foolish. If she continues this on a regular basis, she is jeopardizing her health. A hamburger may run 250 to 400 kcal. The salad will contain less than 50 kcal without dressing, and the dressing could be limited to one table-spoon, or approximately 100 kcal, for a total kcal intake of approximately 400 to 550 kcal. Pies average 100 kcal per one-inch slice.

Most slices are about 3 1/2 inches. A scoop of ice cream on the pie would bring the kcal total up at least another 100 kcal. Although the kcal intakes of the husband and wife will be comparable, the nutrient intakes will not. The wife's will be inadequate. And if the woman is of childbearing age and plans to have children, her future children, as well as she, may suffer from such habits.

WEIGHT CONTROL

Weight control is probably one of the top ten concerns of U.S. adults. Whether for reasons of vanity, health, or both, most people are interested in controlling their weight. It is advisable because overweight may introduce health problems. Cases of diabetes mellitus and hypertension are more numerous among the overweight than among those of normal weight. Overweight individuals are poor risks for surgery, and their lives are generally shorter. They are prone to social and emotional problems because obesity reduces self-esteem.

The causes of overweight are not always known, but the most common cause appears to be energy imbalance. In other words, if one is overweight, chances are that more kcal have been taken in than were needed for energy. Congenital problems and metabolic disturbances may also contribute to overweight.

For those individuals who are overweight simply because of energy imbalance, the problem may be solved by eating less, by increasing the amount of exercise (work) performed, or by eating less combined with increased exercise. Exercise will increase the number of kcal burned. However, unless the exercise is sufficient to burn more kcal than are ingested, exercise alone will not solve the problem. See Table 2-2 for the amounts of

Table 20-1 Nutrient Requirements

	Age (years)	Weight		Height		Protein (g)	Fat-Soluble Vitamins		
		(kg)	(lb)	(cm)	(in)		Vitamin A (µg RE)	Vitamin D (µg)	Vitamin E (mg α-TE)
Males	11–14	45	99	157	62	45	1000	10	8
	15–18	66	145	176	69	56	1000	10	10
	19–22	70	154	177	70	56	1000	7.5	10
	23–50	70	154	178	70	56	1000	5	10
	51+	70	154	178	70	56	1000	5	10
Females	11–14	46	101	157	62	46	800	10	8
	15–18	55	120	163	64	46	800	10	8
	19–22	55	120	163	64	44	800	7.5	8
	23–50	55	120	163	64	44	800	5	8
	51+	55	120	163	64	44	800	5	8
Pregnant						+30	+200	+5	+2
Lactating						+20	+400	+5	+3

Source: Food and Nutrition Board, National Academy of Sciences—National Research Council, 1980

Table 20-2 Mean Heights and Weights and Recommended Energy Intake for Adults

Category	Age (years)	Weight		Height		Energy Needs (with range)		
		(kg)	(lb)	(cm)	(in.)	(kcal)		(MJ)
Males	11–14	45	99	157	62	2700	(2000–3700)	11.3
	15–18	66	145	176	69	2800	(2100–3900)	11.8
	19–22	70	154	177	70	2900	(2500–3300)	12.2
	23–50	70	154	178	70	2700	(2300–3100)	11.3
	51–75	70	154	178	70	2400	(2000–2800)	10.1
	76+	70	154	178	70	2050	(1650–2450)	8.6
Females	11–14	46	101	157	62	2200	(1500–3000)	9.2
	15–18	55	120	163	64	2100	(1200–3000)	8.8
	19–22	55	120	163	64	2100	(1700–2500)	8.8
	23–50	55	120	163	64	2000	(1600–2400)	8.4
	51–75	55	120	163	64	1800	(1400–2200)	7.6
	76+	55	120	163	64	1600	(1200–2000)	6.7
Pregnancy						+300		
Lactation						+500		

Source: Food and Nutrition Board, National Academy of Sciences—National Research Council, 1980

Table 20-1 (*Continued*)

	Water-Soluble Vitamins						Minerals					
Vitamin C (mg)	Thiamin (mg)	Riboflavin (mg)	Niacin (mg NE)	Vitamin B-6 (mg)	Folacin (μg)	Vitamin B-12 (μg)	Calcium (mg)	Phosphorus (mg)	Magnesium (mg)	Iron (mg)	Zinc (mg)	Iodine (μg)
50	1.4	1.6	18	1.8	400	3.0	1200	1200	350	18	15	150
60	1.4	1.7	18	2.0	400	3.0	1200	1200	400	18	15	150
60	1.5	1.7	19	2.2	400	3.0	800	800	350	10	15	150
60	1.4	1.6	18	2.2	400	3.0	800	800	350	10	15	150
60	1.2	1.4	16	2.2	400	3.0	800	800	350	10	15	150
50	1.1	1.3	15	1.8	400	3.0	1200	1200	300	18	15	150
60	1.1	1.3	14	2.0	400	3.0	1200	1200	300	18	15	150
60	1.1	1.3	14	2.0	400	3.0	800	800	300	18	15	150
60	1.0	1.2	13	2.0	400	3.0	800	800	300	18	15	150
60	1.0	1.2	13	2.0	400	3.0	800	800	300	10	15	150
+20	+0.4	+0.3	+2	+0.6	+400	+1.0	+400	+400	+150	+30–60	+5	+25
+40	+0.5	+0.5	+5	+0.5	+100	+1.0	+400	+400	+150	+30–60	+10	+50

energy burned by specific types of work. By far the most effective method of weight loss is increased exercise combined with reduced kcal intake. This will help tone the muscles as the excess adipose tissue is lost. For additional information regarding weight loss diets, see chapter 25.

SUMMARY

Although kcal requirements diminish between the ages of 23 and 50, nutrient requirements do not. Consequently, food must be selected with increasing care as one ages to ensure that nutrient requirements are met without exceeding the kcal requirement.

Overweight can cause health problems. If it is caused by energy imbalance, a program of weight loss should be undertaken. A sensible weight loss program includes exercise. The diet should be based on the Basic Four food groups and eating habits should be improved during the diet so that the lost weight will not be regained later.

Table 20-3 2,000 Kcal Diet

Breakfast		
1/2 cup orange juice	50 kcal	
1 cup dry cereal	100	
1/2 cup skim milk	50	
2 teaspoons sugar	35	
1 slice toast	70	
1/2 tablespoon butter	50	
1 cup black coffee	0	355 kcal
Lunch		
Roast Beef Sandwich:		
3 oz. roast beef	200	
2 slices bread	150	
2 tablespoons mayonnaise	200	
lettuce	10	
1 cup skim milk	100	
1 orange	75	735
Dinner		
3 oz. broiled fish	150	
1 baked potato	100	
1 1/2 tablespoons butter	150	
1/2 cup green peas	50	
tossed salad with		
1 Tbsp. dressing	150	
1 cup skim milk	100	
3/4 cup ice cream	200	950
		2,040 kilocalories

Discussion Topics

1. Why do kcal requirements diminish between the ages of 23 and 50? Why do nutrient requirements not diminish at the same time?
2. How can only an extra 200 kcal a day result in obesity?
3. What would you advise someone who was about to begin an 800-kcal diet?
4. How would you advise your 30-year old sister who boasts about eating only an English muffin and coffee at lunch?
5. Why is overweight inadvisable?
6. Why are middle-aged adults more inclined to overweight than young adults?

Suggested Activities

1. Plan a panel discussion entitled, "How to lose weight during middle age".
2. Write definitions of the terms listed at the beginning of this chapter. Explain their meanings to a 12-year old.
3. Role play a situation where a 50-year old woman has just been advised by her physician to lose 25 pounds. She does not want to and cannot understand why she should. She insists her eating habits have not changed in 25 years. Consider kcal requirement, nutrient requirements, activity, age, and psychology.
4. Using Table A-7 in the appendix, adapt the menus in Table 20-3 to meet the needs of the following people:
   a. a pregnant 18-year old
   b. a 30-year old nursing mother
   c. a man of 40 years
   d. a 45-year old woman who must follow a 1,000 kcal diet.

Review

A. Multiple Choice

1. The number of kcal one needs each day is called one's
   a. nutrient requirement
   b. kcal intake
   c. kcal requirement
   d. nutritional requirement
2. Overweight during middle age is often due to
   a. obesity
   b. hypertension
   c. adipose tissue
   d. energy imbalance

3. The measure of energy in foods eaten is one's
   - a. kcal requirement
   - b. kcal intake
   - c. nutrient requirement
   - d. energy imbalance

4. Overweight can affect one's
   - a. self-esteem
   - b. state of health
   - c. life span
   - d. all of the above

5. Kcal requirements
   - a. increase with age
   - b. decrease with age
   - c. remain unchanged through-out adult life
   - d. none of the above

6. To lose one pound of weight, kcal intake must be reduced by
   - a. 1000 kcal
   - b. 800 kcal
   - c. 3500 kcal
   - d. none of the above

7. During the childbearing years, women's iron requirement is
   - a. higher than men's
   - b. the same as men's
   - c. lower than men's
   - d. none of the above

8. Exercise can
   - a. contribute to weight loss
   - b. tone the muscles
   - c. increase the number of kcal burned
   - d. all of the above

9. Nutrient requirements during adult life generally
   - a. increase with age
   - b. decrease with age
   - c. remain unchanged through-out adult life
   - d. none of the above

10. Women's kcal requirements as compared with men's are generally
    - a. higher
    - b. lower
    - c. the same as
    - d. none of the above

B. Matching

_____	1. adipose tissue	a. extreme overweight
_____	2. hypertension	b. opinion of one's self
_____	3. obesity	c. more or less kcal ingested than needed
_____	4. self-esteem	
_____	5. nutrient requirement	d. nutrients needed by the body
_____	6. nutritional requirements	e. become less
		f. high blood pressure
_____	7. kcal intake	g. energy and nutrient requirement
_____	8. energy imbalance	h. fat
_____	9. kcal requirement	i. amount of energy needed
_____	10. diminish	j. measure of energy in foods eaten
		k. increase

References

Bodinski, Lois H. 1982. *The Nurse's Guide to Diet Therapy*. New York: John Wiley & Sons.

Green, Marilyn L., and Joann Harry. 1981. *Nutrition in Contemporary Nursing Practice*. New York: John Wiley & Sons.

Luke, Barbara. 1984. *Principles of Nutrition and Diet Therapy*. Boston: Little Brown & Co.

Whitney, Eleanor Noss. 1982. *Nutrition Concepts and Controversies*, 2nd ed. West Publishing Co.

Williams, Sue Rodwell. 1984. *Mowry's Basic Nutrition and Diet Therapy*, 7th ed. St. Louis: C. V. Mosby Co.

Chapter 21

DIET DURING THE SENIOR YEARS

VOCABULARY

anorexia	food faddists	nutritional status
arthritis	geriatrics	osteoporosis
cataracts	gerontology	periodontal disease
diabetes mellitus	hypertension	physical stress
emotional stress	menses	skeletal system

OBJECTIVES

After studying this chapter, you should be able to

* Explain the nutritional needs of people 65 and over

* Evaluate the quality of a senior citizen's diet

* Adapt menus to meet the nutritional needs of these people

It is anticipated that by the year 2000, nearly 20 percent of the U.S. population will be 65 or over. Consequently, *gerontology*, the study of aging, is of increasing importance. There is a great deal of experimentation going on that is hoped will explain the causes of aging. It is known that the body's functions slow and that its ability to replace worn cells is reduced during aging. The metabolism rate slows; bones become less dense; eyes do not focus on nearby objects as they once did; the heart and kidneys become less efficient; hearing, taste, and smell become less acute; and the speed of nerve signals is reduced as one ages. Digestion is affected because the secretion of hydrochloric acid in the stomach and bile in the liver are diminished, and the tone of the intestines is reduced, frequently resulting in constipation. The rate of aging varies. Each person is affected by heredity, emotional and physical stress endured, and nutrition. Experiments are underway to learn more precisely the role of nutrition in the aging process.

NUTRITIONAL REQUIREMENTS OF SENIOR CITIZENS

Although the nutritional needs of growth disappear with age, the normal nutritional needs for maintaining a constant state of good health remain throughout life. With one exception, requirements for specific nutrients do not decrease after the age of 50. This one exception is the iron requirement of women

Table 21-1 Recommended Daily Dietary Allowances

	Age (years)	Weight		Height		Protein (g)	Fat-Soluble Vitamins		
		(kg)	(lb)	(cm)	(in)		Vitamin A (μg RE)	Vitamin D (μg)	Vitamin E (mg α-TE)
Males	23–50	70	154	178	70	56	1000	5	10
	51+	70	154	178	70	56	1000	5	10
Females	23–50	55	120	163	64	44	800	5	8
	51+	55	120	163	64	44	800	5	8

Source: Food and Nutrition Board, National Academy of Sciences—National Research Council, 1980

over 50, which decreases by 8 mg with the cessation of menses. See Table 21-1.

The kcal requirement, however, does decrease with age because metabolism slows and activity is reduced. See Table 21-2. If the kcal intake is not reduced, weight will be increased. This additional weight would increase the work of the heart and put increased stress on the skeletal system. It is very important that the kcal requirement not be exceeded, and just as important that the nutrient requirements be fulfilled to maintain a good nutritional status (condition).

FOOD HABITS OF SENIOR CITIZENS

If the established food habits of the older person are poor, such habits will undoubtedly have been a long time in the making. These habits will not be easy to change. Poor food habits that begin during old age can also present problems. Decreased income during retirement, physical disability, and inadequate cooking facilities may cause difficulties in food selection and preparation. Anorexia caused by grief, loneliness, boredom, or difficulty in chewing may decrease food consumption.

Studies indicate that many senior citizens consume diets that are deficient in vitamins A and C, riboflavin, calcium, and sometimes, kcal.

A person's typical daily food intake should be compared with the Recommended Daily Dietary Requirements. Older persons' needs vary considerably, however, so each should be examined by a physician to determine specific requirements.

Any adjustment in food habits requires great tact, and plans for changes must be based on the individual's total situation.

FOOD FADS AND THE ELDERLY

Some older people are consciously or unconsciously searching for eternal life, if not youth. Consequently, they are frequently susceptible to the claims of food faddists who seek to profit from their ignorance. Senior citizens spend money on unnecessary vitamins, minerals, and special honey, molasses, bread, milk, and other foods that may be guaranteed by the salesperson to prevent or cure various diseases. This money could be much more effectively used on ordinary foods that would cost considerably less.

Table 21-1 (*Continued*)

Water-Soluble Vitamins							Minerals					
Vita-min C (mg)	Thia-min (mg)	Ribo-flavin (mg)	Niacin (mg NE)	Vita-min B-6 (mg)	Fola-cin (µg)	Vitamin B-12 (µg)	Cal-cium (mg)	Phos-phorus (mg)	Mag-nesium (mg)	Iron (mg)	Zinc (mg)	Iodine (µg)
60	1.4	1.6	18	2.2	400	3.0	800	800	350	10	15	150
60	1.2	1.4	16	2.2	400	3.0	800	800	350	10	15	150
60	1.0	1.2	13	2.0	400	3.0	800	800	300	18	15	150
60	1.0	1.2	13	2.0	400	3.0	800	800	300	10	15	150

Table 21-2 Mean Heights and Weights and Recommended Daily Energy Intake

Category	Age (years)	Weight		Height		Energy Needs (with range)		
		(kg)	(lb)	(cm)	(in.)	(kcal)		(MJ)
Females	23–50	55	120	163	64	2000	(1600–2400)	8.4
	51–75	55	120	163	64	1800	(1400–2200)	7.6
	76+	55	120	163	64	1600	(1200–2000)	6.7
Males	23–50	70	154	178	70	2700	(2300–3100)	11.3
	51–75	70	154	178	70	2400	(2000–2800)	10.1
	76+	70	154	178	70	2050	(1650–2450)	8.6

Source: Food and Nutrition Board, National Academy of Sciences—National Research Council, 1980

NUTRITION AND CHRONIC DISEASES COMMON TO SENIOR CITIZENS

It is estimated that 80 percent of people over 65 have one or more chronic disease. Examples include osteoporosis, arthritis, cataracts, cancer, diabetes mellitus, hypertension, heart disease, and periodontal disease. The branch of medicine that is involved with diseases of older people is called *geriatrics*.

Osteoporosis

Osteoporosis is a condition in which the amount of calcium in bones is reduced making them porous. It is estimated that up to 50 percent of elderly people have osteoporosis, and the majority of these are women. It is typically unnoticed at its onset, which is usually after menopause, and may not be noticed at all until a fracture occurs. One of its symptoms is a gradual reduction in height. Doctors are not certain of its cause, but it is thought that years of a sedentary life coupled with a diet deficient in calcium, vitamins D, C, and A, fluoride, and protein contribute to it. Some doctors are advising patients to consume 1500 mg of calcium, which would require the daily consumption of over one quart of milk or its equivalent. Calcium tablets could be used instead, but the patient would also require supplementary vitamins A, D, and C, fluoride, and protein. Another possible cause of osteoporosis may be a diet containing excessive amounts of phosphorus, which can speed bone loss. It is known that Americans are ingesting increasing amounts of phosphorus. Sodas and processed foods contain phosphorus and their consumption is increasing as milk consumption is decreasing in the U.S. Some believe that *periodontal disease* may be a harbinger of osteoporosis. Periodontal disease is characterized by bone loss in the jaw, which can lead to loosened teeth and infection in the gums.

Arthritis

Arthritis is a disease that causes the joints to become painful and stiff. It results in structural changes in the cartilage of the joints. A patient with arthritis should be especially careful to avoid overweight because the extra weight adds stress to joints that are already painful. If the patient is overweight, a weight reduction program should be instituted. The regular use of aspirin by these patients may cause slight bleeding in the stomach lining and subsequent anemia, so their diets may require additional iron. Arthritis can greatly complicate a patient's life because it may partially or completely immobilize the patient to the point that shopping, moving around, and cooking become very difficult.

There is no cure to date. Patients should be well informed of this to prevent wasting their money on so-called "cures" of tricksters.

Cataracts

A cataract is a clouding of the lens of the eye, so that light is obstructed and vision is impaired. Cataracts are somewhat common among older people and can be surgically removed. Various research projects continue in an effort to discover possible roles of nutrition in their development, but as yet, there are no definitive results.

Cancer

Research in the role of nutrition in cancer development continues. The American Cancer Society has indicated that diets consistently high in fat may contribute to cancer.

Diabetes Mellitus

Diabetes mellitus is a chronic disease where the body does not produce sufficient amounts of insulin or does not use it effectively for normal carbohydrate metabolism. Diet is very important in the treatment of diabetes and Chapter 24 discusses this treatment in detail.

Hypertension

Hypertension, or high blood pressure, can lead to strokes. It may be associated with diets high in salt. Most Americans ingest from two to six times the amount of salt needed each day. It is thought that the earlier one reduces salt intake, the better her or his chances of avoiding hypertension, particularly if there is a family history of it. Hypertension is discussed in detail in Chapter 26.

Heart Disease

Heart attack and stroke are the major causes of death in the United States. They occur when arteries become blocked (occluded), preventing the normal passage of

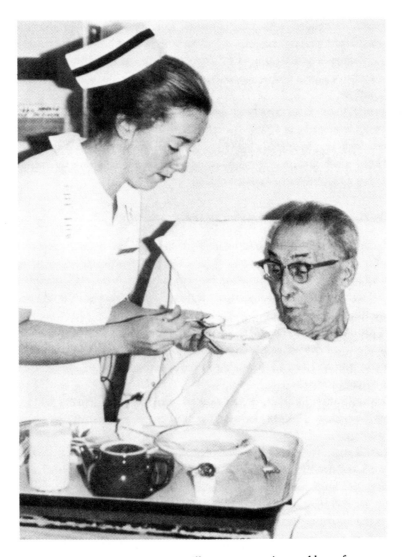

Figure 21-1 Chronic, long-term illnesses are major problems for many senior citizens. *(Reprinted from Grippando, Nursing Perspectives and Issues, 2nd ed., figure 13–5)*

blood. These occlusions are caused by blood clots that form and are unable to pass through an unnaturally narrowed artery. Arteries are narrowed by plaque, a fatty substance containing cholesterol that accumulates in the walls of the artery. This condition is called *atherosclerosis*. It is believed that excessive cholesterol in the diet over many years is a causative factor. The therapeutic diet appropriate for athersclerosis is discussed in Chapter 26.

Current research regarding the role of nutrition in preventing or relieving these dis-

Table 21-3 Suggested Day's Menu Totalling 1640 kcal

Breakfast		Lunch		Dinner	
1/2 cup orange juice	50 kcal	3/4 cup macaroni		1/2 cup pineapple	
poached egg	80	& cheese	300 kcal	juice	75 kcal
2 slices toast	150	sliced tomato	25	3 oz broiled	
1/2 tbsp marg or butter	50	1/2 cup green beans	25	hamburger	200
coffee		1 cup skim milk	100	1/2 cup rice	100
	—	2/3 cup custard	200	shredded lettuce	10
	330 kcal		650 kcal	1 tbsp dressing	75
				1 cup skim milk	100
				sliced banana	100
					660 kcal

eases continues. The effects of nutrition are cumulative over many years. The effects of a lifetime of poor eating habits cannot be cured overnight. When diets have been poor for a long time, prevention of these diseases may not be possible. It may be possible to use nutrition to help stabilize the condition of a patient with one of these diseases, however. The prevention of many of the diseases of the elderly should begin in one's youth.

APPROPRIATE DIETS FOR SENIOR CITIZENS

The diets of senior citizens should be planned around the Basic Four food groups. When special health problems exist, the normal diet should be adapted to meet individual needs. (See Section 5 on Therapeutic diets.)

The federal government provides the states with funds to serve senior citizens hot meals at noon in senior centers across the country. These senior centers become social clubs and are immensely beneficial to the elderly. They provide companionship in addition to nutritious food. Frequently the noon meal at "the center" becomes the focal point

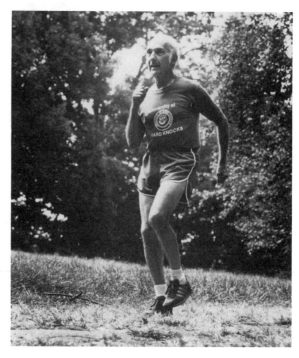

Figure 21-2 Exercising for good health is not limited to the young.

of an older person's day. The federal government also provides transportation to those who are otherwise unable to reach the senior center for the meal. When individuals are completely

Nocturia - night wetting
Protein - for infections
    hurts

CHAPTER 21   DIET DURING THE SENIOR YEARS   231

homebound, arrangements can be made for the meals to be delivered to their homes. In some communities, there are Meals-on-Wheels projects. Participating people pay according to ability. In addition, food stamps are available, and can sometimes be used for the Meals-on-Wheels programs.

SUMMARY

The elderly are becoming an increasingly large segment of the U.S. population and their nutritional needs are of growing concern. It is becoming apparent that many of the chronic diseases of the elderly could be delayed or avoided by maintaining good nutrition throughout life. Nutrient requirements of the elderly do not decrease, but kcal requirements do decrease with age. When food habits of senior citizens must be changed, adjustments require great tact and patience on the part of the nutrition counselor. Older people are easily attracted to food fads that promise good health and prolonged life.

Discussion Topics

edentulous
mechanical
altered
soft/pureed

1. Why are the normal nutrient requirements of people in their seventies the same as those of people in their fifties?
2. Why does the iron requirement usually diminish for women after the age of 50?
3. Why might elderly people suffer from anorexia?
4. How might arthritis affect one's eating habits?
5. In what ways can emotional stress affect eating habits? What kinds of emotional stress do the elderly sometimes suffer?
6. Why are older people inclined to believe food faddists' stories?
7. What is the difference between geriatrics and gerontology?
8. What is periodontal disease and what is its possible significance?
9. What is osteoporosis?
10. Why do kcal requirements diminish as people age?

Suggested Activities

1. Arrange a panel discussion on nutrition for the senior citizen. Consider nutrient requirements, kcal requirements, physical disabilities, food habits, food fads, chronic diseases, appropriate diets, and the means of obtaining them.
2. If possible, visit a nursing home at mealtime. Write your evaluation of the food, and a description of patient reaction(s) to it and to you, the visitor.
3. Role-play a situation where a 75-year old arthritic woman who has just

been widowed, is very depressed and disinterested in food, and is being counseled to eat a nutritious diet.

4. Describe an appropriate response to your 65-year old aunt who has just become captivated by a salesperson in a local health food store, and has announced that she is buying a six-months' supply of vinegar-honey tablets that are guaranteed to prevent arthritis.

5. Plan a talk on nutrition for the Parents' Association of a local high school entitled, "Invest Now for Future Dividends—Eat Well".

6. Adapt the menus in Table 21-3 to meet the kcal requirements of someone who needs 2,000 kcal.

7. Divide the menus in Table 21-3 into the Basic Four food groups and list the foods that do not fit into these groups as well.

Review

A. Completion

1. _Anorexia_ is a condition in which the patient, for psychological reasons, has no appetite or interest in food, and weight loss becomes a concern.

2. _Arthritis_ is a chronic disease in which the joints become painful and stiff.

3. _Cataracts_ result in the clouding of the lens of the eye and impaired vision.

4. _Diabetes_ is a chronic disease that prevents normal production of insulin so that carbohydrate metabolism is affected.

5. _geriatrics_ is the branch of medicine dealing with diseases of the elderly.

6. _gerontology_ is the study of aging.

7. _Hypotension_ is also known as high blood pressure.

8. _health_ is the condition of one's nutrition.

9. _Osteoporosis_ is the disease in which bones become porous.

10. _periodontal_ occurs in the gums and supportive tissue of the teeth.

B. Multiple Choice

1. Gerontology is of increasing interest because it is

   a. the branch of medicine involved with diseases of older people.

   b. the study of nutrition.

c. hoped experimentation in this field will explain the causes of aging.

    d. the study of heart disease.

2. After the age of 50, nutrient requirements generally

    a. increase   c. remain unchanged

    b. decrease   d. none of the above

3. After the age of 50, kcal requirements generally

    a. increase   c. remain unchanged

    b. decrease   d. none of the above

4. The iron requirement for women after the age of approximately 50 generally

    a. increases   c. remains unchanged

    b. decreases   d. none of the above

5. Studies indicate that diets of many senior citizens are deficient in vitamins A, C, riboflavin, and calcium. A simple solution would be to increase their consumption of

    a. yellow vegetables, citrus fruits, and milk.

    b. breads, cereals, and macaroni products.

    c. meats, fish, and eggs.

    d. vegetable oils and wheat germ.

6. Osteoporosis is a disease that causes

    a. poor appetite

    b. a reduction in the number of red blood cells

    c. joints to become painful and stiff

    d. bones to become porous

7. Arthritis is a disease that causes

    a. poor appetite

    b. a reduction in the number of red blood cells

    c. joints to become painful and stiff

    d. bones to become porous

8. Cataracts

    a. may be surgically removed

    b. are caused by excess vitamin D in the diet

    c. cause high blood pressure

    d. always cause anorexia

9. Hypertension is related to diets high in

    a. cholesterol   c. calcium

    b. vitamin D   d. salt

10. Diets high in cholesterol content are thought to contribute to

    a. diabetes mellitus   c. heart disease

    b. hypertension   d. cataracts

C. Essay Questions

1. What factors may contribute to the formation of poor food habits during the senior years?

2. Why are the elderly especially susceptible to food fads?

3. Explain how the cumulative effects of diet are thought to be related to the development of osteoporosis and heart disease.

References

Hui, Y.H. 1983. *Human Nutrition and Diet Therapy*. Monterey, Calif.: Wadsworth Health Sciences Division of Wadsworth Inc.

Iowa Dietetic Association. 1984. *Simplified Diet Manual with Meal Patterns*, 5th ed. Ames: Iowa State University Press.

Robinson, Corinne H., and Marilyn R. Lawler. 1982. *Normal and Therapeutic Nutrition*, 16th ed. New York: McMillan Publishing Company.

Whitney, Eleanor Noss. 1982. *Nutrition Concepts and Controversies*, 2nd ed. St.Paul: West Publishing Co.

Whitney, Eleanor Noss, and Eva May Nunnelley Hamilton. 1984. *Understanding Nutrition*, 3rd ed. St. Paul: West Publishing Co.

Section 5
Therapeutic Diets

Chapter 22

INTRODUCTION TO DIET THERAPY

VOCABULARY

consistency
dietician
diet therapy
energy value

nutrient content
nutrient
   supplement

nutritionally
   adequate
therapeutic diets

OBJECTIVES

After studying this chapter, you should be able to

- Define diet therapy
- Identify roles of the physician and dietitian in diet therapy

Proper nutrition is necessary for maintaining good health, and for building good health during and after an illness. Using nutrition to build good health is called *diet therapy*. Diet therapy means modifying or changing the patient's normal diet to meet requirements created by disease or injury. Sometimes it is simply a matter of changing a nutritionally inadequate diet to a nutritionally adequate diet. More often, diet therapy means the addition or subtraction of specific nutrients and foods in specified amounts to or from a diet, or the modification of their consistencies. Such diets are called *therapeutic diets* and must always be prescribed by a physician. A *dietitian* (specialist in planning diets) plans the meals that fit the physician's prescription.

It can be difficult to convince the patient to eat meals based on a therapeutic diet. People are often reluctant to eat new foods or familiar foods prepared in unfamiliar ways, especially when they are ill. Weakness, exhaustion, illness, loneliness, and self-pity also discourage appetites. Anorexia is not uncommon among hospital patients. Cheerfulness on the part of the person serving the food can improve the patient's attitude and appetite. At times, an explanation of the value of the diet motivates the patient to eat. It is useful to explain that the diet will improve health and general well-being. It is important to help the patient learn to select appropriate foods for the diet. The patient should be encouraged to overcome prejudices about certain foods. Elementary facts of nutrition can be explained in simple language and explanations given so the patient understands the reasons for the diet. The person serving the meal should encourage the patient to eat the prescribed diet. Unless the prescribed food is eaten, it is useless.

When certain foods are consistently refused, the refusal should be discussed with the dietitian and physician. Sometimes, necessary foods that are disliked can be disguised when combined with other foods. Milk, for example can be included in the diet in pudding, ice cream, cheese, cream sauce, soup, or custard. If such measures fail and the patient continues to refuse the needed foods, the physician may prescribe supplements such as calcium and vitamin tablets. Since most people have better appetites when they are rested, it is advisable to serve the most nutritious meals early in the day and to make the evening meals light. (See Chapter 16 for additional information on patients' meals.)

SUMMARY

The treatment of disease through diet is called diet therapy. This therapy consists of the addition or subtraction of certain nutrients or foods in the patient's diet. It is difficult to convince people to change their eating habits. The person serving the meals should be pleasant and able to explain the value of the special diet to the patient.

Discussion Topics

1. What is diet therapy?
2. What is a dietitian?
3. Discuss ways in which the nurse may help solve the problem of friends and relatives bringing food to patients on therapeutic diets.
4. What are food prejudices? Name some and discuss how you might attempt to help the patient overcome them.
5. Why is it important to teach the patient about her or his new diet?
6. Why do people who are ill frequently experience a decrease in appetite? How can the nurse encourage patients to eat well?

Suggested Activities

1. Role-play a situation in which a nurse persuades a middle-aged woman who loves sweets that her carbohydrate-controlled diet can be satisfying. The class should evaluate the "nurse's" tact and ingenuity in persuading the "patient."
2. Plan a visit to a hospital kitchen. If possible, ask the dietitian to explain the various procedures to the class. Discuss this visit in class.

Review

Multiple Choice. Select the *letter* that precedes the best answer.

1. The use of diet to build good health during and after illness is called
   a. diet therapy
   b. dietetics
   c. dietitian
   d. physical therapy

2. Special diets are prescribed by the
   a. nurse
   b. dietitian
   c. physician
   d. physical therapist

3. The planning of special diets is done by the
   a. nurse
   b. physician
   c. dietitian
   d. physical therapist

4. Necessary foods that are disliked can be more easily accepted if they are
   a. disguised in a combination with other foods
   b. highly seasoned with spicy sauces
   c. served for lunch rather than for supper
   d. served frequently throughout the week

5. Basic diets may be modified by changing their
   a. color, flavor, or satiety value
   b. consistency, energy value, or nutrient content
   c. temperatures and serving times
   d. cost and efficiency of preparation

6. A therapeutic diet
   a. is always prescribed by a physician
   b. may add certain nutrients and foods in specified amounts
   c. may subtract certain foods from a diet
   d. all of the above

7. If the patient refuses to eat the necessary foods, the doctor may
   a. prescribe a sedative
   b. prescribe a diet supplement
   c. prescribe both a sedative and a diet supplement
   d. order an injection of calcium

8. A modification in consistency means a change in
   a. texture
   b. flavor
   c. color
   d. satiety value

9. A modification in energy value means a change in
   a. nutrient content
   b. vitamin content
   c. kcal content
   d. all of the above

10. A patient may refuse a therapeutic diet because of
   a. anorexia
   b. ignorance
   c. prejudice
   d. all of the above

References

Bodinski, Lois H. 1982. *The Nurse's Guide to Diet Therapy*. New York: John Wiley & Sons.

Howe, Phyllis Sullivan. 1981. *Basic Nutrition in Health and Disease*. Philadelphia: W.B. Saunders Co.

Williams, Sue Rodwell. 1982. *Essentials of Nutrition and Diet Therapy*. 3rd ed. St. Louis: C.V. Mosby Co.

Williams, Sue Rodwell. 1984. *Mowry's Basic Nutrition and Diet Therapy*, 7th ed. St. Louis: C.V. Mosby Co.

Chapter 23

STANDARD HOSPITAL DIETS

VOCABULARY

ambulatory	diarrhea	milliliter
acute	eggnog	mechanical soft
bouillon	fecal matter	diet
broth	flatulence	postoperative
clear liquid diet	full liquid diet	soft diet
coarse foods	gastrointestinal	standard hospital
condiment	junket	diets
convalescent	light diet	

OBJECTIVES

After studying this chapter, you should be able to

* Identify standard hospital diets and the ways they can be modified

* Identify varying conditions for which these diets may be prescribed

* Identify foods allowed on these diets

STANDARD HOSPITAL DIETS

Health facilities such as hospitals and nursing homes usually have standard diets that simplify their meal planning. Hospitals typically have *liquid*, *soft*, *regular*, and *light* diets.

These basic diets may be modified by changing their consistency, energy value, or nutrient content. For example, a low-calorie diet or a sodium-restricted diet can be prepared as a liquid, soft, light, or regular diet.

The person serving a meal should learn to recognize the types of food allowed in each diet. In some facilities it is the duty of the nurse to double-check the meal tray before it is served.

Regular Diet

A regular diet is a nearly normal diet based on the Basic Four food groups. People on the regular diet require nutrients for health maintenance only, and not for therapy. A regular diet includes a great variety of foods. However, the caloric value of this diet is somewhat lower than for normal diets because the people on it are not normally active, and consequently require fewer calories than the ordinary person. Some patients on the regular diet are advised to limit or avoid highly seasoned foods, hollow calorie foods, and

Table 23-1 A Day's Menu with a Regular Diet Can Include a Wide Variety of Foods

Breakfast	Dinner	Lunch or Supper
Orange Juice	Roast Beef	Poached Egg on Toast
Oatmeal	Mashed Potatoes	Cooked Spinach
Milk-Sugar	Steamed Carrots	Fruit Gelatin
Toast-Butter	Lettuce with French Dressing	Plain Cookie
Coffee or Tea	Bread-Butter	Milk or Tea
	Milk Pudding	
	Milk	

very rich foods such as pastries, heavy cakes, and fried foods. Such foods may cause digestive disturbances, or weight gain in people who are not active. The regular diet is usually intended for the *ambulatory* patient (one who walks).

THE LIGHT DIET

The light diet is an intermediate diet sometimes used between the soft and the regular diets. It is nutritionally adequate.

The light diet is also called the *convalescent diet* because it is primarily used for *convalescent* (recovering from an injury or illness) patients and for those with minor illnesses. The light diet is considered one of the four standard diets. However, some health facilities do not use it because it is so similar to the regular diet.

The important fact to remember concerning the light diet is that the foods must be easy to digest. Foods are simply cooked, with little seasoning, and served without heavy

Table 23-2 Selecting Foods for a Light Diet

FOODS ALLOWED IN LIGHT DIETS	FOODS TO BE AVOIDED
cheddar cheese	rich pastries
tender cuts of beef, lamb, and veal such as steaks, roasts, and chops	heavy salad dressings
bacon, liver	fried foods
all soups	coarse foods such as some very coarse cereals
cooked vegetables and fruits, citrus fruits, bananas, lettuce and tomato salads	fruits and vegetables that are high in cellulose
enriched and whole wheat bread and crackers	foods that cause flatulence
plain cakes	nuts

Table 23-3 Sample Menus for a Light Diet

Breakfast	Dinner	Lunch or Supper
Orange Sections	Vegetable Soup	Tomato Juice
Oatmeal with Cream and Sugar	Roast Lamb	Scrambled Eggs with Cottage Cheese
Buttered Toast	Baked Potato	Asparagus Tips
Jelly	Buttered Carrots	Bread and Butter
Coffee with Cream and Sugar	Lettuce Salad	Orange Sherbet
	Bread and Butter	Tea with Cream and Sugar
	Strawberry Ice Cream	
	Tea with Cream and Sugar	

sauces or spicy seasonings. The diet includes all foods allowed on the soft and liquid diets plus those foods listed in table 23-2.

THE SOFT DIET

The soft diet is very similar to the regular diet except that the texture of the foods has been modified. The soft diet commonly follows a full liquid diet. It may be ordered for *postoperative* (after surgery) cases, for patients with *acute* (severe) infections, gastrointestinal conditions, or chewing problems.

This diet includes liquids and foods that have a soft texture and are easy to digest. The foods allowed are those that contain very little indigestible carbohydrate (cellulose) and no tough connective tissue. As a result, a soft diet leaves little food *residue* (indigestible fiber). Meals in a soft diet are very tender. Most fruits must be cooked, but bananas, orange, or grapefruit sections (with membranes removed) are sometimes allowed. Usually only young, tender, cooked vegetables are served; frequently these are pureed. Cereals are either refined or cooked.

When patients are unable to chew, the *mechanical soft diet* may be ordered. In this diet, all meats are ground and fruits and vegetables are pureed. It may be necessary after facial surgery, or when teeth are missing or inadequate.

Generally, foods on the soft diet are mild flavored, slightly seasoned, or left unseasoned, and are prepared in easily digestible forms. Although this diet nourishes the body, between-meal feedings are sometimes given to increase the energy value.

LIQUID DIETS

A *liquid* diet consists of foods that will pour or are liquid at body temperature. The nutritive value of liquid diets is low and consequently they are usually used only for very limited periods of time. Liquid diets are subdivided into two types—the clear liquid and the full liquid diet.

Clear Liquid Diet

The clear liquid diet consists of liquids that do not irritate the gastrointestinal tract, cause *flatulence* (gas in the stomach or in-

Table 23-4 Selecting Foods in a Soft Diet

FOODS ALLOWED IN SOFT DIET	FOODS TO BE AVOIDED
milk, cream, butter	meat and shellfish with tough connective tissue
mild cheeses such as cottage or cream cheese	coarse cereals
eggs, except fried	condiments (foods used as seasonings, relishes)
tender chicken, fish, sweetbreads, ground beef and lamb	rich pastries and desserts
soup broth and strained cream soups	foods high in cellulose
tender, cooked vegetables or pureed vegetables	fried foods
fruit juices, cooked fruits, bananas, orange and grapefruit sections with membranes removed	raw vegetables and raw fruits (except bananas and citrus fruits with membranes removed)
refined cereals, cooked cereals, spaghetti, noodles, macaroni, enriched white bread, white crackers	nuts and coconut
tea, coffee, cocoa, carbonated beverages	
sherbet, ices, plain ice cream, custard, pudding, junket, gelatin, plain cookies, angel and sponge cake	
salt and some spices in small amounts as allowed by the physician	

Table 23-5 Sample Menu for a Soft Diet

Breakfast	Dinner	Lunch or Supper
Orange Juice	Cream of Tomato Soup	Apple Juice
Cream of Wheat with Milk and Sugar	Broiled Ground Beef Patty	Creamed Chicken with Peas and Noodles
Buttered Toast	Mashed Potatoes with Butter	Baked Squash
Tea or Coffee with Cream and Sugar	Green Beans	Bread and Butter
	Bread and Butter	Custard
	Stewed Peaches	Tea with Cream and Sugar
	Milk	

Note: Between meals the patient may have malted milk, milkshakes, eggnog, or cocoa.

Table 23-6 Sample Menu for a Clear Liquid Diet

Breakfast	10 a.m.	Dinner	3 p.m.	Lunch or Supper	9 p.m.
Apple Juice Tea with Sugar	Tomato Juice	Beef Bouillon Gelatin Tea with Sugar	Grape Juice	Chicken Broth Fruit Ice Tea with Sugar	Beef Bouillon

testines), or stimulate peristalsis. A clear liquid diet passes through the body easily and does not create residue. Therefore, this diet is used when the amount of *fecal matter* (waste material) in the colon must be kept at a minimum. The clear liquid diet may be used after surgery. The diet may also be ordered to replace fluids lost through vomiting or diarrhea.

The clear liquid diet is composed mainly of water and carbohydrates. It is only a temporary diet since it is nutritionally inadequate. Its use is typically limited to 24—36 hours. The meals, which are small and frequent, are usually served every two, three, or four hours. It is usually followed by the full liquid diet.

Full Liquid Diet

The full liquid diet contains all foods in the clear liquid diet and additional, more nutritious foods as well.

The full liquid diet includes many milk-based foods that make this diet more nutritious than the clear liquid diet. Compared to a regular diet, however, the nutritive value of a full liquid diet is low. The caloric value of the full liquid diet may be increased by adding

Table 23-7 Foods Allowed in a Clear Liquid Diet

apple and tomato juice
fat-free broths or bouillon (clear soups)
plain gelatin
fruit ice
ginger ale and carbonated water (if permitted by physician)
tea or black coffee with sugar

lactose (milk sugar) or corn syrup to the beverages. Its protein content may be increased by adding dried milk or commercial protein substitutes to whole milk. In addition, the physician may prescribe a vitamin supplement. A minimum serving of 180 to 240 milliliters (six to eight ounces) is usually given every two or three hours.

This diet may be given to patients who have acute infections; to patients who have difficulty chewing; to those who have had heart attacks; and to patients with gastrointestinal disturbances.

SUMMARY

The standard hospital diets include liquid, soft, regular, and light. Each diet may be

Table 23-8 Sample Menus for a Full Liquid Diet

Breakfast	10 a.m.	Dinner	3 p.m.	Lunch or Supper	9 p.m.
Strained Orange Juice Strained Oatmeal Gruel with Cream and Sugar Coffee or Tea with Cream and Sugar	Tomato Juice	Strained Cream of Chicken Soup Plain Gelatin with Sweetened Whipped Cream Milk Tea with Cream and Sugar	Eggnog	Apple Juice Beef Broth Vanilla Ice Cream Milk Coffee or Tea with Cream and Sugar	Cocoa

modified by changing its consistency, energy value, or nutrient content. The regular diet is comparable to the average well-balanced diet but limited in caloric value, hollow calorie foods, highly seasoned foods, and very rich foods.

The clear liquid diet consists only of nonirritating liquids and is nutritionally inadequate. It may be used following surgery. The full liquid diet provides more nourishment than the clear liquid diet, but it is still low in nutritional value. It ordinarily is prescribed to follow the clear liquid diet. It is used for patients who cannot chew, patients with severe infections, for heart attack victims, and for patients with gastrointestinal disturbances.

The soft diet nourishes the body. It includes foods that are liquid or semisolid with soft textures, very little indigestible carbohydrate, and no tough connective tissue. It may be ordered for postoperative patients, for patients with severe infections, or for patients with gastrointestinal or chewing problems.

The light (convalescent) diet is an intermediate diet between the soft and regular diets. It is nutritionally adequate. The light

Table 23-9 Foods Allowed in a Full Liquid Diet

all clear liquids

fruit and vegetable juices

strained soups (cream or water based)

strained, cooked cereals

custard

ice cream

puddings

junket (sweetened, flavored, thickened milk dessert)

sherbet

milk, cream, buttermilk

cocoa

eggnog

carbonated beverages

diet is a standard diet but is not used in all health facilities because it is so similar to the regular diet. It is used for convalescent patients and those with minor illnesses. The light diet contains only foods that are easily digested.

Case Study—An Elderly Woman with a Bone Fracture

Mrs. J. was hospitalized with a fractured hip. She was very thin and although her doctor considered her hip bone to be somewhat osteoporotic, her surgery had been uneventful and her incision was healing normally. She had had many visitors—friends as well as her husband and children—and was scheduled for discharge two weeks after her operation. She was listless and pale, however, and seemed to grow increasingly depressed, weeping more and more frequently. Her physician prescribed iron tablets because her hemoglobin count was somewhat low. The dietician was asked to interview her because the nurses reported that she scarcely touched her trays. The dietician discovered that Mrs. J. suffered from periodontal disease and could not manage to chew the bacon, meat, and toast on her trays.

Case Study Questions

1. What diet should the dietician suggest for Mrs. J?
2. Is this diet nutritionally adequate?
3. How could its kilocalorie content be increased without changing its texture?
4. How could the nutrient content of this diet be improved?
5. What advice should the dietician give Mrs. J. so that she could improve her iron absorption?
6. What possible conclusion could one draw regarding Mrs. J.'s diet history?

Discussion Topics

1. What are the usual standard hospital diets? If anyone in the class has eaten or seen any hospital diets, ask that person to describe them.
2. Describe the regular hospital diet? How can it differ from a normal diet?
3. Why is the calorie count sometimes lower on the regular hospital diet than on a normal diet?
4. When is the light diet used? Why is it not included in the diets of all hospitals?
5. What type of foods are included in the light diet?
6. Would the light diet be generally suitable for healthy geriatric patients? For children? Is it nutritionally adequate?

7. Many people have unknowingly been on a self-imposed light diet at home. Under what conditions might this have occurred?

8. Describe a soft diet. Does it nourish the body? When may it be prescribed?

9. What kinds of foods are allowed in the soft diet?

10. Why are between-meal feedings sometimes given to patients on the soft diet?

11. What are condiments and why are they excluded from the soft diet?

12. Name the conditions for which a soft diet may be prescribed.

13. What is indigestible carbohydrate? Why should it be limited in a soft diet? Name several foods that contain a large proportion of indigestible carbohydrate. Name foods containing very little.

14. What are food "membranes?" Why should such membranes be omitted from the soft diet?

15. Why are patients on the clear-liquid diet fed so frequently? Why is it only a temporary diet?

16. How does the full liquid diet differ from the clear liquid diet?

17. What is an eggnog? How can calories be added to an eggnog?

18. How can protein be added to cream soup and cocoa?

19. What is bouillon? How is it prepared?

20. What is junket? If anyone in the class has tasted it, ask that person to describe it.

21. Mr. Brown has recently had a stroke that paralyzed his right side. Why do you think a liquid diet has been prescribed for Mr. Brown?

Suggested Activities

1. Make a chart of the diets discussed in this chapter and include the foods allowed in each. Compare the charts and correct if necessary. The charts should be kept for reference.

2. Plan a daily menu for each of the diets in this chapter. Compare menus and correct them if necessary.

3. Adapt the menus for the regular diet to suit a 40-year-old woman. How might the diet be changed if the patient were a 16-year-old boy with a broken leg?

4. In some hospitals, regular diets do not include rich, high calorie foods. Substitute other foods or methods of preparation to make the regular diet that follows more appropriate:

Deep-fried Fish Fillets
French Fried Potatoes
Green Peas
Lettuce with Oil and Vinegar
Bread and Butter
Pecan Pie with Whipped Cream
Milk

5. Make a list of the foods eaten yesterday. Circle those foods that would not be allowed on the light diet.
6. Adapt the following menu to make it appropriate for a patient on a light diet.

Breakfast	Dinner	Lunch or Supper
Orange Juice	Roast Beef	Pepper Steak
2 Fried Eggs	Mashed Potato	Cooked Spinach
Danish Pastry	Steamed Carrots	Fruit Gelatin
Coffee or Tea	Lettuce	Pecan Roll
with	with	Milk or Tea
Milk-Sugar	Creamy Garlic Dressing	
	Whole Wheat Bread	
	Milk Pudding	
	Milk	

7. Adapt the following menu to suit the needs of a patient on a soft diet:

Fresh Fruit Cup
Oatmeal with Milk and Sugar
Bran Muffin and Butter
Tea with Sugar

8. Write your dinner menu for last night. Adapt it to suit a patient on the soft diet.
9. Find recipes that are suitable for these standard hospital diets.
10. Begin a Therapeutic Diet Recipe File in which recipes are coded according to the diet in which they are allowed. Code them by using a special color dot in the upper right-hand corner of each recipe or use the initials of the diet. Many of the recipes may be suitable for several different diets.
11. Observe demonstrations of the electric blender and the food processor. Practice using them and cleaning them.

12. Prepare one or more of the meals on the menu. Evaluate each in terms of nutritive content, flavor, aroma, color, shape, appearance, texture, and satiety value.

Review

A. Multiple Choice. Select the *letter* that precedes the best answer.

1. The standard hospital diets are usually
   a. liquid, soft, regular, and light
   b. soft, light, and salt-free
   c. low fat, regular, soft, and normal
   d. liquid, soft, and diabetic

2. Regular diets usually limit
   a. pastries and fried foods
   b. all fats
   c. broiled and boiled foods
   d. meats and meat products

3. Regular diets are based on
   a. individual doctors' prescriptions
   b. low calorie foods only
   c. all-vegetable diets
   d. the Basic Four food groups

4. The ambulatory patient is one who
   a. cannot walk
   b. can walk
   c. has no teeth
   d. arrives in an ambulance

5. The light diet is also called the
   a. soft diet
   b. full liquid diet
   c. invalid diet
   d. convalescent diet

6. The light diet is
   a. always one of the standard hospital diets
   b. more restrictive than the soft diet
   c. very similar to a regular diet in some health facilities
   d. rarely used for obese patients

7. The light diet, if used, is typically given
   a. after the full liquid diet and before the soft diet
   b. after the regular diet and before the soft diet
   c. after the soft diet and before the regular diet
   d. immediately after surgery

8. The light diet is given to
   a. newborns
   b. patients recovering from an illness
   c. patients preparing for surgery
   d. all patients over 60

9. Foods included in the light diet must be
   a. coarse
   b. easy to chew
   c. from health food stores
   d. easy to digest

10. The soft diet
    a. is a standard diet in health facilities
    b. is always served to children under 12 years old
    c. is similar to a high-residue diet
    d. does not nourish as well as a full liquid diet

11. A major difference between the regular and the soft diet is the
    a. nutrient content
    b. texture of the foods
    c. energy values
    d. satiety value of the foods

12. It is not unusual for the soft diet to be
    a. ordered to precede the clear liquid diet
    b. ordered to precede the full liquid diet
    c. ordered to succeed the full liquid diet
    d. used in place of the clear liquid diet

13. The soft diet is sometimes ordered for
    a. preoperative patients
    b. postoperative patients
    c. comatose patients
    d. all of these

14. The following would not be included in a soft diet:
    a. ground beef
    b. leg of lamb
    c. roast chicken
    d. baked pork chops

15. Cellulose is
    a. a complete protein
    b. an indigestible carbohydrate
    c. a saturated fat
    d. an essential mineral

16. The clear liquid diet consists of liquids that do not
    a. irritate
    b. cause flatulence
    c. stimulate peristalsis
    d. all of these

17. The clear liquid diet
    a. replaces lost body fluids
    b. provides a nutritionally adequate diet
    c. includes any food that pours
    d. is never used after surgery

18. The following group of foods would be allowed on a clear liquid diet:
    a. cream of chicken soup, coffee, and tea
    b. tomato juice, sherbet, and strained cooked cereal
    c. raspberry ice, beef bouillon, and apple juice
    d. tea, coffee, and eggnog

19. The full liquid diet
    a. is always nutritionally adequate
    b. is followed by a clear liquid diet
    c. does not include milk in any form
    d. is sometimes given patients with acute infections
20. The full liquid diet
    a. is given all patients on the first day of their hospital stay
    b. includes no protein foods
    c. includes no highly fibrous foods
    d. is commonly given immediately after surgery
21. The caloric value of the full liquid diet
    a. is always adequate
    b. cannot be varied
    c. may be increased by adding lactose or corn syrup
    d. is usually 3000 calories per day
22. The protein content of the full liquid diet
    a. can be increased by adding lactose to beverages
    b. can be increased by adding dried milk to beverages
    c. cannot be varied
    d. is always adequate
23. The clear liquid diet
    a. is given all patients with chewing difficulties
    b. may be used after surgery
    c. includes milk foods
    d. is nutritionally adequate
24. One of the reasons for giving the clear liquid diet is to
    a. rest the teeth and gums
    b. cause weight reduction
    c. activate the colon
    d. reduce peristalsis
25. Eggnog and beef bouillon are
    a. allowed on both liquid diets
    b. not allowed on either liquid diet
    c. allowed only on the clear liquid diet
    d. allowed on the full liquid diet

References

Iowa Dietetic Association. 1984. *Simplified Diet Manual with Meal Patterns*, 5th ed. Ames: Iowa State University Press.

Massachusetts General Hospital Dietary Department. 1976. *Diet Manual*. Boston: Little Brown & Co.

Mayo Clinic, Rochester Methodist Hospital and St. Mary's Hospital. 1981. *Mayo Clinic Diet Manual, a Handbook of Dietary Practices*. Philadelphia: W.B. Saunders Co.

University of Iowa Hospitals and Clinics. 1979. *Recent Advances in Therapeutic Diets*. Iowa City: Iowa State University Press.

Williams, Sue Rodwell. 1981. *Nutrition and Diet Therapy*, 4th ed. St. Louis: C.V. Mosby Co.

Chapter 24

DIET IN THE TREATMENT OF DIABETES MELLITUS

VOCABULARY

acidosis	exogenous insulin	IDDM
arterial	free diet	insulin reaction
aspartame	genetic	ketones
chemical method	predisposition	ketonuria
of regulation	glycosuria	NIDDM
chronic	hormone	polydipsia
clinical method	hyperglycemia	polyphagia
of regulation	hypoglycemia	polyuria
diabetes mellitus	hypoglycemic	renal
diabetic coma	agents	saccharin
endogenous insulin	insulin	weighed diet
exchange lists	insulin coma	vascular system

OBJECTIVES

After studying this chapter, you should be able to

* Describe diabetus mellitus

* Name the symptoms of diabetes mellitus

* State the function of insulin

* Explain three types of diabetic diets

* Explain how non-metabolized glucose is excreted

Diabetes mellitus is a chronic (of long duration) disease in which the body's metabolism of carbohydrate and consequently, protein and fat, is disturbed because of inadequate production or inadequate use of the hormone, *insulin*. Insulin controls glucose metabolism and is secreted by the islets of Langerhans in the pancreas. Current research indicates that another pancreatic hormone, *glucagon*, also plays a part in diabetes mellitus, but its specific role remains controversial.

The causes of diabetes mellitus are not confirmed, but while the tendency to it is inherited, environmental factors may also contribute to its occurrence. For example,

viruses or obesity may precipitate the disease in people who are genetically predisposed.

Diabetes mellitus is a very serious disease. It causes deterioration of the vascular system, creating an increased susceptibility to arterial, heart, and kidney disease, blindness, and skin infections. It is the third-ranking cause of death in the United States, with an estimated 5 percent of the population suffering from it.

The World Health Organization indicates that the prevalence of the disease is increasing worldwide, especially in areas showing improvement in living standards.

SYMPTOMS OF DIABETES MELLITUS

Symptoms of diabetes mellitus usually include weakness, fatigue, loss of weight, *polydipsia* (excessive thirst), *polyuria* (excessive production of urine), and *polyphagia* (increased appetite).

In uncontrolled diabetes, where the supply of insulin is inadequate, the glucose that is not metabolized accumulates in the blood. This is called *hyperglycemia* (abnormally large amounts of sugar in the blood). When hyperglycemia exceeds the renal threshold (kidneys' capacity to reabsorb the sugar), *glycosuria* (excessive sugar in the urine) occurs and sugar is excreted. The kidneys need extra fluids to excrete this sugar. Consequently, fluid is drawn from body cells and polydipsia and polyuria result. The patient also experiences polyphagia because the food that is eaten is not metabolized normally.

Because the diabetic patient cannot use carbohydrate for energy, increasing amounts of fat are oxidized. The liver breaks down the fatty acids to *ketones*. In healthy people, ketones are subsequently broken down to carbon dioxide and water, yielding energy.

In diabetes mellitus, fatty acids break down faster than the body can handle them. They collect in the blood (*ketonemia*) and must be excreted in the urine (*ketonuria*). Ketones are acids that lower blood pH, causing *acidosis*. Acidosis may lead to *diabetic coma*, which can result in death if the patient is not treated quickly with fluids and insulin.

TYPES OF DIABETES MELLITUS

There are two types of diabetes mellitus—*insulin dependent diabetes mellitus* (IDDM), and *non-insulin dependent diabetes mellitus* (NIDDM).

IDDM was formerly classified as juvenile-onset diabetes mellitus. It occurs between the ages of 1 and 40, and includes from 10—20 percent of all diabetes cases. These patients secrete little, if any insulin and thus become insulin dependent, requiring both insulin and a carefully controlled diet. This type of diabetes occurs suddenly, exhibiting many of the symptoms described in the preceding section. It can be difficult to control.

NIDDM was previously called adult-onset diabetes. It usually occurs after the age of 35. Its onset is gradual. It is common for the patient to have no symptoms and to be totally ignorant of her or his condition until it is discovered accidentally during a routine urine or blood test. This type of diabetes can usually be controlled by diet, or diet and oral *hypoglycemic agents*. Hypoglycemic agents stimulate the pancreas to produce insulin. It is less severe than IDDM. Eighty-five percent of NIDDM patients are overweight. Consequently, these patients are typically placed on weight-reduction diets until their weights reach an acceptable level.

TREATMENT OF DIABETES MELLITUS

The ultimate goal of treatment is the control of blood glucose levels so that food can be metabolized and the patient provided with sufficient energy. Treatment is usually begun when urine and blood tests indicate that sugar is present, or when any of the previously discussed symptoms occur.

The treatment may be by diet alone, or by diet combined with insulin or a hypoglycemic agent. It should relieve symptoms, allow the

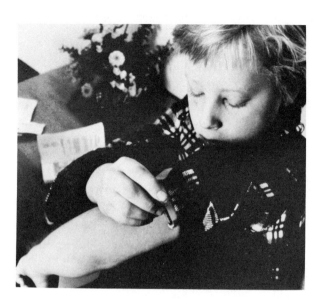

Figure 24-1 Self-injection into the upper arm (*Reprinted from Reiss and Melick, Pharmacological Aspects of Nursing Care, figure 31-5*)

patient to live a normal life, and prevent or delay the physical complications common to diabetes mellitus.

There are three basic types of therapeutic diets prescribed for diabetic patients. Physicians vary as to the type of diet prescribed, depending on their philosophy and experience. Each diet may be modified to meet the requirements of other physical conditions such as cardiac, renal, or gastro-intestinal problems.

The Weighed Diet

The weighed diet is based on a very conservative approach to the treatment of diabetes. The glucose levels are rigidly controlled by carefully weighed food portions, urine tests during the day, and the use of insulin or hypoglycemic agents, whose dos-

ages may be adjusted as needed throughout the day. This treatment of diabetes is called the *chemical method of regulation*.

The Unweighed or "Free" Diet

The unweighed diet is based on a very liberal approach to the treatment of diabetes. Patients are allowed to choose their foods (except for sugar and high-sugar foods). If this diet is not successful in controlling the diabetes, they are placed on insulin.

This treatment is known as the *clinical method of regulation*.

Diet Based on Exchange Lists

Exchange lists are the most commonly used method of diet therapy for diabetic patients. They may also be used to control calories and fats.

In this method of diet therapy, foods are grouped into six major lists. Each list includes measured amounts of foods that contain approximately equal amounts of calories, carbohydrates, proteins, fats, vitamins, and minerals. This means that any one food within a particular list may be substituted for any other food *within that particular list* and still provide the patient with the prescribed types and amounts of nutrients and kcal. The types and amounts of nutrients and the number of kcal are not the same on different lists.

List 1 contains milk and milk products.
List 2 contains all nonstarchy vegetables.
List 3 contains all fruits and fruit juices.
List 4 contains breads, cereals, pasta, starchy vegetables, and prepared foods such as biscuits, muffins, crackers, french-fried potatoes, potato chips, pancakes and waffles.
List 5 contains meats.

List 6 contains fats.

When the exchange lists are used, the diet is prescribed by the physician who determines the total energy requirement of the patient. This is done by evaluating age, size, sex, and activities. The nurse or physician may then direct the patient to the dietitian who plans the diet.

Diets based on the exchange lists are individualized. The diet is planned in consultation with the patient. Considerations include

- where meals will be eaten,
- the time the meals are usually eaten,
- personal and family food likes and dislikes,
- the amount of money typically allotted to food,
- the entire life-style of the patient.

The plan is carefully devised so that about 50 percent of the total caloric intake will be obtained from the consumption of carbohydrates, 15 percent from proteins, and 35 percent from fats. All of these nutrients are provided by foods that provide sufficient vitamins and minerals as well.

To determine the specific amounts of carbohydrate, protein, and fat in a patient's diet, the percentage requirement for each of these nutrients in the diet is multiplied by the total daily kcal requirement and the resulting answer is divided by the number of kcal per gram of each nutrient. For example, if a patient is on an 1800 kcal diet, the following calculations would be made:

Carbohydrate (50%)—1800 kcal × .50 = 900 ÷ 4 (kcal per gram of carbohydrate) = 225 grams of carbohydrate

Protein (15%)—1800 kcal × .15 = 270 ÷ 4 (kcal per gram of protein) = 67.5 grams of protein

Fat (35%)—1800 kcal × .35 = 630 ÷ 9 (kcal per gram of fat) = 70 grams of fat.

The total energy requirements for adult diabetic patients who are not overweight will be the same as for nondiabetic individuals. When patients are overweight, a reduction in kcal will be built into the diet plans. If the total daily intake is 1000 kcal or less, vitamin and mineral supplements may be ordered.

The diet is given in terms of exchanges rather than as particular foods. For example, the menu pattern for breakfast may include 1 fruit exchange, 1 meat exchange, 2 bread exchanges, and 2 fat exchanges. The patient may choose the desired foods from the exchange lists for each meal but must adhere to the specific exchange lists named and the specific number of exchanges on each list. In this way, the patient has variety in a simple yet controlled way. Table A-6 in the Appendix contains these Exchange Lists for Meal Planning.

TEACHING THE DIABETIC PATIENT

Dietary Adjustments

It is important to point out to the diabetic patient that one can live a near-normal life if the diet is followed, medication is taken as prescribed, and time is allowed for sufficient exercise and rest. The importance of eating all of the prescribed food must be emphasized. It

Table 24-1 Foods Usually Omitted in Diabetic Diets

sugar	honey
cookies	condensed milk
pies	jam
candy	chewing gum
syrup	jelly
cakes	soft drinks

Table 24-2 Foods Usually Allowed in Diabetic Diets

coffee	parsley
tea	nutmeg
bouillon without fat	lemon
unsweetened gelatin	mustard
unsweetened pickles	chili powder
salt	onion salt or powder
pepper	horseradish
red pepper	vinegar
paprika	mint
garlic	cinnamon
celery salt	lime

is important for meals to be eaten at regular times so that the insulin-sugar balance can be maintained. It is imperative that the patient learn to carefully read all labels on commercially prepared foods. This is necessary to avoid eating or drinking anything that may contain an unknown amount of sugar. It must be explained that prepared foods with unknown amounts of sugar added are not allowed because they upset the insulin-sugar balance. Adjustments must be made in the shopping, cooking, and eating habits so the diet plan can be followed. Family meals can be simply adapted for the diabetic diet. For example, sugar and flour can be omitted from the patient's portions, and lemon juice, herbs, and spices can be substituted for rich sauces on salads, vegetables, and meats. The diabetic patient soon learns which exchange lists are to be included at each meal and at snack times, and the foods within each exchange list.

Alcohol

Alcohol is not recommended for diabetic patients. Its use must be approved by the physician. Some diabetic patients who use hypoglycemic agents cannot tolerate alcohol. When used, its kcal content must be included in the diet plan. It is also advisable to use distilled alcohol products such as gin, vodka, rum, rye, scotch, or bourbon rather than fermented products such as beer and wine because the latter contain carbohydrates.

Diabetic Foods

The use of diabetic or dietetic foods is generally a waste of money and can be injurious to the patient. Very often the containers of foods will contain the same ingredients as containers of foods prepared for the general public, but the cost is typically higher for the diabetic foods. The inherent danger for diabetic patients is that some may not read the labels on the food containers and so may think that the food can be used with abandon when in reality it may be used, but only in specified amounts. The food will usually contain carbohydrates, fat, or protein. The diabetic patient must use these only in specified amounts so that they are balanced by the insulin or hypoglycemic agent.

It is advisable for the diabetic patient to use foods prepared for the general public, but to avoid those packed in syrup or oil. Today many food manufacturers prepare foods both in syrup or water as well as in oil or water. The important thing is for the diabetic patient to *read the label* on all food containers purchased.

Artificial Sweeteners

The artificial sweeteners available today are saccharin and aspartame. Saccharin has been shown to produce cancer in rats, but not in humans. Aspartame is the generic name for a relatively new artificial sweetener. It is a protein and consequently does not require insulin for metabolism. It contains 4 kcal per gram and is approximately 200 times sweeter than sugar. It has been approved by the FDA, and the American Diabetes Association has given its approval for its use "in moderation".

Insulin

The insulin given diabetic patients is prepared from the pancreas glands of cattle and pigs. Its production is carefully controlled. Insulin must be given by injection because it is a protein and if swallowed, would be digested and so would not reach the bloodstream as the complete hormone. Once insulin treatment is begun, it is generally continued throughout the life of the patient.

There are various types of insulin available. They differ in the length of time required to act, and in how long they continue to act. Consequently, they are classified as *rapid*, *intermediate*, and *long-acting*. Those most commonly used are intermediate-acting types that work within 2—8 hours and are effective

for 24—28 hours. Typically, one injection of intermediate-acting insulin is given daily.

The insulin that is injected into the body is called *exogenous* as opposed to *endogenous*, which is produced in the body. Because the exogenous remains in the blood, the patient must take in food on a regular basis. It appears that exercise enhances glucose utilization in a diabetic patient, so if the patient increases daily exercise to any significant degree, she or he must increase food intake or decrease the insulin for the day.

Insulin Reactions

When patients do not eat the prescribed diet but continue to take the prescribed insulin, *hypoglycemia* (subnormal level of blood sugar) can result. This is called an insulin reaction or hypoglycemic episode, and may lead to *insulin coma*. Symptoms include headache, blurred vision, tremors, confusion, poor coordination, and eventual unconsciousness. Insulin reaction is dangerous because if frequent or prolonged, brain damage can occur. If patients are conscious, they can be treated by giving hard candy, a sugar cube, or a beverage containing sugar. If the patient is unconscious, intravenous treatment of dextrose and water is given. It is advisable for the diabetic patient to carry identification explaining the condition so that people do not think she or he is drunk when in reality the person is experiencing an insulin reaction.

SUMMARY

The diabetic diet is used in treating diabetes mellitus, a metabolic disease caused by the improper functioning of the pancreas that results in inadequte production or utilization of insulin. If the condition is left un-treated, the body cannot use glucose properly and serious complications leading to death may occur. Treatment includes diet, medica-tion or both. Diabetic diets are prescribed by the physician and planned by a diet counselor after consultation with the patient.

Case Study—Diabetes Mellitus

Karen W. is a 20-year-old college student who, early in her fall term, began to experience polyuria, combined with poly-dipsia and polyphagia. She felt weak and tired most of the time. She expressed a slight concern about this to her friend one day, but her friend only laughed, saying, "How can you possibly worry about being sick? You're tired because you study when you should be sleeping. And you have the best appetite I have ever seen." This was all true. Karen did study a great deal, and she was usually hungry.

However, when Karen's parents ar-rived for a weekend visit early in October, they were shocked to see how thin she had become. Karen agreed to see a doctor on Monday. The doctor took her history and tested her blood and urine.

Case Study Questions

1. What type of diabetes mellitus do Karen's symptoms suggest?
2. Does this type of diabetes usually require insulin or hypoglycemic agent?
3. The doctor put Karen on a 2400-kcal diet and sent her to a nutrition counselor to plan her meals, using the Exchange Lists. What questions should this counselor ask Karen before beginning her meal plans?
4. What food items should Karen be careful to avoid?
5. What food items can Karen eat without concern?
6. Determine the number of grams of protein, carbohydrate, and fat Karen should have each day.
7. Plan a day's menus for Karen, using the Exchange Lists.
8. Why will Karen's doctor want to see her again after she has been on her new diet for just a few days?
9. Karen's dormitory is having an International Food Festival running for the next six weeks, featuring typical meals of various countries on Friday nights. This Friday there will be a Swedish dinner including the following foods. Karen is not familiar with some of these foods. Which should she avoid? Why? Which could she eat? Why?
   Mixed, Fresh Vegetables with Sourcream Horseradish Dip
   Pickled Herring
   Boiled Shrimp with Lemon Wedges
   Swedish Meat Balls

Baked Ham
Roast Pork with Prunes
Flatbread
Rye bread
Boiled Potatoes
Beet Salad
Pound-type Cake with Whipped Cream
Cookies
Lingonberry Sauce

Discussion Topics

1. Describe diabetes mellitus. Explain why it is a serious disease?
2. What is insulin? What is its use? Why can it not be taken orally?
3. What is the function of oral hypoglycemic agents? For which type of diabetes are they usually prescribed?
4. Explain the differences between IDDM and NIDDM.
5. Describe the symptoms of IDDM. Include the following terms: hyperglycemia, renal threshold, glycosuria, polydipsia, polyuria, polyphagia, ketones, ketonuria, acidosis.
6. Name the six Exchange Lists and explain how they are used.
7. Explain why it is essential that diabetic patients read labels on foods.
8. Why should a diabetic patient avoid adding flour to foods during the cooking process?
9. Why are "dietetic" foods not recommended for diabetic patients?
10. Explain how an insulin reaction may occur.
11. Why must a diabetic patient's tray be checked carefully after meals?

Suggested Activities

1. Ask a physician or registered nurse to speak to the class on diabetes mellitus and its treatment.
2. Ask a diet counselor to explain and demonstrate the planning of diabetic diets using the exchange lists.
   a. Observe the diet counselor planning a 1200-calorie and a 1500-calorie diabetic diet using the exchange lists.
   b. Observe the diet counselor adapting a normal, 2400-calorie daily menu to suit the needs of the diabetic patient on a 1500-calorie diet.

3. Find recipes suitable for the diabetic diet and add them to the diet recipe file.
4. Prepare and serve a meal as planned in activity 2. Evaluate it in terms of nutritive content, flavor, aroma, color, shape, appearance, texture, and satiety value.
5. Visit a local supermarket and compare regular and "dietetic" containers of food in terms of cost, kcal, and nutrient content.

Review

A. Multiple-multiple Choice. Select the *letter* that precedes the best answer.

1. Diabetes mellitus is a metabolic disorder
   1. caused by malfunction of the pancreas gland
   2. for which a diabetic diet may be ordered
   3. in which sugar accumulates in the blood
   4. for which a regular diet is adequate
   5. that is very contagious
      a) all   b) 1,2,3   c) 4,5   d) 1,2,4,5

2. The metabolism of glucose
   1. depends on insulin secreted by the islets of Langerhans
   2. depends on enzymes present in pancreatic juice
   3. is inefficient if diabetes is left untreated
   4. is directly related to secretions from the thyroid gland
      a) 1,3,4   b) all   c) 2,3   d) 1,3

3. Diabetes mellitus is treated by
   1. administration of insulin
   2. exclusion of foods that contain glucose
   3. administration of thyroxine
   4. use of a diabetic diet
      a) 1,3,4   b) 1,4   c) all   d) 1,2,3

4. When considering diets to be used in the management of diabetes, the doctor may order
   1. unweighed or "free" diet
   2. weighed diet
   3. diet based on exchange lists

    4. elimination diet
      a) 1,2,3   b) 1,3,4   c) 2,3,4   d) all

5. The diabetic diet is
    1. also prescribed for hyperthyroidism
    2. based on age, size, sex, and activity
    3. always a low calorie diet
    4. part of the medical treatment for diabetes mellitus
      a) 1,2,3   b) 2,4   c) 1,3,4   d) all

6. When an excessive amount of glucose accumulates in the blood, the condition
    1. is called hyperglycemia   4. is known as acidosis
    2. leads to glycosuria   5. leads to insulin coma
    3. contributes to polydipsia
      a) all   b) 1,2,4   c) 1,3,4,5   d) 1,2,3

7. Diabetic coma
    1. is called acidosis   4. causes polyuria
    2. is caused by excessive insulin   5. is caused by insufficient
    3. is preceded by ketonuria   insulin
      a) 1&2   b) 2,3,4   c) 1,3,5   d) 1,2,4

8. NIDDM
    1. usually occurs before the age of 40
    2. usually occurs after the age of 35
    3. usually requires insulin
    4. can usually be controlled by diet and hypoglycemic agent
    5. occurs more often than IDDM
      a) 2,4,&5   b) 1,2,&3   c) 2,3,4   d) 1,4,&5

9. Hypoglycemic agents
    1. have exactly the same effect as insulin
    2. cannot be used for patients over 40
    3. stimulate the pancreas to produce insulin
    4. are used for NIDDM patients
    5. must be injected into the vascular system
      a) 1,2,&3   b) 1,2,&5   c) 3&4   d) 4&5

10. Diabetic diets based on the Exchange Lists regulate amounts of
    1. carbohydrate   4. fat
    2. kcal   5. fiber
    3. protein
      a) 1,2,3,&5   b) 1,2,3,&4   c) 1,3,4,&5   d) 1,2,3,&5

B. Matching

_____ 1. acidosis	a.	long standing
_____ 2. aspartame	b.	subnormal level of glucose in blood
_____ 3. chronic	c.	artificial sweetener
_____ 4. endogenous insulin	d.	insulin injected into the body
_____ 5. glycosuria	e.	diabetic coma
_____ 6. hyperglycemia	f.	relating to the kidneys
_____ 7. ketonuria	g.	hormone essential for metabolism of glucose
_____ 8. polydipsia	h.	excessive thirst
_____ 9. renal	i.	excessive hunger
_____10. polyuria	j.	excessive production of urine
_____11. exogenous insulin	k.	excessive glucose in the blood
_____12. hypoglycemia	l.	relating to the vascular system
_____13. insulin	m.	insulin produced in the body
_____14. ketones	n.	excessive sugar in the urine
_____15. polyphagia	o.	ketones in the urine
	p.	dismantled parts of fatty acids

References

American Diabetes Association and American Dietetic Association. 1980. *Family Cookbook*. Englewood Cliffs, N.J.: Prentice-Hall Inc.

Bodinski, Lois H. 1982. *The Nurse's Guide to Diet Therapy*. New York: John Wiley & Sons.

U.S. Department of Agriculture. *Composition of Food*. 1963, 1975.

Eschleman, Martin M. 1984. *Introductory Nutrition and Diet Therapy*. Philadelphia: J. B. Lippincott Co.

Krause, Marie V., and L. Kathleen Mahan. 1979. *Food, Nutrition and Diet Therapy*, 6th ed. Philadelphia: W.B. Saunders Co.

Chapter 25

DIETS FOR WEIGHT CONTROL

VOCABULARY

amphetamines	fad diets	jejunoileal bypass
average weight	gastric bypass	normal weight
calipers	hyperthyroidism	obesity
crash reducing	hypothyroidism	overweight
diets	ideal weight	standard weight
desired weight	ileum	underweight
diuretics	jejunum	

OBJECTIVES

After studying this chapter, you should be able to

- Explain the dangers of overweight

- Explain the dangers of underweight

- Identify foods suitable for high-kcal diets and those suitable for low-kcal diets

- Adapt family menus to meet the needs of people on low-kcal or high-kcal diets.

One must understand some commonly used terms before discussing weight control. *Normal weight* can be translated to read *average*, *ideal*, *desired*, or *standard*. It means the weight appropriate for the maintenance of good health. *Overweight* is defined as weight 10—20 percent above average. *Obesity* is defined as excessive body fat, with weight 20 percent above average. *Underweight* is weight 10—15 percent below average. Body weight is composed of fluids, organs, fat, muscle, and bones so there is large variation among people. In addition to height, one's general frame size (small, medium, or large) is a critical factor in determining desired weight. For example,

a 6'2" man with a 44" chest, 36" arms, and 8 1/2" wrists will weigh more than a 6'2" man with a 40" chest, 35" arms, and 7 1/2" wrists because he has more body tissue.

The National Research Council has summarized desirable weights for women and men, using data collected from insurance company statistics on weight as related to longevity. See Table 25-1. Some people may weigh more than is indicated on the tables and still be in good physical condition. Professional football players, because of the amount of muscle they develop, are examples of this. However, when they retire and reduce their physical activity, that same muscle may

Table 25-1 Suggested Desirable Weights for Heights and Ranges for Adult Males and Females

Height[a]		Weight[b]							
		Men				Women			
in.	cm	lb		kg		lb		kg	
58	147	—		—		102	(92–119)	46	(42–54)
60	152	—		—		107	(96–125)	49	(44–57)
62	158	123	(112–141)	56	(51–64)	113	(102–131)	51	(46–59)
64	163	130	(118–148)	59	(54–67)	120	(108–138)	55	(49–63)
66	168	136	(124–156)	62	(56–71)	128	(114–146)	58	(52–66)
68	173	145	(132–166)	66	(60–75)	136	(122–154)	62	(55–70)
70	178	154	(140–174)	70	(64–79)	144	(130–163)	65	(59–74)
72	183	162	(148–184)	74	(67–84)	152	(138–173)	69	(63–79)
74	188	171	(156–194)	78	(71–88)	—		—	
76	193	181	(164–204)	82	(74–93)	—		—	

SOURCE: Bray, 1975
[a]Without shoes.
[b]Without clothes. Average weight ranges in parentheses.

change to fat. If their weight remains the same, they will then be considered overfat because the proportion of fat will have become too high. Some may weigh just what the chart indicates they should and yet be overfat because too great a percentage of the weight is made up of fat.

To measure body fat, an instrument called a *caliper* is used. Because the fat under the skin on the stomach and the upper arm is representative of the percentage of overall body fat, it is usually measured when knowledge of the percentage of body fat is required. If it is more than 1 1/2 inches, one is considered overweight. If it is under 1/2 inch, one is considered underweight.

Generally, it is accepted that if one's weight at the age of 25 is normal, that is the weight one should remain. Being slightly underweight throughout life appears to increase longevity. The final determination of desirable weight depends on common sense.

One can usually see when one is overweight. Table 25-2 lists mean (intermediate point of those surveyed) weights and heights.

OVERWEIGHT AND OBESITY

Overweight is a serious health hazard. It puts extra strain on the heart, lungs, muscles, bones, and joints, and increases the susceptibility to diabetes mellitus and hypertension. It increases surgical risks, shortens the life span, and causes emotional problems.

Causes

The most common cause of overweight is energy imbalance. People eat more than they need. Excess weight may accumulate during and after middle age because people reduce their activity and metabolism slows with age. Consequently weight accumulates unless kcal

Table 25-2 Mean Heights and Weights

Category	Age (years)	Weight (kg)	Weight (lb)	Height (cm)	Height (in.)
Infants	0.0–0.5	6	13	60	24
	0.5–1.0	9	20	71	28
Children	1–3	13	29	90	35
	4–6	20	44	112	44
	7–10	28	62	132	52
Males	11–14	45	99	157	62
	15–18	66	145	176	69
	19–22	70	154	177	70
	23–50	70	154	178	70
	51–75	70	154	178	70
	76+	70	154	178	70
Females	11–14	46	101	157	62
	15–18	55	120	163	64
	19–22	55	120	163	64
	23–50	55	120	163	64
	51–75	55	120	163	64
	76+	55	120	163	64

Source: Food and Nutrition Board, National Academy of Sciences—National Research Council, 1980

intake is reduced. A thyroid gland dysfunction called *Hypothyroidism* is rarely the cause of obesity.

Hypothyroidism is a condition in which the basal metabolism rate is lowered, consequently the number of kcal needed for energy is reduced. Unless corrected, this can result in excess weight.

Dietary Treatment of Obesity

Obviously, if the most common cause of overweight is overeating, the solution is to reduce one's food intake. This is seldom easy. To accomplish it, a weight-reduction (low-kcal) diet must be undertaken. For the diet to be effective, one must have a *genuine* desire to lose weight.

The best weight-reduction diet is the normal diet planned around the Basic Four food groups, but with the kcal content controlled. If necessary, its consistency can also be adapted to meet individual needs by using a food processor or a blender.

A reduction of 3500 kcal will result in a weight loss of one pound. Physicians frequently recommend that no more than two pounds of weight be lost in one week. To accomplish this, one must reduce one's weekly kcal intake by 7,000, or daily intake by 1,000. Diets should not be reduced below 1000 kcal per day or the dieter will not receive the required nutrients. The diet should consist of 15—20 percent protein, 45—50 percent carbohydrate, and 30—35 percent fat, in other words, normal proportions of nutrients, but in reduced amounts. The number of meals and snacks each day is not important so long as the total number of kcal is not exceeded.

There is no magic way of losing weight and maintaining the reduced weight, but there is a key to it. That key is revised eating habits. In fact, unless eating habits are truly revised, it is very likely that the lost weight will be regained once the weight reduction has been accomplished because at that point the dieter may be euphoric about the weight loss and forget its cost. The cost of slimness is eating less than one might prefer.

The dieter must learn to "eat lean". It is useful to learn the kcal values of favorite foods, and to consider this before indulging. Kcal counting is not necessary, however, if one learns a basic list of foods that are allowed on low-kcal diets because of their low-kcal values, and another list of foods that should be avoided because of their high-kcal values. The high-kcal foods should be avoided during the diet, and except for very special occasions, after the diet.

Table 25-3

Foods Allowed in a Low-Kcal Diet	Foods to Avoid on a Low-kcal Diet	
skim milk, buttermilk	cream soups	nuts
cottage cheese and other skim milk cheeses	cream sauces	jellies/jams
eggs, except prepared with fat	cream in any form	fatty meats
lean beef, lamb, veal, pork, chicken, turkey, fish	gravies	salad dressing
clear soups	rich desserts	cakes
whole grain or enriched bread as allowed by doctor	sweet drinks/sodas	cookies
vegetables should be low in carbohydrate	alcoholic beverages	pastries
fresh fruits and those canned without sugar	candy	oily fish
coffee or tea, without milk and sugar		whole milk
salt, pepper, herbs, garlic, and onions		

In addition, one should remember that the following foods must be used very judiciously:

- butter or margarine—one tablespoon contains 100 kcal
- sugar—one teaspoon contains 16 kcal
- crackers—kcal contents vary, but may run from 15 for a soda cracker to 50 for a graham cracker

Substitutions of foods with very low kcal contents should be made for those with high kcal contents whenever possible. The following are examples:
- skim milk for whole milk
- yogurt for sour cream
- lemon juice and herbs for heavy salad dressings
- fruit for rich appetizers or desserts
- consomme or boullion instead of cream soups

Cooking methods should be considered. Broiling, baking, roasting, poaching, or boiling are the preferred methods because they do not require the addition of fat, as frying does. Skimming of fat from the tops of soups, meat dishes, and vegetables reduces their fat content as does trimming fat from meats before cooking. The addition of extra butter or margarine to foods should be avoided. Water-pack canned foods rather than those in oil or syrup should be used.

Generally, "diet" or "dietetic" foods are not advisable. Frequently their kcal contents are not much different from the same food in a normal pack, although they are more expensive. Diet sodas may pacify the appetite for some dieters, but may cause diarrhea. Until there is certainty that the artificial sweeteners are not dangerous to health, their use seems unwise.

Some foods that may be eaten with relative disregard for kcal content (provided they are served without additional calories) are listed in Table 25-4.

Patience and encouragement are needed throughout the ordeal of the diet. Temptation is everywhere, and the dieter should be forewarned. Just one piece of chocolate cake could set the diet back for half a day (400—500 kcal) and lower resistance to future temptation. Breaking the diet one day will make it seem easy to break it a second day, and so on. Fresh vegetables and drinks of water may be used to harmlessly prevent or assuage the hunger pains that are bound to appear. A short

Table 25-4 Low-Kcal Foods

black coffee	cauliflower
plain tea or tea with lemon	broccoli
cantaloupe	celery
strawberries	cucumbers
lettuce	red and green peppers
cabbage	bean sprouts
asparagus	mushrooms
tomatoes	spinach
zucchini	

walk or a few minutes of exercise may help to turn the dieter's thoughts from food.

Exercise

Exercise is an excellent adjunct to any weight loss program because it helps tone the muscles. Rarely can it replace the actual diet. The dieter should be made aware of the number of kcal burned by specific exercises so as to avoid overeating after the workout. See Table 2-2, giving numbers of kcal required for specific activities.

Fad Diets

Many of the countless fad reducing diets regularly published in magazines and books are *crash-reducing diets*. This means they are intended to cause a very rapid rate of weight reduction. Often fad diets require the purchase of expensive foods. Others are part of a weight loss plan including exercise with special equipment. Expensive food items and equipment can add to the burden of dieting.

A crash diet usually does result in an initial rapid weight loss. However, the weight loss is thought to be caused by a loss of body water rather than body fat. Sudden weight loss of this type is followed by a plateau period, that is, a period in which weight does not decrease. Disillusionment is apt to occur during this period and this may cause the dieter to go on an "eating binge." This can result in regaining the weight that was lost and sometimes more.

Some popular reducing diets severely limit the foods allowed, providing a real danger of nutrient deficiencies over time, and their restricted nature makes them very boring. Some provide too much cholesterol and fat, contributing to atherosclerosis. Some contain an excess of protein, which puts too great a demand on the kidneys. The powdered varieties of weight-loss diets available are not only expensive and inconvenient (if one is not at home to prepare them), they can be life threatening if they fail to supply sufficient potassium for the heart.

These diets ultimately fail because they defeat the dual purpose of the dieter, which is to lose weight and prevent its returning. To accomplish this, eating habits must be changed and crash diets do not do this.

Surgical Treatment of Obesity

When obesity becomes morbid (life endangering), and the individual lacks the self-control to reduce weight by dieting, surgery may be indicated. Two of the surgical procedures used for this include the *jejunoileal bypass* and the *gastric bypass*. In the former, the *jejunum* (the middle section of the small intestine) is surgically attached to a very small section of the *ileum* (the last part of the small intestine). This results in fewer nutrients being absorbed and consequent loss of weight.

Some obese people believe that such a procedure would be their salvation, believing that following it, they could eat as much as they wanted and still lose weight. It may not be salvation. Common complications of this type of surgery include diarrhea and consequent electrolyte and fluid imbalances, liver

Table 25-5 Sample Menu for a Low Calorie Diet—1200 Calories

Breakfast	Dinner	Lunch or Supper
Orange Juice (1/2 cup = 55 cal.)	Half Grapefruit (45 cal.)	Sliced Chicken (1/2 breast = 3 oz. at 155 cal.)
Poached Egg (80 cal.)	Lean Roast Beef (3oz. = 125 cal.)	Asparagus on Lettuce (4 spears = 10 cal. + lettuce leaves at 5 cal.) with
Whole Wheat Toast (1 sl. = 60 cal.)	Baked Potato (90 cal.)	Cottage Cheese (2 oz. = 50 cal.)
Butter (1 tsp. = 33 cal.)	Cooked Carrots (1/2 cup = 23 cal.)	Bread (1 sl. = 60 cal.)
Skim Milk (1/2 cup = 45 cal.)	Lettuce and Tomato Salad (1/8 head lettuce = 8 cal. 1/2 tomato = 20 cal.)	Butter (1 tsp. = 33 cal.)
Black Coffee	Bread (1/2 sl. = 30 cal.)	Cantaloupe (1/2 melon = 45 cal.)
	Butter (1 tsp. = 33 cal.)	Black Coffee or Tea
	Strawberries (1 cup fresh = 55 cal.)	
	Skim Milk (1/2 cup = 45 cal.)	
	Black Coffee or Tea	

problems, kidney stones, and bone disease—the last probably caused by reduced absorption of minerals and vitamins.

The gastric bypass is a procedure in which the stomach is stapled so that only a part of it is attached to the jejunum where absorption occurs. This reduced stomach capacity reduces the amounts of food that can be eaten. Post surgery complications (nausea and vomiting) are fewer than with jejunoileal bypass surgery, but there is comparatively less weight lost.

Pharmaceutical Treatment of Obesity

Amphetamines (pep pills) have been used in the treatment of obesity because they depress the appetite. However, it has been learned that their effectiveness is reduced within a relatively short time, and they can become habit-forming. They are rarely prescribed now.

Thyroid hormone has been used also, but it is considered to be dangerous to medicate an otherwise healthy thyroid gland.

Some people believe that *diuretics* (medications that cause frequent urination) and laxatives promote weight loss. They do, but only of water. They do not cause a reduction of body fat, which is what the dieter is really seeking. An excess of either could be dangerous because of possible upsets in fluid and electrolyte balance. They should not be used on any frequent or regular basis without the supervision of a physician.

UNDERWEIGHT

Dangers

Underweight may cause complications of pregnancy and various nutritional deficiencies. It is thought to lower one's resistance to infections and, if carried to the extreme, can cause death.

Causes

Underweight may be caused by inadequate consumption of food because of depression, anorexia nervosa, or poverty. It may also be caused by excessive activity, the tissue wasting of certain diseases, poor absorption of nutrients, infection, or *hyperthyroidism* (A condition in which the basal metabolism rate is increased and consequently the number of kcal needed for energy is increased. Unless corrected, it results in weight loss.).

Treatment

Underweight is treated by a high-kcal diet, or by a high-kcal diet combined with psychological counseling if the condition is psychological in origin as, for example, in depression or anorexia nervosa. In many cases a high-kcal diet will be met with resistance. It can be as difficult for an underweight person to gain weight as it is for an overweight person to lose it.

The diet should be based on the Basic Four food groups and can be easily adapted from the regular, family menus, or to a soft textured diet. The total number of kcal prescribed per day will vary from person to person, depending upon the person's activity, age, size, sex, and physical condition.

If the individual is to gain one pound a week, 3500 kcal in addition to the individual's basic normal weekly kcal requirement are prescribed. This means an extra 500 kcal must be taken in each day. If two pounds of weight gain per week are required, an additional 7000 kcal each week, or an addition of 1000 kcal each day are necessary. This diet cannot be immediately accepted at full kcal value. Time will be needed to gradually increase the daily kcal value. In this diet, there is an increased intake of foods rich in carbohydrates, some fats, and proteins. Vitamins and minerals are supplied in adequate amounts. If there are deficiencies of some vitamins and minerals, supplements are prescribed.

Nearly all nutritious foods are allowed in the high-kcal diet, but easily digested foods (carbohydrates) are recommended. Because an excess of fat can be distasteful and spoil the appetite, fatty foods must be used with discretion. Fried foods are not recommended. Bulky foods should be used sparingly. Bulk takes up stomach space that could be better used for more concentrated, higher kcal foods.

Those requiring this diet frequently have poor appetites so meals should be made

Table 25-6 Sample Menu for a High-K cal Diet—3000 Calories

Breakfast	Dinner	Lunch or Supper
Orange Juice (1 cup = 110 cal.)	Sirloin Steak (4 oz. = 230 cal.)	Grapefruit Juice (1/2 cup = 50 cal.)
Oatmeal (1 cup = 130 cal.) with Milk and Sugar (1/2 cup milk = 80 cal. +2 tbsp. sugar = 90 cal.)	Baked Potato (90 cal.) with Butter* (1 tbsp. = 100 cal.)	Lamb Chop (150 cal.)
Soft Cooked Egg (80 cal.)	Lima Beans (1/2 cup = 95 cal.)	Mashed Potatoes (3/4 cup = 145 cal.)
Bacon* (2 sl. = 90 cal.)	Lettuce and Tomato Salad (1/8 head lettuce = 8 cal. +1/2 tomato at 20 cal.)	Cooked Carrots (1/2 cup = 23 cal.)
Whole Wheat Toast (1 sl. = 60 cal.) with Butter* (2 tsp. = 66 cal.)	Salad Dressing* (1 tbsp. commercial "French" type = 65 cal.)	Celery-Apple Salad (1 stalk celery = 5 cal. +1/2 apple at 35 cal. +1 tbsp. mayonnaise at 100 cal.)
Coffee with Milk and Sugar (2 tbsp. milk = 20 cal. +1 tbsp. sugar = 45 cal.)	Roll and Butter (200 cal.)	Bread and Butter (125 cal.)
	Chocolate Ice Cream (1/2 cup = 160 cal.)	Baked Apple (apple = 70 cal. +2 tbsp. sugar at 90 cal.)
	Coffee	Milk (160 cal.)
		Coffee or Tea

Snack		Snack	
1/2 cup Milk (80 cal.) 1 cookie (100 cal.)		1/2 cup Milk (80 cal.) 2 Graham Crackers (55 cal.)	

*If patient tolerates the fat

especially appetizing. Favorite foods should be served, and portions of all foods should be small to avoid discouraging the patients. Many of the extra calories needed may be consumed as snacks between meals, unless these snacks reduce the patient's appetite for meals and consequently reduce the total kcal intake. In some cases, the patient may consume more calories each day if the number of meals is reduced, thereby increasing the appetite for each meal served. When the causes of underweight are psychological, therapy is required before the diet is begun, and the diet counselor and therapist may well need to consult one another before and during treatment. Foods to be avoided in a high-kcal diet are foods the patient dislikes, fatty foods, and bulky, low-calorie foods.

SUMMARY

Excessive weight endangers health and should be lost by the use of a restricted-kcal diet based on the Basic Four food groups. Such a diet helps the dieter revise eating habits and avoid regaining the lost weight. Excess weight is usually caused by energy imbalance. Exercise is beneficial to weight loss regimes, but rarely can replace the restricted-kcal diet. Fad diets are expensive, boring, and conducive to nutritional deficiencies. They ultimately fail because they do not revise eating habits.

Underweight is also dangerous to health and psychological counseling as well as a high-kcal diet may be required for proper treatment.

Case Study—Weight Control

Marilyn E. was finding it increasingly difficult to breathe after any sort of exertion. Her knees were giving her a great deal of pain and she was ashamed of her shape. She was 5'6", of medium build, and weighed 180 pounds. Her friend convinced her to see a doctor. The doctor examined her and advised her to lose 60 pounds. He told her that her breathing would be easier and her knees should give her no trouble if she were lighter. He put her on a low-kcal diet.

Marilyn could not understand why she was so heavy. She never ate breakfast—"just coffee and Danish after I get to the office". Furthermore, she did not always eat lunch, but usually had coffee and doughnuts with the people in her office around 4 P.M. Dinner was usually a sandwich at the local coffee shop where they baked delicious pies. She admitted to sometimes having more than one slice. She said she seldom snacked on anything except cookies and soda. Marilyn's favorite activity was watching T.V.

Case Study Questions

1. How many pounds a week has Marilyn probably been told to lose?
2. How long should she expect this to take?
3. How many kcal each day will she have to omit from her diet?
4. Approximately how many kcal did Marilyn probably ingest each day on her pre-diet regime?
5. What should Marilyn's first step be in beginning her diet?
6. When Marilyn visits her parents, they always have her favorite meal—leg of lamb with gravy, mashed potatoes, lima beans, coleslaw and apple pie with whipped cream and pecans. How many kcal would an average-sized meal of these foods total? What can Marilyn say to her parents?
7. How can Marilyn improve her breakfast habits?
8. How can Marilyn improve her lunch habits? She does not feel she has a great deal of money.
9. What should Marilyn be told about her evening meal? Her snacks?
10. What snacks could Marilyn have on her low-kcal diet? Why?
11. Will Marilyn ever be able to eat her favorite apple pie again?
12. Marilyn admits that while she likes meats and vegetables, she does not know how to cook. What advice can she be given?
13. Plan a week's menu for Marilyn who is on a 1200-kcal diet. What questions should Marilyn be asked before the menus are planned? Why?

Discussion Topics

1. Discuss *overweight*, *obesity*, and *underweight*. Tell how someone may be overweight according to the height/weight charts and still be considered to be in good physical condition. What factors contribute to the determination of one's correct weight?
2. What are some causes of overweight? Discuss why some people eat more than they need. Discuss how this can be prevented or changed.
3. Explain why revised eating habits are essential to an effective weight loss program.
4. Describe three cooking methods that are preferred for people on low-kcal diets, and explain why they are preferred.
5. Name ten foods that should be avoided during a weight-loss program. Tell why.
6. Name ten foods that may be used without concern as to kcal during a weight loss program. Explain why.
7. In addition to its high kcal content, how could a slice of chocolate cake be detrimental to a weight-loss diet?
8. Describe the use of exercise during a weight-loss program. Could it be used in lieu of the diet? Why?
9. Describe one or two popular reducing diets. Could such a diet have any effect on the nutrition of those people who subscribe to it? If so, what? Ask if anyone in the class has used such a diet. If so, ask that person to describe the diet, the physical effects felt during the diet, and the ultimate result.
10. Explain why a high-kcal diet could be unpleasant for a patient.
11. Discuss the causes and dangers of underweight.

Suggested Activities

1. Using table A-7, The Nutritive Values of Foods, in the Appendix, look for caloric values of 10 familiar foods. Make two lists. On the left, list which of the ten foods would be suitable for a high-calorie diet. On the right, list those foods suitable for a low-calorie diet.
2. Make a list of foods eaten yesterday. Circle those foods that would not be suitable for a low-calorie diet. Explain why.
3. Find recipes that are suitable for the high-calorie diet and others that are suitable for the low-calorie diet. Add these to the special diet recipe file.

4. Adapt a sample menu for the 1200-calorie diet in this chapter to make it suitable for a regular 2400-calorie diet. Adapt it for a high-calorie diet (3000 calories). Use table A-7 for caloric values of foods.

5. Plan a day's menu for a 1200-calorie diet. Compare menus with other class members and correct them if necessary. Adapt them for a 3,000-kcal diet.

6. Prepare at least one of the meals on the planned menu, and evaluate it in terms of nutritive content, flavor, aroma, color, shape, appearance, texture, and satiety value, as well as kcal value.

Review

A. Multiple Choice. Select the *letter* that precedes the best answer.

1. The general type of foods that should be avoided in the high-kcal diet are
   - a. fatty foods
   - b. foods the patient likes
   - c. breads and cereals
   - d. coffee and tea

2. In the high-kcal diet, the energy value
   - a. is increased
   - b. is decreased
   - c. is reduced to minimal levels
   - d. remains the same as on the regular diet

3. The low-kcal diet may be prescribed for
   - a. obesity
   - b. anorexia nervosa
   - c. hyperthyroidism
   - d. severe allergies

4. In the low kcal diet, the energy value
   - a. remains the same as for the regular diet
   - b. is decreased
   - c. is increased
   - d. should equal that of the clear-liquid diet

5. A proper weight reduction plan allows for loss of
   - a. 1 to 2 pounds per day
   - b. 1 to 2 pounds per week
   - c. 3 to 5 pounds per week
   - d. 15 to 20 pounds per month

6. Popular crash-reducing diets
   - a. are always effective and totally harmless
   - b. are very useful for teenagers
   - c. result in a slow, even loss of weight
   - d. are potentially hazardous

7. Normal weight may be
   a. defined as ideal
   b. considered average
   c. greater than the amounts indicated on the height/weight charts in some cases
   d. all of the above

8. A caliper is used
   a. to measure the amount of weight to be lost
   b. to determine the percentage of body fat
   c. to determine the percentage of muscle tissue
   d. only in cases of gross obesity

9. The most common cause of overweight is
   a. hypothyroidism   c. energy imbalance
   b. hyperthyroidism   d. all of the above

10. The dysfunction of the thyroid gland in which the basal metabolism rate is lowered and the need for kcal is reduced is called
    a. hypothyroidism   c. energy imbalance
    b. hyperthyroidism   d. none of the above

11. The dysfunction of the thyroid gland in which the basal metabolism rate is raised and the need for kcal is increased is called
    a. hypothyroidism   c. energy imbalance
    b. hyperthyroidism   d. either a or b

12. To lose two pounds per week, one's weekly kcal intake must be reduced by
    a. 500   c. 3500
    b. 1500   d. 7000

13. To lose one pound per week, one's weekly kcal intake must be reduced by
    a. 500   c. 3500
    b. 1500   d. 7000

14. The "key" to losing weight and maintaining the reduced weight is
    a. skipping lunch
    b. fasting one day each week
    c. revised eating habits
    d. assiduously counting kcal each meal

15. Strawberries, buttermilk, poached egg, and whole wheat toast would
    a. be allowed on a kcal-restricted diet
    b. not be allowed on a low-kcal diet
    c. constitute an excellent breakfast for someone on a high-kcal diet
    d. not be a nutritious breakfast for someone on a weight-controlled diet

16. Baking, roasting, broiling, boiling, and poaching are recommended for
   a. low-kcal diets only
   b. high-kcal diets only
   c. both high- and low-kcal diets
   d. none of the above
17. Large green salads with creamy dressings are
   a. recommended for low-kcal diets
   b. recommended for high-kcal diets
   c. recommended for either low- or high-kcal diets
   d. not recommended for either low- or high-kcal diets
18. Fad diets are not recommended as reducing diets because they
   a. can create nutritional deficiencies
   b. can contribute to atherosclerosis
   c. do not alter eating habits
   d. may be responsible for all of the above
19. The jejunoileal bypass
   a. prevents food from reaching the large intestine
   b. reduces the stomach capacity
   c. reduces the absorption capacity of the small intestine
   d. is highly recommended for obese patients
20. Amphetamines are
   a. an excellent method of maintaining a depressed appetite
   b. interchangeable with diuretics
   c. frequently used today
   d. dangerously habit forming
B. Complete the following statements.
   1. The high-calorie diet is one in which the energy value is _____.
   2. The patient requiring a _____ calorie diet usually has a poor appetite; therefore, serving sizes should be _____.
   3. When the thyroid gland is overactive and raises the metabolism rate, the condition is called _____.
   4. The diet ordered for a patient with an overactive thyroid gland is the _____.
   5. Bulky foods such as fresh fruits and vegetables are usually advisable for _____ calorie diets.
   6. A type of milk recommended for patients on the low-calorie diet is _____ or _____.
   7. Steak, lima beans, and ice cream are examples of food allowed on the _____ calorie diet.
   8. Lean meat, strawberries, and skim milk are examples of foods recommended for the _____ calorie diet.
   9. Underweight caused by anorexia nervosa will probably require _____ in addition to a high-kcal diet.

10. The surgical procedure that is used to reduce stomach capacity is called the _____.

References

Bland, Jeffrey. 1983. *Medical Applications of Clinical Nutrition*. New Canaan, Ct.: Keats Publishing Co.

Berland, Theodore. 1980. *Rating the Diets*. Consumer Guide.

Corbin, Cheryl. 1980. *Nutrition*. New York: Holt Rinehart & Winston.

Eschelman, Marian M. 1984. *Introductory Nutrition and Diet Therapy*. Philadelphia: J.B. Lippincott Company.

Greenwood, M.R.C., ed. 1983. *Obesity*. New York: Churchill Livingstone.

Long, Patricia J., and Barbara Shannon. 1983. *Focus on Nutrition*. Englewood Cliffs, N.J.: Prentice Hall Inc.

Luke, Barbara. 1984. *Principles of Nutrition and Diet Therapy*. Boston: Little Brown & Co.

U.S. Department of Agriculture. 1963, 1975. *Composition of Foods*.

Chapter 26

DIETS FOR DISEASES OF THE CARDIO-VASCULAR SYSTEM

VOCABULARY

angina pectoris
asymptomatic
arteriosclerosis
atherosclerosis
brine
cardiac disease
cardiovascular
  disease
cerebral accident
cholesterol
compensated heart
  disease
congestive heart
  failure

coronary occlusion
decompensated
  heart disease
diuretics
edema
endocardium
fatty acids
hyperlipidemia
hypertension
hypokalemia
intima
lipoproteins
lumen
MSG

myocardial
  infarction
myocardium
pericardium
polyunsaturated
  fats
saturated fats
sodium chloride
triglycerides
unpalatable
vascular disease

OBJECTIVES

After studying this chapter, you should be able to

- Explain why sodium is limited in some cardiovascular conditions

- Explain why cholesterol is limited in some cardiovascular conditions

- Identify foods that are limited or prohibited in low-sodium diets

- Identify foods suitable for a low-cholesterol diet

- Adapt family meals to meet the requirements of heart patients on low-cholesterol or on low-sodium diets

- Explain why some heart patients are put on kcal-restricted diets

Cardiovascular disease affects the heart and blood vessels. It is the leading cause of death and permanent disability in the United States today. The grief and economic distress it causes are staggering. Organizations, especially the American Heart Association, are promoting programs designed to detect and treat cardiovascular disease in its early stages to reduce its devastating impact on society.

Heart disease exists in several forms. *Primary cardiac disease* is caused by congenital deformities of the heart that can often be surgically corrected. *Secondary cardiac disease* is caused by infections such as rheumatic fever or syphilis, or by vascular disease such as arteriosclerosis or hypertension.

Cardiac disease may be acute (sudden) or chronic (of long standing). *Myocardial infarction* (heart attack) is an example of the acute form. Chronic heart disease causes an increased loss of heart function over time. If the heart can maintain circulation, the disease is classified as *compensated*. Compensation may require that the heart beat unusually fast; consequently the heart enlarges. If the heart cannot maintain circulation, the classification is *decompensated*. The heart muscle (*myocardium*), the valves, the lining (*endocardium*), the outer covering (*pericardium*), or its blood vessels may be affected by the disease.

MYOCARDIAL INFARCTION

Myocardial infarction is caused by the blockage of a coronary artery supplying blood to the heart. The heart tissue denied blood because of this blockage, dies.

Following the attack, the patient is given nothing by mouth until the physician evaluates her or his condition. A liquid diet of 500—800 kcal is recommended for the first 24 hours. Following that, meals for the next five to ten days are small and frequent, with a kcal total of 1000—1200. Meals consist of 45 percent carbohydrate, 20 percent protein, and 30—35 percent fat, mainly polyunsaturated. Sodium may be limited, depending upon the patient's condition. Foods should not be extremely hot or cold. They should be easy to chew and digest, and contain little roughage. Anything containing caffeine is usually prohibited because caffeine increases the heart rate. After recovery, the patient may be put on a sodium-restricted, fat-controlled, or a low-kcal diet, depending on her or his condition.

CONGESTIVE HEART FAILURE

Congestive heart failure is an example of decompensation, or severe heart disease. In this situation, when damage is extreme and the heart cannot provide adequate circulation, the amount of oxygen taken in and carbon dioxide released is insufficient for body needs. Shortness of breath and chest pain occur with activity. Also, because of the reduced circulation, tissues retain fluid that would normally be carried off by the blood. Sodium builds up, and more fluid is retained, resulting in *edema*. This adds to the heart's burden. In advanced cases when edema reaches the lungs, death can ensue. Diuretics to aid in the excretion of water and sodium, and a sodium-restricted diet may be prescribed. The patient's blood potassium will then be carefully watched to prevent *hypokalemia* (low blood potassium) which can upset the heartbeat. This can occur during treatment with diuretics. Fruits can help counter this situation, especially oranges, bananas, and prunes because they are excellent sources of potassium and contain only negligible amounts of sodium.

HYPERTENSION

Hypertension is abnormally high blood pressure. It is considered a symptom of other vascular or kidney disease. It has been estimated that as many as 20 percent of U.S. adults suffer from it, with members of the black race more prone to it than others. Sufferers may be *asymptomatic* (without symptoms) or there may be symptoms including headache, dizziness, edema, fatigue and fainting. It is treated with anti-hypertensive drugs, diuretics, and diet therapy.

Heredity is a predisposing factor. Relatives of people with hypertension should have their blood pressure checked regularly. Obesity is also a predisposing factor in hypertension, and weight reduction usually reduces the blood pressure. Consequently, patients are sometimes placed on weight reduction diets. Excessive use of ordinary table salt is also considered a contributory factor in hypertension. Table salt is over 40 percent sodium, a mineral essential in regulating the water balance in the body. When sodium is consumed in normal quantities by healthy people, it is beneficial. However, when this balance is upset, and sodium and fluid collect in body tissue causing edema, extra pressure is placed on the blood vessels. To alleviate this condition, a sodium-restricted diet, probably accompanied by diuretics, is prescribed. When the sodium content in the diet is reduced, the water and salts in the tissues flow back into the blood to be excreted by the kidneys. In this way, the edema is relieved. The amount of sodium to be restricted is determined by the physician on the basis of the patient's condition.

Dietary Treatment of Cardiovascular Conditions Causing Edema

The sodium-restricted diet is a regular diet in which the amount of sodium is limited. Nutritionists estimate that the average person on an unrestricted diet consumes about 6000 milligrams of sodium each day. This is greatly in excess of bodily needs, which are thought to be 400 mg. Blood pressure is usually reduced in hypertensive people when their salt intake is restricted because fluid retention is reduced.

Foods that are relatively low in sodium are used. They are prepared and served without salt or with very little salt added. Foods that contain relatively large amounts of sodium are allowed in very limited quantities or omitted entirely. It is not possible to have a diet totally free of salt since foods and water naturally contain sodium. Meats, fish, poultry, dairy products, and eggs all contain substantial amounts of sodium naturally. Cereals, vegetables, and fruits contain very small amounts of sodium assuming no additions of sodium-containing products.

Sodium is often added to foods during their processing and cooking. The food label usually indicates the addition of sodium to commerical food products. The following sodium compounds are frequently added to foods.[1]

- *Salt* (sodium chloride)—used in cooking or at the table, and in canning and processing.
- *Monosodium glutamate* (called MSG, and sold under several brand names)—a seasoning used in home, restaurant, and hotel cooking, and in many packaged, canned, and frozen foods.
- *Baking powder*—used to leaven quick breads and cakes.
- *Baking soda* (sodium bicarbonate)—used to leaven breads and cakes; sometimes added to vegetables in cooking or used as an "alkalizer" for indigestion.
- *Brine* (table salt and water)—used in processing foods to inhibit growth of bacteria; in cleaning or blanching vegetables and fruits; in freezing and canning

[1]"Your Mild Sodium-Restricted Diet." American Heart Association (New York, 1969), pp. 8–9

certain foods; and for flavor, as in corned beef, pickles, and sauerkraut.

- *Di-sodium phosphate*—present in some quick-cooking cereals and processed cheeses.
- *Sodium alginate*—used in many chocolate milks and ice creams for smooth texture.
- *Sodium benzoate*—used as a preservative in many condiments such as relishes, sauces, and salad dressings.
- *Sodium hydroxide*—used in food processing to soften and loosen skins of ripe olives, hominy, and certain fruits and vegetables.
- *Sodium propionate*—used in pasteurized cheeses and in some breads and cakes to inhibit growth of mold.
- *Sodium sulfite*—used to bleach certain fruits in which an artificial color is desired, such as maraschino cherries and glazed or crystallized fruit; also used as a preservative in some dried fruit, such as prunes.

Since the amount of sodium in tap water varies in different communities, the local department of health or heart association should be consulted if this information is needed.

Some medicines contain sodium. A patient on a sodium-restricted diet should always get the doctor's permission before using any medication or salt substitute.

The American Heart Association has devised three sodium-restricted diets: (1) the mild sodium-restricted diet, (2) the 1000 milligram sodium diet and (3) the 500 milligram sodium diet. In these diets, foods are divided into seven lists. Each list includes a specific group of foods as shown in table 26-1. The foods on each of these lists are listed as

Table 26-1 Sodium-Restricted Diet Lists

Lists 1 and 1A: Milk
List 2: Vegetables
List 3: Fruits
List 4: Bread
List 5: Meat
List 6: Fat
List 7: Free Choice

units, as are the foods allowed on the diabetic diet lists discussed in chapter 24.

In any particular diet, a specified number of units is allowed from each list and arranged into personally planned menus. The units are carefully calculated so that each unit in any specific list has the same number of calories and the same amounts of carbohydrates, fats, and proteins as any other unit in that list. It is important that the patient use the exact number of units from each list on the diet that his physician prescribes.

Each of the low-sodium diets planned by the American Heart Association is further subdivided into the 1200-calorie diet, the 1800-calorie diet, and the unrestricted-calorie diet. The doctor decides which one of these diets is best suited for the patient.

The Mild Sodium-Restricted Diet

On the mild sodium-restricted diet, the patient may use approximately half the salt previously used. This is assuming that the patient uses the average amount of added table salt in her or his diet. Salt may not be added to canned or processed foods that have already been salted during preparation. Baking soda may be used only in baking and not in cooking

Table 26-2 Sample Menu for the 1800-Calorie, Mild Sodium-Restricted Diet

Breakfast	Lunch	Dinner
2 Medium Prunes with 2 tbsp. Juice 3/4 cup Puffed Wheat 1 cup Milk 1 slice Toast 1 small pat Butter Coffee or Tea as desired	2 oz. Broiled Liver Baked Acorn Squash with 1 small pat Butter Cabbage Slaw with Caraway Seeds, Green Pepper and Vinegar 2 medium Muffins 1 small pat Butter Apricot Bread Pudding made with 1 slice Bread, 1/4 cup Milk, 4 dried Apricot halves, 1 small pat Butter Coffee or Tea as desired	Baked Casserole of Beef with Whipped Potato Topping made with 3 oz. cooked Beef, 1/2 cup broth from Beef, 1/2 cup Potato Green Beans Tomato and Cucumber Salad on Lettuce Leaf with 1 Tbsp. French Dressing* 2 medium Rolls 1 small pat Butter* 1/2 Grapefruit Coffee or Tea as desired
Mid-morning snack	**Mid-afternoon snack**	**Evening snack**
1/2 cup Milk	1 small Orange	1 small sliced Banana* with 1/4 cup Milk

*selected as free choice

vegetables or relieving indigestion. Very salty foods such as pickles, olives, ham, canned soups, and meats should be avoided.

The sample menu in table 26-2 is taken from the booklet, "Your Mild Sodium-Restricted Diet," published by the American Heart Association (1969).

The 1000 Milligram Sodium Diet

The patient on the 1000 milligram sodium diet may not consume more than 1000 milligrams of sodium daily. The diet is calculated so that half the sodium allowed is found in the foods selected and the other half (1/4 teaspoon) comes from the salt that the patient adds to food. It is important that the sodium content of the drinking water be included in the calculations for this diet.

Canned vegetables and vegetable juices must be low-sodium dietetic. The American Heart Association suggests that the patient have an individual salt shaker and that 1/4 teaspoon of salt be measured into it each day.

Baked products must not include regular baking powder or baking soda (sodium bicarbonate). Appropriate substitutions are 1 1/2 teaspoons low-sodium baking powder for 1 teaspoon regular baking powder and equal amounts of potassium bicarbonate for baking soda.

The 500 Milligram Sodium Diet

The 500 milligram sodium diet is the most restrictive of the three low-sodium diets. In some cases, however, even this diet allows the patient too much sodium. If this is the case, the patient may be advised to follow a 250 milligram sodium diet. When the 250 milligram sodium diet is ordered, the American Heart Association advises using the 500 milligram diet but with the substitution of low-sodium milk for regular milk.

Because of the relatively high sodium content of milk and meat, only two milk units and five meat units are allowed daily. Canned vegetables and vegetable juices must be low-sodium dietetic. Baked products must not include common baking powder or baking soda. If tap water contains more than 5 milligrams sodium per 8-ounce cup, the patient must use distilled water for cooking and drinking.

Adjustment to Sodium Restriction

Sodium-restricted diets range from "different" to "tasteless" because most people are accustomed to salt in their food. It may be difficult to understand the necessity of following such a diet, particularly if it must be followed for the remainder of one's lifetime. Cheerfulness, tact, and understanding are essential in impressing the patient with the importance of the diet. For variety, there are numerous herbs, spices, and flavorings that are allowed on sodium-restricted diets. Salt substitutes and low-sodium dietetic foods are available. The patient must understand, however, that these should be used only with the approval of the physician.

ATHEROSCLEROSIS

Arteriosclerosis is the general term for vascular disease in which arteries "harden" or become thickened, making the passage of blood difficult and sometimes impossible. *Atherosclerosis* is the form of arteriosclerosis that occurs most frequently in developed countries. It affects the inner lining of arteries (the *intima*) where deposits of lipoproteins and other fatty materials build up over time, thickening and weakening artery walls. These deposits are called *plaque*. Plaque deposits gradually reduce the size of the *lumen* (tube area) of the artery, and consequently the amount of blood flow. The heart, like all muscles, reacts with pain to an inadequate blood supply. Such a cardiac reaction is called *angina pectoris* and should be considered a warning. When the flow of blood is stopped in a coronary artery because of a thickened artery wall, *coronary occlusion* (blood clot) occurs, and myocardial infarction results. If this occurs in the brain, *cerebral accident* (stroke) occurs.

Studies indicate that *cholesterol* in the diet is related to coronary artery disease. Cholesterol is a necessary part of body cells and a component of fats. The human body produces it. It is also found in animal food products. Cholesterol is stored in the liver and is carried by the blood to the cells as needed. It is known that dietary cholesterol and the type of fatty acids (saturated or polyunsaturated) affect *hyperlipidemia*, which is an increased concentration of blood lipids, especially cholesterol and triglycerides (Triglycerides are combinations of fatty acids and glycerol.). Foods containing saturated fats increase one's serum (blood) cholesterol while polyunsaturated fats tend to reduce it.

Hypertension (high blood pressure), smoking, hyperlipidemia, diabetes mellitus, obesity, male sex, heredity, age (risk increases with age), personality type, and sedentary living are contributory factors in atherosclerosis. Obviously, some of these are beyond one's control, but some are not. Diet can alleviate obesity, hypertension, and greatly reduce hyperlipidemia. A sedentary lifestyle can be changed. One can stop smoking. It would seem that one could considerably reduce one's risk of atherosclerosis.

Dietary Treatment of Atherosclerosis

The American Heart Association has recommended reducing cholesterol and triglycerides in the blood to prevent the fatty deposits on artery walls. Dietary cholesterol, saturated fats, and total fat in the diet should be decreased to achieve this goal. The AHA suggests that adult diets contain less than 300 mg of cholesterol per day, that saturated fats provide no more than 10 percent of total kcal, and that total fat in the diet not exceed 30—35 percent of total kcal.

Cholesterol is found only in animal tissue. The following foods are rich sources of it:

- muscle meats
- organ meats
- animal fats
- eggs
- whole milk
- cream
- butter

See Table 26-3 for specific amounts in particular foods.

Saturated fats are found in all animal fats, coconut, and chocolate. They are usually solid at room temperature. Unsaturated or polyunsaturated fats are derived from plants (except for coconut and chocolate) and fish, and are usually liquid at room temperature.

Physicians vary in their choice of dietary treatment of atherosclerosis. Some limit cholesterol (low-cholesterol diet) and some limit all fats, in varying amounts (low-fat or fat-restricted diets). Fat-controlled diets may be deficient in fat-soluble vitamins as a result of the decreased fat intake. Consequently a vitamin supplement may be prescribed for a patient on a fat-controlled diet.

Low-Fat Diet

The low-fat (also called fat-restricted) diet contains a specific, maximum amount of fat.

The exact amount of fat contained in the average diet is difficult to determine. However, it is believed by some experts that the average diet contains 155 grams of fat.[1] A low-fat diet may contain a maximum of 70 grams of fat, 50 grams of fat, 30 grams of fat, or 20 grams of fat. Obviously, a diet this low in fat will seem very unusual and *unpalatable* (unpleasant tasting) to some patients. Special understanding and patience will be required. Information regarding the fat content of foods and methods of preparation that minimize the amount of fat in the diet should be given. No foods that are high in fat are permitted. Foods must be prepared without the addition of any fat. All visible fat must be removed from

---

[1]Dorothea Turner, Handbook of Diet Therapy. Chicago: University of Chicago Press. 1970

Table 26-3 Cholesterol Content of Foods*

Item No. (A)	Item (B)	Amount of cholesterol in —		
		100 grams edible portion (C)	Edible portion of 1 pound as purchased (D)	Refuse from item as purchased (E)
		Milligrams	*Milligrams*	*Percent*
1	Beef, raw:			
a	with bone	70	270	15
b	without bone	70	320	0
2	Brains, raw	>2,000	>9,000	0
3	Butter	250	1,135	0
4	Caviar or fish roe	> 300	>1,300	0
	Cheese:			
5	Cheddar	100	455	0
6	Cottage, creamed	15	70	0
7	Cream	120	545	0
8	Other (25% to 30% fat)	85	385	0
9	Cheese spread	65	295	0
10	Chicken, flesh only, raw	60	. . . .	0
11	Crab:			
a	In shell	125	270	52
b	Meat only	125	565	0
12	Egg, whole	550	2,200	12
13	Egg white	0	0	0
	Egg yolk:			
14	Fresh	1,500	6,800	0
15	Frozen	1,280	5,800	0
16	Dried	2,950	13,380	0
17	Fish:			
a	Steak	70	265	16
b	Fillet	70	320	0
18	Heart, raw	150	680	0
19	Ice Cream	45	205	0
20	Kidney, raw	375	1,700	0
21	Lamb, raw:			
a	with bone	70	265	16
b	without bone	70	320	0
22	Lard and other animal fat	95	430	0
23	Liver, raw	300	1,360	0
24	Lobster:			
a	Whole	200	235	74
b	Meat only	200	900	0
	Margarine:			
25	All vegetable fat	0	0	0
26	Two-thirds animal fat, one-third vegetable fat	65	295	0
	Milk:			
27	Fluid, whole	11	50	0
28	Dried, whole	85	385	0
29	Fluid, skim	3	15	0
30	Mutton:			
a	with bone	65	250	16
b	without bone	65	295	0
31	Oysters:			
a	In shell	≧200	≧ 90	90
b	Meat only	≧200	>900	0
32	Pork:			
a	With bone	70	260	18
b	Without bone	70	320	0
33	Shrimp:			
a	In Shell	125	390	31
b	Flesh only	125	565	0
34	Sweetbreads (thymus)	250	1,135	0
35	Veal:			
a	With bone	90	320	21
b	Without bone	90	410	0

*Letters *a* and *b* designate items that have the same chemical composition for the edible portion but differ in the amount of refuse. The data in column C applies to 100 grams of edible portion of the item, although it may be purchased with the refuse indicated in column E and described or implied in column B. Source: U.S. Department of Agriculture *Composition of Foods,* Agriculture Handbook No. 8, 1963 Agricultural Research Service

Table 26-4 Selecting Foods for a Low-Fat (30 gram) Diet

FOODS ALLOWED IN A LOW-FAT DIET	FOODS TO BE AVOIDED
skim milk, buttermilk, and yogurt made from skim milk	cream and whole milk
cottage cheese and skim milk cheese	cheeses except uncreamed cottage cheese
eggs, but limited in number according to amount of fat allowed in diet	all fats unless a minimum amount of butter or margarine is allowed
butter and margarine — usually limited to 1 Tbsp. or less daily and excluded entirely in very low fat diets	commercially prepared soups or any soups made with whole milk or cream
very lean fish, fowl, and meats — amount limited by physician according to the total amount of fat allowed in diet	fatty meats such as pork, bacon, ham, goose, duck, and fatty fish
fat-free soup broth	desserts except for those on the allowed list
any vegetables; and fruits	chocolate, nuts, coconut
any breads and cereals that contain less than 1 gm of fat per serving	salad dressings, salad oils, gravies
gelatin, angel cake, cereal puddings made with skim milk, ices	fried foods
coffee, tea, carbonated beverages	
jelly, honey as desired	

Table 26-5 Sample Menu for a Low-Fat (30 gram) Diet

Breakfast	Dinner	Lunch or Supper
Orange Juice	2 oz. Chicken	Tomato Juice
Cream of Wheat with 1 Tbsp. Sugar and 1 Cup Skim Milk	Boiled Potato	Uncreamed Cottage Cheese on Fruit Salad*
1 Slice Toast	Baked Squash with 1 Tbsp. Honey	2 Slices Toast with 2 Tbsp. Honey
1 Tbsp. Jelly	Lettuce Salad	Angel Cake
Coffee	1 Slice Bread	1 Cup Milk
	1 Tbsp. Jelly	Tea
	Canned Peaches	
	1 Cup Milk	
	Tea	

*No Avocado

meats. Foods must not be fried. Skim milk must be used instead of whole milk. Sometimes this diet is also restricted in fiber content. The Exchange Lists devised for diabetic patients can sometimes be used by patients on fat-restricted diets (see Chapter 24).

The Low-Cholesterol Diet

The low-cholesterol diet is modified by type and amount of fat allowed. In the low-cholesterol diet, protein requirements are met by lean muscle meats, fish, skim milk, and skim milk cheeses. All visible fats should be removed and the use of bacon and fatty luncheon meats should be restricted. Organ meats, egg yolks, and shellfish are used in very limited quantities because of their high cholesterol content. Skim milk is used instead of whole milk. Desserts containing whole milk, eggs, and cream are avoided. Margarine containing liquid vegetable oil is substituted for butter, and liquid vegetable oils are used in cooking.

Chapter 3, Carbohydrates and Fats, may be reviewed for additional information.

SUMMARY

Cardiovascular disease represents the leading cause of death in the United States. It may be acute as in myocardial infarction, or chronic as in hypertension and atherosclerosis. Hypertension is a symptom of other disease and is thought to affect 20 percent of the U.S. population. Weight loss, if the patient is overweight, and a salt-restricted diet are typically prescribed.

Atherosclerosis is a vascular disease in which the arteries are narrowed by fatty deposits, reducing blood flow. Angina pectoris, myocardial infarction, and cerebral accident can result. Because cholesterol is associated with atherosclerosis, a low-cholesterol diet, or a fat-restricted diet may be prescribed.

By maintaining one's weight and activities at a healthy level, limiting salt and fat intake, and avoiding smoking, one can reduce the risks of heart disease.

Case Study—Heart Conditions

Joe G., a lawyer, married with two teen-aged children, suffered a myocardial infarction last week. He was lucky. His doctor told him that with time, rest, and an appropriate diet he should be able to regain his strength and live a normal life.

Immediately following the M.I., Joe was put on a liquid diet, then a soft diet, and now is allowed a regular diet, with kcal and cholesterol controlled.

His doctor told Joe that he had atherosclerosis and that he was 20 pounds overweight.

He explained the reasons for the low-cholesterol diet, described the diet, and told Joe that he should follow it for the rest of his life. He also explained the dangers of the excess weight and said that after losing 20 pounds, Joe should not have to continue the low-kcal diet.

Joe was very surprised by all of this. He weighs exactly the same as when he was a quarterback at the University, 20 years ago. He and his wife had considered themselves "health freaks" in regard to diet. They always ate a good breakfast with bacon, or ham and eggs. They never sent their children off to school having only cereal. They all have good meat sandwiches at noon, enjoy steaks, chops and fish—especially shrimp and lobster–at their evening meals.

They use real butter and whole milk that they buy at the local health food store so they know it is healthy. They do not indulge in sweets, but they usually have ice cream at bedtime.

Case Study Questions

1. Joe's diet had averaged 3500 kcal each day. The doctor put him on a 2500 kcal diet. How much weight will Joe lose each week? How many weeks will Joe require to lose 20 pounds?
2. Why was Joe put on a low-cholesterol diet? Would it harm his wife and children to eat the same foods Joe does on this diet? Explain your answer.
3. What foods should Joe avoid on his low-kcal, low-cholesterol diet? Must he continue to avoid these foods after he has lost 20 pounds? Are there any acceptable foods that might be substituted for these foods?

   Joe's favorite food is steak, but he understands that he can have it only occasionally now. How should it be prepared before it is cooked? How should it be cooked? Why? Joe enjoys a baked potato with sour cream with the steak. Can he still have this? Explain.

   Joe enjoys lobster with melted butter. Is this advisable for him now?
6. Do you think Joe will have any problems adjusting to his new diet? Why?
7. What may happen to Joe if he disregards his doctor's dietary advice?
8. Plan a day's menu for Joe when he gets home from the hospital. Adapt it for his family.

Discussion Topics

1. Why are sodium-restricted diets prescribed for patients with hypertension or heart failure?
2. What precautions might one take to prevent hypertension? Atherosclerosis? Explain your answers.
3. What may occur in severe myocardial infarction? What causes myocardial infarction?
4. Describe the dietary progression following a myocardial infarction.
5. What are diuretics? How could they be harmful? How could this danger be avoided?

6. What is edema? How is it related to cardiovascular diseases?

7. Are sodium-restricted diets nutritious? Why

8. If a class member knows anyone who must follow a sodium-restricted diet, discuss that person's initial reaction to this diet. Has this person become accustomed to it?

9. Why is it impossible to prepare a diet absolutely free of salt?

10. Why may a sodium-restricted diet be unpleasant for a patient?

11. Why are potato chips and peanuts not allowed on sodium-restricted diets?

12. Why is table salt restricted in sodium-restricted diets?

13. Name and describe the fat-controlled diets discussed in this chapter. For what heart condition might such diets be ordered? What foods would be prohibited? Restricted?

14. In what respect are fat-controlled diets modified? Is the patient apt to notice these modifications?

15. Are low-fat diets nutritious? If not, what nutrient(s) may be lacking? Why?

16. What is cholesterol? How is it associated with atherosclerosis? What has been published recently in newspapers and magazines concerning cholesterol and heart problems?

17. Why is skim milk allowed on low-fat diets when whole milk is not?

18. Discuss the differences between saturated and polyunsaturated fats. In what foods is each of these fats predominantly found?

19. What is hyperlipidemia? How is it related to atherosclerosis?

Suggested Activities

1. Find recipes suitable for low-fat diets and for a low-cholesterol diet. Compare recipes and check one another's for correctness. Suggest alternate ingredients for any that are not suitable for these diets.

2. Make a list of the foods eaten yesterday. Circle those foods that would not be allowed on a low-cholesterol diet and suggest satisfactory substitutions.

3. Plan a day's menu for a low-fat (70 gram) diet, using Table A-7 in the Appendix.

4. Plan a day's menu for a low-cholesterol diet.

5. Prepare at least one of these meals and evaluate it in terms of nutritive content, flavor, aroma, color, shape, appearance, texture, and satiety value.

6. Visit a local supermarket. List the foods containing sodium compounds. Suggest substitutes for these foods for patients on sodium-restricted diets.

7. Find recipes suitable for sodium-restricted diets.

8. List the foods eaten yesterday. Circle those that would not be allowed on the mild sodium-restricted diet. Make appropriate substitutions for a patient on a mild sodium-restricted diet.

9. Plan a day's menu for a patient on the unrestricted calorie, mild sodium-restricted diet. Use Tables A-3 and A-7 in the Appendix.

10. Prepare and evaluate at least one of the meals on the menu and evaluate it in terms of nutritive content, flavor, aroma, color, shape, appearance, and satiety value.

11. Mary Jones was placed on a low-fat diet containing no more than 70 grams fat. She wants to order the following breakfast. Would this be acceptable? Explain your answer and, if necessary, suggest alternate foods that would be acceptable.

Sliced Avocado
Poached Egg with Ham in Cheese Sauce
on English Muffin
Coffee with Cream

12. John Brown has been told that he has atherosclerosis and must follow a low-cholesterol diet. He is visiting his aunt who is serving the following meal. Which of the foods can John eat and which must he avoid? Why? Can he eat certain parts of any of the foods? If so, which? Why?

Cream of Broccoli Soup
Roast Chicken
Mashed Potatoes with Gravy
Lima Beans with Butter
Green Salad with Vinegar and Oil Dressing
Rolls and Butter
Milk
Angel Food Cake with Whipped Cream
and Strawberries

13. Susan Smith has developed hypertension and has been placed on a Mild Sodium-Restricted Diet. She has planned the following dinner for her daughter's graduation party. Which of the foods can she eat and which must she avoid?

Fresh Fruit Cup
Baked Ham
Potato Chips
Fresh Frozen Broccoli Chunks Baked in
Canned Cream of Chicken Soup
Homemade Coleslaw
Rolls and Butter
Pickles and Olives
Chocolate Cake with Peppermint Ice Cream

Review

A. Multiple-multiple Choice. Select the *letter* that precedes the best answer.

1. Sodium
   1. is an essential vitamin   p. 283
   2. regulates the water balance in the body
   3. adds flavor to foods
   4. is found in table salt
      a) 1, 2, 3   b) 1, 3, 4   c) 2, 3, 4   (d) all

2. Sodium is found in
   1. most foods
   2. water
   3. baking soda and baking power
   4. brine
      a) 1, 2, 3   b) 2, 3, 4   c) 1, 3, 4   (d) all

3. In the 1000 milligram and 500 milligram sodium diets,
   1. baked products containing baking powder and baking soda cannot be used
   2. canned vegetables and vegetable juices must be low-sodium dietetic
   3. the amount of sodium in tap water must be considered
   4. only low-sodium milk is allowed
      a) 1, 2   b) 3, 4   c) 2, 3, 4   (d) 1, 2, 3

4. Herbs, spices, and flavorings may
   1. be used in sodium-restricted diets
   2. never be used in sodium-restricted diets
   3. detract from the blandness of sodium-restricted diets
   4. be used only in the mild sodium-restricted diet
      (a) 1, 3   b) 2   c) 4   d) 3, 4

5. On the mild sodium-restricted diet, the patient may
   1. use approximately 1/2 the salt previously used
   2. not add salt to processed food
   3. use baking soda in baked foods
   4. not have pickles and ham
       a) 1, 2, 3   b) 2, 3, 4   c) 1, 4   d) all

6. A sodium-restricted diet may be ordered for patients with
   1. edema
   2. hypertension
   3. congestive heart failure
   4. atherosclerosis
       a) 1, 2, 3   b) 2, 4   c) 1, 4   d) all

7. When water accumulates in body tissues,
   1. the condition is called edema
   2. a sodium-restricted diet may be prescribed
   3. It is a definite symptom of myocardial infarction
   4. salt is completely eliminated from the diet
       a) 1, 3   b) 2, 3, 4   c) 1, 2   d) all

8. Monosodium glutamate and table salt
   1. are not allowed in any sodium-restricted diet
   2. both contain sodium
   3. are commonly used in food processing
   4. occur naturally in all foods
       a) 1, 3, 4   b) 2, 3   c) 3, 4   d) all

9. Table salt
   1. is 100 percent sodium
   2. is over 40 percent sodium
   3. contains only negligible amounts of sodium
   4. must be restricted in sodium-restricted diets
       a) 1, 3, 4   b) 2, 3, 4   c) 2, 4   d) 2, 3

10. In a low-cholesterol diet
    1. eggs are used freely
    2. skim milk is used instead of whole milk
    3. lean muscle meats and fish are permitted
    4. vegetable oils are permitted
        a) 1, 2, 3   b) 2, 3, 4   c) 1, 3, 4   d) all

11. The amount of fat allowed in the low-fat diet is
    1. reduced   3. eliminated completely
    2. increased   4. the same as in a regular diet
        a) 1, 3   b) 1 only   c) 2 only   d) all

12. Persons on a low-fat diet will
    1. need information regarding the fat content of foods
    2. need information regarding cooking methods for their diets
    3. never be allowed butter or magarine
    4. probably find the diet somewhat unpalatable
        a) 1, 3, 4   b) 1, 2, 3   c) 1, 2, 4   d) all

13. Foods allowed in a low-fat diet include
    1. all cheeses
    2. cooked vegetables
    3. refined cereals
    4. limited amounts of lean meats
        a) 1, 3, 4   b) 2, 3, 4   c) 1, 3, 4   d) all

14. When preparing foods for the low-fat diet,
    1. very small amounts of fat may be added
    2. visible fats must be removed from meats
    3. skim milk is never used
    4. no frying is permitted
        a) 1, 4   b) 2, 3, 4   c) 2, 4   d) all

15. On the low-cholesterol diet, saturated fats are
    1. reduced
    2. eliminated
    3. increased
    4. unchanged from that of the regular diet
        a) 1, 2   b) 2 only   c) 1 only   d) all

16. Saturated fats are usually
    1. solid at room temperature   3. found in animal foods
    2. liquid at room temperature   4. derived from plants
        a) 1, 3   b) 2, 3   c) 1, 4   d) all

17. Polyunsaturated fats are usually
    1. solid at room temperature   3. found in animal foods
    2. liquid at room temperature   4. derived from plants
        a) 1, 3   b) 2, 4   c) 1, 4   d) all

18. When the heart muscle reacts with pain because of inadequate blood supply after activity, the condition is called
    1. cerebral accident
    2. edema
    3. hypertension
    4. angina pectoris
        a) 1, 3   b) 2, 3   c) 3 only   d) 4 only

19. Some examples of blood lipids are
    1. triglycerides
    2. lumens
    3. cholesterol
    4. plaques
       a) 2, 3 (b) 1, 3 c) 1, 2 d) 3, 4

20. Bacon, potato chips, cheddar cheese, and sour cream would be acceptable for the following diets
    1. low cholesterol
    2. 500-milligram sodium diet
    3. mild-sodium diet
    4. none of the above
       a) 1, 3 b) 2, 3 c) 1, 2, 3 (d) 4 only

References

Biology book of choice

Encyclopedia of choice

American Dietetic Association. 1981. *Handbook of Clinical Dietetics*. New Haven: Yale University.

American Heart Association. 1969. *Your Mild Sodium-Restricted Diet.*

American Heart Association. 1969. *Your 1000 Mg. Sodium-Restricted Diet.*

American Heart Association. 1968. *Your 500 Mg. Sodium-Restricted Diet.*

Krause, Marie, and Kathleen L. Mahan. 1979. *Food, Nutrition, and Diet Therapy*, 6th ed. Phildelaphia: W.B. Saunders Co.

Iowa Dietetic Association, 1984. *Simplified Diet Manual with Meal Patterns*, 5th ed.

U.S. Department of Agriculture. 1963, 1975. *Composition of Foods*.

University of Iowa Hospitals and Clinics. 1979. *Recent Advances in Therapeutic Diets*. Iowa City: Iowa State University Press.

Chapter 27
DIETS FOR RENAL DISEASE

acid-ash foods   hematuria   renal calculi
alkaline-ash foods   hyperkalemia   trauma
capillaries   nephritis   urea
creatinine   nephrolithiasis   uremia
cystine   nephron   ureters
cysts   nephrosclerosis   uric acid
dialysis   osteomalacia
filtrate   polycystic kidney
glomerulonephritis   disease
glomerulus   purines

OBJECTIVES

After studying this chapter, you should be able to

- Explain why protein is sometimes increased or decreased for renal patients

- Explain why sodium and water are sometimes restricted for renal patients

- Explain why potassium and phosphorus are sometimes restricted for renal patients

- Explain why kcal are sometimes restricted for patients with renal disease

- Adapt family meals to meet the needs of patients with renal disease

The kidneys are intricate and efficient processing systems that excrete wastes, maintain volume and composition of body fluids, and secrete certain hormones. To accomplish these tasks, they filter the blood, cleansing it of waste products and recycling other usable substances so that the necessary constituents of body fluids are constantly available.

Each kidney contains approximately one million working parts called *nephrons*. Each nephron contains a filtering unit called a *glomerulus* in which there is a cluster of specialized capillaries (tiny blood vessels connecting veins and arteries). Approximately 180 liters of *filtrate* (substance to be filtered) is processed each day. As the filtrate passes through the nephrons, the kidneys are able to concentrate or dilute it to meet the body's needs. This enables the kidneys to maintain both the composition and the volume of body fluids and consequently, fluid balance, acid-base balance, and electrolyte balance. The waste materials are sent via two tubes called the *ureters* from the kidneys to the bladder from which they are excreted as urine. These include end products of protein metabolism (urea, uric acid, creatinine, ammonia, and sulfates), excess water, dead renal cells, and toxic substances. The recycled materials are resorbed by the blood. They include amino acids, sodium, glucose, potassium, vitamins, and water.

The kidneys synthesize and secrete certain hormones as needed. For example, it is the kidneys that make the final conversion of vitamin D so that it can play its role in the absorption of calcium. The kidneys create stimulation which causes the bone marrow to produce red blood cells.

TYPES OF RENAL DISORDERS

Kidney disorders may be initially caused by infection, degenerative changes, cardiovascular disorders, cysts (growths), renal calculi (stones), or trauma (surgery, burns, poisons). When they are severe, renal failure may develop. It may be acute or chronic. Acute renal failure occurs suddenly and may last a few days or a few weeks. It can be expected in some situations so preventive steps may be taken. It is usually reversible. Chronic renal failure develops slowly with the number of functioning nephrons constantly diminishing. When renal tissue has been destroyed to the point that the kidneys are no longer able to filter the blood, excrete wastes, or recycle nutrients as needed, *uremia* occurs. Uremia is a condition in which protein wastes that should normally have been excreted are instead circulating in the blood. Symptoms include nausea, headache, coma, and convulsions. Severe renal failure will result in death unless mechanical dialysis (filtration) is begun or a kidney transplant is performed.

Nephritis is a general term referring to the inflammatory diseases of the kidneys. Nephritis may be caused by infection, degenerative processes, or vascular disease.

Glomerulonephritis is a nephritis affecting the capillaries in the glomeruli. It may occur acutely in conjunction with another infection and be self-limiting, or it may lead to serious renal deterioration.

Nephrosclerosis is the hardening of renal arteries. It is caused by arteriosclerosis and hypertension. Although it usually occurs in older people, it sometimes develops in young diabetics.

Polycystic Kidney Disease is a relatively rare, hereditary disease. Cysts form and press on the kidneys. The kidneys enlarge and lose function. Although people with this condition have normal kidney function for many years, renal failure may develop near the age of 50.

Renal Calculi or Nephrolithiasis is a condition in which stones develop in the kidneys, the ureters, or the bladder. The size varies from that of a grain of sand to much larger. Some remain at their point of origin and others move. While the condition is sometimes asymptomatic, symptoms may include *hematuria* (blood in the urine), infection, obstruction and, if the stones move, intense pain. The stones are classified according to their composition—calcium, uric acid, cystine (amino acid), and oxalic acid. They are associated with metabolic disturbances and immobilization of the patient.

Dietary Treatment of Renal Disease

The dietary treatment of renal disease can be extremely complicated. It is intended to reduce the amount of excretory work demanded of the kidneys while assisting them in maintaining fluid, acid-base, and electrolyte balance. Patients require sufficient protein to prevent malnutrition and muscle wasting. Too much, however, will contribute to uremia. Typically, the patient with chronic renal failure will have protein and sodium, and possibly potassium and phosphorus, restricted.

It is essential that renal patients receive sufficient kcal—35 to 40 kcal per kilogram of body weight—unless they are overweight. Energy. requirements should be fulfilled by carbohydrates and fat. The fats must be polyunsaturated to prevent or check hyperlipidemia. If the energy requirement is not met by carbohydrates and fat, ingested protein or body tissue will be metabolized for energy. Either would increase the work of the kidneys because protein increases the amount of nitrogen waste the kidneys must handle. The diet may limit protein to 20 grams. The specific amount of protein allowed is calculated according to the patient's GFR (glomerular filtration rate) and weight. Other times, protein may be increased in an effort to increase blood protein, and the requirement may go as high as 125 grams.

Sodium may be limited if the patient tends to retain it. Retained sodium and water could result in edema, hypertension, and congestive heart failure. Fluids are typically restricted for renal patients.

Calcium supplements may be prescribed if the kidneys are unable to absorb calcium. In addition, vitamin D may be added and phosphorus limited, to prevent *osteomalacia* (soft-ening of the bones due to excessive loss of calcium). Phosphorous appears to be retained in patients with kidney disorders, and a disproportionately high ratio of phosphorus to calcium tends to increase calcium loss from bones.

Potassium may be restricted in some patients because *hyperkalemia* (high blood potassium) tends to occur in renal failure. Excess potassium can cause cardiac arrest. Because of this danger, renal patients should not use salt substitutes or low-sodium milk because the sodium in these products is replaced with potassium. Potassium restriction can be especially difficult for a renal patient who probably must also limit sodium intake. Potassium is particularly high in fruits—one of the few foods a patient on a sodium-restricted diet may eat without concern.

Renal patients often have an increased need for vitamins B, C, and D. Supplements are often given. Vitamin A should not be given because the blood level of vitamin A tends to be elevated in uremia. If a patient is receiving antibiotics, a vitamin K supplement may be given. Otherwise, supplements of vitamins E and K are not necessary. Iron is commonly prescribed since anemia frequently develops in renal patients.

Diet During Dialysis

Dialysis patients lose some protein and vitamins and should be given supplements of them. It appears these patients do not metabolize fats normally, causing hyperlipidemia. Consequently, polyunsaturated fats rather than saturated should be chosen. Bone disease is common among dialysis patients and the problem is compounded by the additional protein they need, since most protein foods contain large amounts of phosphorus.

Diet After Kidney Transplant

Because cardiovascular disease is a significant cause of death among transplant patients, and because triglycerides and cholesterol levels are typically high among them, polyunsaturated fats (rather than saturated fats) are recommended. Carbohydrates are also restricted because they tend to raise triglyceride levels. Sodium is somewhat restricted and if weight loss is necessary, kcal are also restricted. A high protein diet of about 1.5 to 2 grams per kilogram of body weight is recommended. This may average about 120 grams. Calcium is increased to 1200 mg.

Dietary Treatment for Renal Calculi

Because the causes of renal calculi have not been confirmed, treatment of them may vary. Generally, however, large amounts of fluid—at least half of it water—are helpful in diluting the urine, as is a well-balanced diet. Once the stones have been analyzed, specific diet modifications may be indicated.

Alkaline-ash and acid-ash diets are sometimes used in an effort to change the pH of the urine and consequently, the incidence of stones. In these diets foods are labeled by the ash they leave after oxidation. If the ash is acid, the food is labeled *acid-ash*; if alkaline, it is labeled *alkaline-ash*. Foods that cause the urine to become acidic (a pH below 7) are called acid-ash and those that cause the urine to become alkaline (a pH above 7), alkaline-ash. Both diets become very tedious and difficult to follow.

Calcium Stones

About two-thirds of the kidney stones formed contain calcium. If the patient has a history of calcium stones this mineral is restricted in the diet, but not usually to less than 600 mg per day. Obviously, foods rich in calcium will have to be limited.

Table 27-1

Acid-ash foods	Alkaline-ash foods
Meats, fish, poultry, eggs	Milk, cream
Breads, cereals, macaroni, rice, crackers, cakes, cookies	Almonds, chestnuts
corn, lentils	Coconut
Peanuts, brazil nuts, filberts, walnuts	Vegetables, except corn and lentils
Cranberries, plums, prunes	Fruits, except plums, prunes, cranberries

Neutral foods
Coffee, tea
Butter, margarine, cooking oils
Sugar, syrup, honey, plain candy
Tapioca

Table 27-2 Calcium Content of Common Dairy Products

1 cup whole milk	291 mg Calcium
1 cup skim milk	302 mg Calcium
1/2 cup ice cream	90 mg Calcium
1 oz. wedge cheddar cheese	204 mg calcium
1/2 cup cottage cheese	70 mg calcium
1 oz process cheese	174 mg calcium
1 cup eggnog	330 mg calcium

Uric Acid Stones

When the stones contain uric acid, purine-rich foods may be restricted. Purines are the end products of nucleoprotein metabolism and are found in all meats, fish, and poultry. Organ meats, anchovies, sardines, meat extracts, and broths are especially rich souces of them.

Oxalic Acid Stones

Stones containing oxalic acid are thought to be partially caused by a diet especially rich in oxalic acid, which is found in nuts, chocolate, tea, citrus fruits, rhubarb, and spinach. Evidence also indicates that deficiencies of

Table 27-3 Purine-rich Foods

Avoid	Limit
liver	meats
kidneys	fish
sweetbreads	poultry
brains	meat soups
heart	
anchovies	
sardines	
meat extracts	
boullion	
broth	

pyridoxine, thiamin, and magnesium may contribute to the formation of oxalic acid kidney stones.

Cystine Stones

Cystine is an amino acid. Cystine stones may form when the cystine concentration in the urine becomes excessive due to a hereditary metabolic disorder. The usual practice is to increase fluids and recommend an alkaline-ash diet.

The High-Protein Diet

The high-protein diet is a regular diet with increased protein content. The protein is provided by normal protein-rich foods and may be further increased by the addition of skim milk powder to soups, cream sauces, gravies, and baked products. It is highly nutritious, but does contain large amounts of phosphorus and sodium.

The Low-Protein Diet

When a low-protein diet is prescribed, it is important that the protein be equally distributed among the three meals. This diet con-

Table 27-4 Foods Included in a High-Protein Diet

milk: 3 to 4 cups
cheeses
eggs
lean meats, fish, and poultry
vegetables
fruits
cereals (whole grain or enriched) and breads as desired

Table 27-5 Sample Menu for a High-Protein Diet

Breakfast	Dinner	Lunch or Supper
Orange Juice	Roast Chicken	Ground Round Steak
Scrambled Eggs	Baked Potato	Asparagus
Bacon	Green Peas	Tomatoes on Lettuce
Toast	Lettuce Salad	Bread and Butter
with	Bread and Butter	Fresh Fruit Cup
Butter and Jelly	Custard	Milk
Milk	Milk	Tea
Coffee		with
with		Cream and Sugar
Cream and Sugar		

Table 27-6 Selecting Foods for a Low-Protein (30 Gram) Diet

FOODS ALLOWED IN A LOW-PROTEIN (30 GRAM) DIET	FOODS NOT ALLOWED IN A LOW-PROTEIN (30 GRAM) DIET
milk: 1/2 cup per day	milk, other than the 1/2 cup allowance (or its equivalent)
soups: permitted if made from allowed foods	
meats, fish, poultry, cheese: 2 oz	high protein cereals
1 egg	legumes
vegetables: any except corn, lima beans, peas	baked products containing eggs and milk
fruits: any	
bread: one serving of cereal, bread, potato, or potato substitute	
butter, margarine, cooking oils, salad dressings	
coffee, tea, carbonated beverages	
fruit ice, plain hard candy	
salt, herbs, spices, pickles	

Table 27-7 Sample Menu for a Low-Protein (30 Gram) Diet

Breakfast	Dinner	Lunch or Supper
Orange Juice	Pineapple Juice	Apple Juice
Soft Cooked Egg	1 oz. Roast Beef	1 oz. Roast Chicken
Rice Cereal with 1/2 Cup Milk and Sugar	Baked Squash with Butter	Asparagus with Butter
Coffee	Baked Apple with Sugar	Sliced Tomatoes
	Tea	Fruit Cup
		Tea with Sugar

tains insufficient protein, minerals, vitamins, and in some cases, kcal.

SUMMARY

The kidneys rid the body of wastes, maintain fluid balance, and secrete hormones. When they are damaged by disease or injury, the entire body is affected. Diet therapy for renal disorders can be extremely complex because of the multifaceted nature of the kidneys' functions. Untreated severe kidney disease can result in death unless dialysis or kidney transplant is undertaken.

Case Study—Renal Disease

Laura E. had been experiencing a frequent need to urinate the past few days. When she did urinate she felt a burning sensation. The problem seemed to be getting worse. On the fifth day she felt quite ill with chills and fever and called her doctor. After examining Laura and testing her urine, her doctor told her she had nephritis and admitted her to the hospital. Laura was put on antibiotics. She began to feel better in a few days, and was discharged in a week.

Case Study Questions

1. Why did the doctor want Laura's blood and urine tested regularly during her illness?
2. Why was there no salt on Laura's meal trays?
3. Why was Laura given a vitamin supplement?
4. Laura's appetite was rather poor during her hospital stay. Why did the nurse urge her to "clean" her plate?
5. The nurse also urged Laura to drink her milk. Laura could not understand this because when her aunt had been in the hospital with nephrosclerosis, she had been allowed only low-sodium milk. Explain this to Laura.

6. Judging from Laura's rapid recovery, what do you think may have caused her nephritis?

Discussion Topics

1. Discuss the three main tasks of the kidneys.
2. Define *nephrons* and explain what they do.
3. Discuss some causes of kidney disease.
4. What is nephritis? glomerulonephritis? nephrosclerosis?
5. Why is diet therapy of renal disease so complex?
6. Discuss why protein is sometimes increased in renal disease and at other times decreased.
7. Why are sodium and water sometimes restricted in renal disease?
8. Why is potassium sometimes restricted in renal disease? What is hyperkalemia?
9. Why is phosphorous sometimes restricted in renal disease?
10. Why might kcal be restricted in renal disease?
11. What are three common nutritional problems of dialysis patients?
12. What is nephrolithiasis? How is it treated?

Suggested Activities

1. Using outside sources, prepare a short report on the functions of the circulatory system, the liver, and the kidneys in eliminating nitrogenous waste products from the body.
2. Find recipes that are suitable for high-protein and low-protein diets.
3. List the foods eaten yesterday. Compute the protein by using table A-7 in the Appendix. Compare the total proteins with the total given for someone your age and sex in table A-1. Would such a diet meet the requirements of the low-protein diet? The high-protein diet? Does it contain adequate protein for you?
4. Plan a day's menu for a high-protein diet. Plan a day's menu for a low-protein diet by adapting the high-protein menus and correct if necessary. Adapt them to suit the needs of your family.
5. Prepare at least one meal on each of the menus. Evaluate each in terms of nutritive content, flavor, aroma, color, shape, appearance, texture, and satiety value.
6. Using table A-7 in the Appendix, compute the protein in the sample high-protein diet menu in this chapter.

7. Plan a day's menus for a patient on a calcium-restricted (600 mg.) diet. Adapt the menus to suit her or his family's needs.
8. Plan a day's menus for a patient who must limit her or his intake of oxalic acid. Adapt it to suit her family's needs.

Review

Multiple Choice. Select the letter that precedes the best answer.

1. The kidneys maintain the body's
   a. acid-base balance
   b. electrolyte balance
   c. fluid balance
   d. all of these
2. The specialized part within each nephron that actually filters the blood is called the
   a. ureter
   b. filter
   c. glomerulus
   d. capillary bunch
3. Kidney disorders may be caused by
   a. cysts
   b. infections
   c. burns
   d. all of these
4. When renal tissue has been destroyed to the point that it can no longer filter the blood, the following occurs:
   a. nephritis
   b. nephrosclerosis
   c. uremia
   d. nephrolithiasis
5. The general term referring to the inflammatory diseases of the kidneys is
   a. nephritis
   b. nephrosclerosis
   c. uremia
   d. nephrolithiasis
6. The term referring to the hardening of renal arteries is
   a. nephritis
   b. nephrosclerosis
   c. uremia
   d. nephrolithiasis
7. The rare hereditary disease causing cysts to develop on the kidneys is called
   a. nephritis
   b. glomerulonephritis
   c. renal calculi
   d. polycystic kidney disease
8. The condition in which stones develop in the kidneys, ureters, or bladder is called
   a. nephritis
   b. nephrolithiasis
   c. polycystic kidney disease
   d. glomerulonephritis
9. Because its nitrogenous wastes contribute to uremia, the following nutrient may be restricted in diets of renal patients.
   a. carbohydrate
   b. saturated fat
   c. protein
   d. vitamin A

10. Saturated fats may be restricted in the diets of renal patients because they
    a. contribute to uremia
    b. increase hypercalcemia
    c. contribute to hyperlipidemia
    d. contribute to hypertension

11. Sodium and water may be restricted in the diets of renal patients because they
    a. contribute to uremia
    b. increase hypercalcemia
    c. contribute to hyperlipidemia
    d. contribute to hypertension

12. If osteomalacia occurs in renal patients, the following nutrient may be prescribed
    a. potassium
    b. protein
    c. calcium
    d. phosphorus

13. In a case of hyperkalemia, the following nutrient may be restricted
    a. potassium
    b. protein
    c. calcium
    d. phosphorus

14. Fruits are an especially rich source of
    a. potassium
    b. protein
    c. calcium
    d. phosphorus

15. Because anemia may be present in renal patients, the following nutrient may be prescribed
    a. phosphorus
    b. carbohydrate
    c. calcium
    d. iron

16. The vitamins renal patients may have an increased need for are
    a. the water-soluble vitamins
    b. the fat-soluble vitamins
    c. only the B vitamins
    d. vitamins E and A

17. An excess of the following nutrient can compound bone loss in renal patients
    a. phosphorus
    b. carbohydrate
    c. calcium
    d. iron

18. Acid-ash foods include
    a. meats
    b. dairy foods
    c. vegetables, except corn and lentils
    d. fruits, except cranberries, plums, and prunes

19. Purine-rich foods include
    a. meats
    b. dairy foods
    c. vegetables, except corn and lentils
    d. fruits except cranberries, plums, and prunes

20. An example of nitrogenous waste found in the urine is
    a. ureter
    b. uremia
    c. urea
    d. all of these

References

Biology book of choice

Encyclopedia of choice

Howard, Roseanne B, and Nancie H. Herbold. 1982. *Nutrition in Clinical Care*, 2nd ed. New York: McGraw Hill Book Company.

Iowa Dietetic Association. 1984. *Simplified Diet Manual with Meal Patterns*, 5th ed. Ames: Iowa State University Press.

Krause, Marie, and Kathleen L. Mahan. 1979. *Food, Nutrition and Diet Therapy*, 6th ed. Philadelphia: W.B. Saunders Co.

U.S. Department of Agriculture. 1963, 1975. *Composition of Foods*.

University of Iowa Hospitals and Clinics. 1979. *Recent Advances in Therapeutic Diets*. Iowa City: Iowa State University Press.

Chapter 28

DIETS FOR DISEASES OF THE GASTRO-INTESTINAL SYSTEM

OBJECTIVES

After studying this chapter, you should be able to

- Explain the uses of diet therapy in the gastrointestinal disturbances discussed here

- Identify the foods in the therapeutic diets discussed

- Adapt normal diets to meet the requirements of patients with these conditions

The gastrointestinal tract is where digestion and absorption of food occurs.

The primary organs include the mouth, esophagus, stomach, small and large intestine. The liver, gall bladder, and pancreas are accessory organs that are also involved in these processes. Some disturbances affecting the gastrointestinal tract are discussed here along with appropriate diet therapy.

DISORDERS OF THE PRIMARY ORGANS

Dyspepsia

Dyspepsia or indigestion is a condition of discomfort in the digestive tract that may be physical or psychological in origin. If physical, it may be due to rushed eating, over-rich foods, or it may be a symptom of another problem, such as appendicitis, kidney, gallbladder or colon disease. Psychological stress can affect stomach secretions, thereby triggering dyspepsia. If there is no underlying disease, improved eating habits should help the patient overcome the condition. A bland diet is sometimes prescribed. This not only eliminates irritating foods, but may also contribute to improved eating habits.

The Bland Diet

The definition of *bland* is "mild or soothing." The bland diet includes foods that are prepared simply, and have little connective tissue or fiber. Bland foods do not increase the production of stomach acid, and are mild-flavored. Therefore, the bland diet should not irritate the gastrointestinal tract chemically or mechanically. Currently, its effectiveness is somewhat doubted among physicians.

The foods allowed depend on the type of disturbance being treated and the judgment of the physician. Often the bland diet begins as a full liquid diet and then very soft foods are introduced gradually. The temperatures of the foods served should be moderate. The size and frequency of the meals prescribed depend upon the physician's evaluation.

Hiatus Hernia

Hiatus hernia is a condition in which a part of the stomach protrudes through the *diaphragm* (a muscular sheet separating the abdominal cavity from the chest cavity) into the thoracic cavity. This prevents the food

Table 28-1 Selecting Foods for a Bland Diet

FOODS ALLOWED IN A BLAND DIET	FOODS TO BE AVOIDED
milk, cream, buttermilk, yogurt	coarse foods
cottage cheese and cream cheese, mild American cheese if combined with another food	fried foods
butter and margarine	usually coffee and tea
eggs, except fried	highly seasoned foods
very tender roast, broiled, and boiled beef, lamb, veal, chicken, fish, liver, and sweetbreads	? condiments
refined cereals, macaroni, spaghetti, noodles, white bread, rolls, crackers	pastries and candies
cream soups and broths	raw fruits and vegetables (except bananas, fruit juices, lettuce and tomatoes without seeds)
cooked, mild-flavored vegetables without coarse fibers or strings	alcoholic and carbonated beverages
orange, prune, peach, and pear juice, ripe banana, applesauce, baked apple (no skin), canned fruits including skinless apricots, white cherries, peaches and pears. (Orange juice should be served during or after the meal.)	smoked and salted meats and fish; pork
	avocados, nuts, olives, coconut
custard, pudding, gelatin, junket, sponge cake, plain cookies, vanilla ice cream. (The patient should eat ice cream slowly so that it is body temperature when it reaches the stomach.)	whole grain breads and cereals
decaffeinated coffee, weak tea if permitted by physician	

Table 28-2 Sample Menu for a Bland Diet

Breakfast	Dinner	Lunch or Supper
Cream of Wheat with Apricot Puree and Cream and Sugar	Cream of Tomato Soup	Poached Eggs on White Toast
	Baked Fillet of Sole	Creamed Spinach
Buttered White Toast	Baked Potato with Butter	Pear Juice
Orange Juice	Tender Green Peas	Baked Apple
Milk	White Bread and Butter	Milk
	Canned Peaches	
	Milk	
10 a.m. Eggnog	**3 p.m.** Weak Cocoa	**9 p.m.** Milk

from moving normally along the digestive tract, although it does mix somewhat with the gastric juices. Sometimes the food will move back into the esophagus, creating a burning sensation ("heartburn"), and sometimes food will be regurgitated into the mouth. This condition can be very uncomfortable. The problem can sometimes be alleviated by serving small, frequent meals so that the amount of food in the stomach is never large. It may also be helpful if patients avoid lying down soon after eating. When they do lie down they may be more comfortable sleeping with their heads and upper torso somewhat elevated. If discomfort cannot be controlled, surgery may be necessary.

Peptic Ulcers

An ulcer is an erosion of the mucous membrane. Peptic ulcers may occur in the stomach (*gastric ulcer*) or the duodenum (*duodenal ulcer*). Their cause is not entirely clear, but it is thought that an abnormally high secretion of hydrochloric acid by the stomach coupled with an anxious personality-type may contribute to their development. They are treated with antacids and rest, in addition to diet therapy.

In the past, diet therapy typically began with the Sippy Diet, which originally included hourly servings of milk and cream only, and was later liberalized to include some soft foods. It is rarely used today because while whole milk does initially neutralize the gastric acid, the protein it contains stimulates the stomach to secrete additional acid. When it is used, whole or skim milk are now advised because of the danger of atherosclerosis from the cream. Generally, the diet therapy for peptic ulcers has been vastly liberalized and the effectiveness of soft or bland diets has become controversial.

Sufficient protein should be provided, but not in excess because of its ability to stimulate gastric acid secretion. It is recommended that patients receive no less than .8 gram of protein per kilogram of body weight. However, if there has been blood loss, this may be increased to 1 or 1.5 grams per kilogram of body weight.

Although fat inhibits gastric secretions, because of the danger of atherosclerosis, the amount of fat in the diet should be kept to a maximum of 80—100 grams per day. Carbohydrates have little effect on gastric acid secretion.

While coarse foods were previously prohibited ulcer patients because it was thought that the roughage irritated the ulcer, this is now under question. Spicy foods were also previously excluded, but the value of this is now also being questioned, and appears to depend largely on each individual's tolerances. However, the following food items were more often found to be irritating than others: black pepper, chili powder, nutmeg, mustard, and vinegar.

There are indications that a regular diet of small, frequent feedings, consisting of foods that do not irritate the individual are as effective as a strict bland diet, and more nutritious. However, the following food items should not be allowed an ulcer patient:

- Coffee, with or without caffeine
- tea
- caffeine in any form
- alcohol

Coffee, tea, or anything containing caffeine stimulates gastric secretion. Alcohol and aspirin irritate the mucous membrane of the stomach, and cigarette smoking decreases the secretion of the pancreas that buffers gastric acid in the duodenum.

Diverticulosis/Diverticulitis

Diverticulosis is an intestinal disorder characterized by little pockets forming in the sides of the intestines. When food collects in these pockets instead of moving on through the intestines, bacteria may subsequently breed, and inflammation and pain can result, causing *diverticulitis*. If a diverticulum ruptures, surgery may be needed. This condition is thought to be caused by diet lacking in sufficient fiber.

Food residue or *fiber* is that part of food the body cannot digest and; therefore, it is ultimately evacuated in the feces. If there is little food residue, there is little fecal matter for the body to evacuate. If there is a great deal of food residue, the amount of fecal matter is increased. The average diet is thought to contain 2—5 grams of fiber.

Diet therapy for diverticulitis may begin with a clear liquid diet (see Chapter 23), followed by a low-residue or even minimum-residue diet, and very gradually (over several weeks) progressing to a high-fiber diet. The bulk provided by the high-fiber diet increases stool volume, reduces the pressure in the colon, and shortens the time the food is in the intestine, giving bacteria less time to grow. However, the word *gradually* must be noted regarding the introduction of a high-fiber diet. If a high-fiber diet is introduced abruptly, gas and discomfort may develop. For some people, regular use of the high-fiber diet may relieve symptoms of diverticulosis.

The High-Fiber Diet

The high-fiber diet includes foods containing large amounts of fiber. It should provide 5—6 grams of fiber each day. The recommended foods for this diet include

Table 28-3 Sample Menu for a High-Fiber Diet

Breakfast	Dinner	Lunch or Supper
Stewed Prunes	Baked Pork Chops	Fresh Fruit Cup
Bran Cereal	Baked Potato	Roast Beef Sandwich on
with	Fresh Corn	Cracked Wheat Bread
Milk and Sugar	Green Salad	with
Whole Wheat Toast	with	Lettuce and Tomato
with	Oil and Vinegar	Coleslaw
Marmalade	Dressing	Carrot Cake
Coffee	Whole Grain Bread	Milk
	with Butter	Coffee or Tea
	Fresh Pineapple	
	Milk	
	Tea	

coarse cereals, wheat bran, whole wheat and rye flours, all fruits, raw vegetables, and legumes. This diet is nutritionally adequate.

The Low-Residue Diet

The low-residue diet is intended to reduce the normal work of the intestines by reducing food residue. It consists of foods that provide no more than two grams of fiber each day.

The Minimum-Residue Diet

The minimum-residue diet is extremely restricted. Because of the severe limitations of foods allowed, this diet may be inadequate in vitamins and minerals. If this diet must be

Table 28-4 Sample Menu for a Low-Residue Diet

Breakfast	Dinner	Supper or Lunch
Strained Orange Juice	Chicken Broth	Tomato Juice
Cream of Rice Cereal	Ground Beef Patty	Macaroni and Cheese
with	Boiled Potato	Green Beans
Milk and Sugar	Baked Squash	White Bread and Butter
White Toast	Lettuce with	Lemon Sherbet
with	Oil and Vinegar	Tea with Milk and Sugar
Butter and Jelly	Gelatin Dessert	
Coffee with	Milk	
Cream and Sugar		

Table 28-5 Low-Residue Foods

FOODS ALLOWED IN LOW-RESIDUE DIET	FOODS TO BE AVOIDED
milk, buttermilk (limited to two cups daily)	fresh or dried fruits and vegetables
cottage cheese and some mild cheeses as flavoring	
butter and margarine	whole grain breads and cereals
eggs, except fried	
tender chicken, fish, sweetbreads, ground beef, and ground lamb (meats must be baked, boiled or broiled)	nuts, seeds, legumes, coconut, and marmalade
soup broth	fibrous meat
cooked, mild-flavored vegetables without coarse fibers, vegetable juices, fruit juices, applesauce, canned fruits including white cherries, peaches, and pears; pureed apricots, prunes and plums, citrus fruits without membranes	
refined breads and cereals, white crackers, macaroni, spaghetti, and noodles	
custard, sherbet, vanilla ice cream, junket, and *cereal puddings* when considered as part of the 2-cup milk allowance; plain gelatin, angel cake, sponge cake, and plain cookies	
coffee, tea, cocoa, carbonated beverage	
salt, sugar, small amount of spices as permitted by the physician	

Table 28-6 Minimum-Residue Foods

FOODS ALLOWED IN A MINIMUM-RESIDUE DIET		FOODS TO BE AVOIDED
1 cup or less milk	refined breads and cereals white crackers	whole fruits and vegetables
cottage cheese if tolerated	macaroni, spaghetti, and noodles	fried foods
butter and margarine		coarse, whole-grain breads and cereals; quick breads
eggs, except fried	sherbet, gelatin, plain cake and plain cookies	
tender chicken and fish; ground beef and lamb	tea, coffee (if physician permits)	fibrous meats
soup broth		sometimes milk
vegetable juice	small amounts of salt and sugar	nuts, seeds, legumes
fruit juice except prune		

used for a period of time, the physician may prescribe vitamin and mineral supplements. The modifications made for the minimum-residue diet can be seen in table 28-6.

Ulcerative Colitis

Ulcerative colitis is a disease of the colon characterized by numerous ulcerated areas. It's cause is not known. It is sometimes thought to be an autoimmune disease, that is, a condition caused by the body's own defenses turning against itself. Viruses, milk intolerance and even anxiety are also suspected factors in its development. There may be cramping and frequent, semi-liquid stools containing mucus and blood. Patients may be anemic, generally malnourished, and underweight. Diet therapy is intended to restore the patient to a good nutritional status and reduce irritation to the colon. When there is severe ulcerative colitis, *parenteral feedings* (directly into the superior vena cava; see Chapter 29) may be necessary until the patient is able to tolerate food through the gastrointestinal tract. A minimal- or low-residue diet that is also high in protein (see Chapter 27) and high kcal (see Chapter 25) may be used. This is best divided into six meals instead of three because the ingestion of large meals is apt to stimulate the bowels. As the patient begins to regain health, the diet may be increasingly liberalized to suit the patient's tastes while maintaining good nutrition.

Celiac Disease

Celiac disease, also called *non-tropical sprue* or *celiac sprue*, is a disorder characterized by malabsorption. Symptoms include diarrhea, weight loss, and general malnutri-tion. Stools are usually foul smelling, light colored, and bulky. The cause is unknown, but it has been found that the elimination of *gluten* (a protein found in grains) from the diet gives relief. Untreated, it leads to decreased absorption of all nutrients, hence the malnutrition and weight loss.

The Gluten-Controlled Diet

A gluten-controlled diet is used in the treatment of celiac disease. If the patient is underweight, the diet should also be high in kcal, carbohydrates and protein. In addition, fat may be restricted until bowel function is normalized. Vitamin and mineral supplements may be prescribed.

DISORDERS OF THE ACCESSORY ORGANS

Cirrhosis and Hepatitis

The liver is of major importance to, and plays many roles in, metabolism. Except for a few of the fatty acids, all of the nutrients that are absorbed in the intestines are transported to the liver. The liver dismantles some of these nutrients, stores others, and uses some to synthesize other substances. The liver determines where amino acids are needed and synthesizes some proteins, enzymes, and urea. It changes the simple sugars to glycogen, provides glucose to body cells, and synthesizes glucose from amino acids if needed. It converts fats to lipoproteins and synthesizes cholesterol. It stores iron, copper, zinc, and magnesium as well as the fat-soluble vitamins and B vitamins. The liver synthesizes bile and stores it in the gallbladder. It detoxifies many substances such as barbiturates and morphine.

Table 28-7 Sample Menu for a Minimum-Residue Diet

Breakfast	Dinner	Supper or Lunch
Strained Orange Juice	Pineapple Juice	Tomato Juice
Poached Egg on White Toast	Ground Beef	Minced White Poached Fish
	Buttered Noodles	Macaroni with Butter
Coffee or Tea	Toast with Butter	White Bread and Butter
	Plain Gelatin	Lemon Sherbet
	Tea	Tea

Liver disease may be acute or chronic. Early treatment can usually lead to recovery.

Cirrhosis is a general term referring to all types of liver disease characterized by cell loss. Although the liver does regenerate, the replacement during cirrhosis does not match the loss. Cirrhosis may be caused by congenital defects, viral infections, or alcoholism. In addition to the loss of cells during cirrhosis, there is fatty infiltration and *fibrosis* (development of tough, stringy tissue). These developments prevent the liver from functioning normally. Blood flow through the liver is upset

Table 28-8 High-Kcal, High-Protein, Low-Residue Diet Menu

Breakfast	Snack	Lunch
Orange Juice	Beef Broth	Baked Chicken
Poached Egg	Soda Crackers	Macaroni
White Toast		Pureed Green Beans
Butter and Jelly		Rolls & Butter
Coffee with Milk and Sugar		Lemon Chiffon Pie
		Tea with Milk and Sugar
Snack	**Dinner**	**Snack**
Eggnog	Ground Beef Patty	Cookies
	Mashed Potato	Pineapple Juice
	Mashed Acorn Squash	
	Bread & Butter	
	Apple Sauce with Sponge Cake	
	Coffee with Milk & Sugar	

Contains 3,000 kcal
130 grams protein
Approximately 2.2 grams crude fiber

Table 28-9 Diet for Gluten Control—Foods to Allow and Foods to Avoid

Food Groups	Allow	Avoid
Beverage	Coffee; tea; decaffeinated coffee; pure instant coffee*; carbonated beverages; artificially flavored fruit drinks	Cereal beverage; coffee beverages containing cereal grains; root beer†
Meat	Pure meat, fish, fowl, and eggs; guaranteed pure meat cold cuts,* frankfurters,* and sausage*; aged cheese; cottage cheese; cream cheese; peanut butter; soybeans; peanuts	Commercially prepared meat and egg products,† breaded meats, meat loaf, and meat patties; processed cheese†; cheese foods† and dips†; texturized or hydrolyzed vegetable protein products†
Fat	Butter; margarine; cream; vegetable oil; shortening; nuts; olives; mayonnaise; gravies and sauces made with allowed thickening agents	Nondairy cream substitutes†; commercial salad dressing†; commercially prepared gravies and sauces
Milk	Milk; yogurt	Commercial chocolate milk; malted milk; instant milk drinks†; hot cocoa mixes†
Starch	Specially prepared bread and other baked products made with the following flours: corn, rice, potato, soybean, wheat starch	Any homemade or commercially prepared baked goods or mixes containing wheat (except wheat starch), oats, rye, graham, barley, buckwheat pancakes†, bran, or wheat germ; commercially prepared and corn muffins†; gluten bread
	Corn and rice cereals‡	Cereals containing wheat, oats, rye, barley, bran, wheat germ, graham, bulgur, or millet
	Potatoes; rice; hominy grits; low-protein wheat starch pastas	Commercial rice mixes; pasta, noodle, spaghetti, and macaroni products
	Snack foods, chips, and wafers made only of rice, corn, or potato; corn tortillas; popcorn	Crackers, chips,† and other snack foods†
	Thickening agents: corn flour, cornstarch, cornmeal, potato flour, potato starch, wheat starch, soybean starch, arrowroot starch, tapioca, gelatin	All others
Vegetable	All except those in "Avoid" column	Any commercially prepared with cheese sauce† or cream sauce; canned baked beans
Fruit	All except those in "Avoid" column	Commercially prepared pie fillings†; thickened fruit†
Soup	Homemade broth, vegetable, or cream soups thickened with allowed flours or starches	Commercially prepared soup,† soup mixes,† bouillon,† and broth†; any containing barley, pasta, or noodles
Dessert	Gelatin; meringues; custard; cornstarch, rice, and tapioca puddings; specially prepared desserts made of allowed flours and cereal-free baking powder; junket	Commercially prepared desserts and mixes: cookies, cakes, pie, piecrust, pastries, pudding; ice cream†; sherbet†; ice cream cones

Table 28-9 (*Continued*)

Food Groups	Allow	Avoid
Sweets	Sugar; honey; jelly; jam; molasses; corn syrup; pure maple syrup; pure baking chocolate; pure cocoa; coconut	Flavored syrups†; chocolate and other commercial candies†
Miscellaneous	Salt; pepper; other spices and herbs; dry yeast; food coloring and extracts	Prepared catsup,† mustard,† and horseradish†; bottle meat sauces†; soy sauce†; pickles†; seasoning mixes†; cake yeast†; chewing gum†; baking powder†
	Wine; rum; brandy; vermouth; cognac	Beer; ale; alcoholic beverages distilled from cereal grains
Food labeling:	The patient should be advised to read product labels carefully and avoid sources of gluten: wheats, oats, rye, barley, bran, wheat germ, bulgur, millet, graham, durham, and malt. Possible sources of gluten in processed foods include stabilizers, emulsifiers, cereal additives, and vegetable protein. If there is any doubt, the product should be avoided until absence of gluten is verified by the manufacturer or by a brand name list prepared by the research unit of a hospital or university.	

*Check label carefully to be sure gluten is not an ingredient.

†Avoid unless absence of gluten is verified by the manufacturer or by special brand name product lists.

‡Ready-to-eat corn and rice cereals may contain a small amount of malt as flavoring, but the amount usually is well tolerated.

(By permission of Mayo Foundation.)

and a form of hypertension, anemia, and hemorrhage in the esophagus may occur. The normal metabolic processes will also be disturbed to such a degree that in severe cases, death may result.

The dietary treatment of cirrhosis provides at least 35—40 kcal and 1 gram of protein per kilogram of body weight. Vitamins and minerals—especially iron—are very important, and supplements may be needed. In advanced cirrhosis 50—60 percent of the kcal should be from carbohydrates, and feedings should total 5 or 6. In some forms of cirrhosis, patients are unable to tolerate fat well, so it may be restricted to approximately 30 grams (see Chapter 26). In another form, the patients may not tolerate protein well so it may be restricted. Sometimes cirrhosis causes *ascites*

(an accumulation of fluid in the abdomen). In such a case, salt and fluids may be restricted (see Chapter 26). If there is bleeding in the esophagus, fiber may be restricted to prevent irritation of the tissue. No alcohol is allowed.

Hepatitis is an inflammation of the liver. *Necrosis* (tissue death due to loss of blood supply) occurs and the liver's normal metabolic activities are constricted. It may be acute or chronic. There may be bile *stasis* (stoppage or slowing) and decreased blood albumin levels. Patients experience nausea, fatigue, diarrhea, and anorexia. Weight loss may be quite pronounced. Hepatitis may be caused by viruses or toxic agents.

Diet therapy is a very important aspect of the treatment. During early treatment, a full liquid diet (see Chapter 23) may be prescribed. However, if the patient will not accept food by mouth, tube feedings may be necessary (see Chapter 29). As the patient improves and accepts food, the diet should be well balanced, and provide 35—40 kcal per kilogram of body weight. Carbohydrates should provide 50 percent of the kcal, fats 35 percent, and protein 15 percent—unless there has been serious necrosis as may occur in severe hepatitis. In such a case, the liver may only be able to cope with very small amounts of protein, so it may be restricted. Frequent, small meals are thought to be better than three large meals for these patients.

Patients with liver disease require a great deal of encouragement because their anorexia and consequent feelings of general malaise can be quite severe. Their recovery takes patience and time.

Cholecystitis and Cholelithiasis

The dual function of the gallbladder is the concentration and storage of bile. After bile is formed in the liver, the gallbladder concentrates it to several times its original strength, and stores it until needed. Fat in the duodenum triggers the gallbladder to contract and release bile into the common duct for the digestion of fat in the small intestine. If this flow is hindered there may be pain.

Cholecystitis (inflammation of the gallbladder) and *cholelithiasis* (gallstones) may inhibit the flow of bile and cause pain. Cholecystitis can cause changes in the gallbladder tissue which in turn can affect the cholesterol (a constituent of bile), causing it to harden and form stones. It is also thought that chronic overindulgence in fats may contribute to gallstones because the fat stimulates the liver to produce more cholesterol for the bile, which is necessary for the digestion of fat. In addition to pain, which may be severe, there may be indigestion and vomiting, particularly after the ingestion of fatty foods. Treatment may include medication to dissolve the stones as well as dietary treatment. If medication does not succeed, surgery to remove the gallbladder (*cholecystectomy*) may be indicated. Diet therapy includes a low-fat diet of 40—60 grams per day, and for the obese, weight loss. In addition, some patients benefit from a low-fat, bland diet (see Chapter 26 for fat-controlled diets). The particular foods allowed depend upon the patient's tolerance of them.

Pancreatitis

In addition to the hormone, insulin, the pancreas produces enzymes that are important in the digestion of protein, fats, and carbohydrates. When food reaches the duodenum, the pancreas sends its enzymes to the small intestine to aid in digestion.

Pancreatitis is an inflammation of the pancreas. It may be caused by tumors, stomach surgery, alcoholism, biliary tract disease, or severe protein-calorie malnutrition. It may be acute or chronic. Abdominal pain, nausea, and steatorrhea (fat in the stool) are symptoms. Inadequate digestion, malabsorption (particularly of fat soluble vitamins), and weight loss occur, and in cases where the islets of Langerhans are destroyed, diabetes mellitus may result. Diet therapy is intended to reduce pancreatic secretions and bile. Just as fat stimulates the gallbladder to secrete bile, protein and hydrochloric acid stimulate the pancreas to secrete its juices and enzymes. During acute pancreatitis, the patient is nourished strictly parenterally. Later, when the patient is able to tolerate oral feedings, a liquid diet consisting mainly of carbohydrates is given because, of these three nutrients, carbohydrates have the least stimulatory effect on pancreatic secretions.

As recovery progresses, small, frequent feedings of carbohydrates and protein with little fat, are given. The fat is restricted because of the deficiencies of pancreatic lipase. The protein may also be restricted. Antacids may be used to help neutralize gastric acid.

The therapeutic diet for pancreatitis may be a fat-restricted regular or bland diet. Vitamin supplements may be given. Alcohol is forbidden in all cases.

SUMMARY

Disturbances of the gastrointestinal tract require a wide variety of therapeutic diets. Dyspepsia and peptic ulcers may be helped by the use of a bland diet. Diverticulosis may be treated with a high-fiber diet while diverticulitis is better treated with a gradual progression from clear liquid to the high-fiber diet. Ulcerative colitis may require a low-residue diet combined with high protein and high kcal. Cirrhosis requires a substantial balanced diet with occasional restrictions of fat, protein, salt, or fluids. Diet therapy for hepatitis may range from parenteral to a full, well-balanced diet, although protein may be restricted, depending upon the patient's condition. Cholecystitis and cholelithiasis require a low-fat diet alone, or combined with a bland diet. Pancreatitis diet therapy ranges from parenteral to a regular diet, with fat restricted.

Case Study—Gastrointestinal Disease

Mr. F. was a highly successful man, having reached nearly the top position in his company by the age of 43. He worked long and effectively, taking time for neither breakfast nor lunch, unless there was an obligatory business luncheon. When people asked him how he managed to accomplish so much on so little food, he answered that "black coffee and nervous energy" propelled him.

Since his latest promotion to a situation far from his family, he has worked harder than usual, finding unexpected problems in the new position and at home. Recently he has felt unusually tired and even faint at times, and occasionally his stool was tarry. He felt he lacked the time to see a doctor.

Last Friday, he decided to work just a bit past 5, but after the others in the office had left he felt so weak he decided to rest on his couch awhile. The next thing he knew, he was gagging and vomiting blood. The cleaning lady called an ambulance, however, and help soon arrived.

Mr. F. was told he had a gastric ulcer, he would not be released from the hospital for at least a week, he would have to rest—meaning no work—for at least another few weeks, and his eating habits would have to be improved.

The first day he was given a modified Sippy diet and by the second day was put on a bland diet. By the end of the week spicy foods, coffee, and tea were restricted and, of course, no alcohol would be allowed in his diet for a long time.

Case Study Questions

1. What may have contributed to Mr. F.'s ulcer?
2. Did the recent move have any effect on the ulcer? Explain.
3. What could have happened if the cleaning lady had not come by?
4. Why is rest an important element in the treatment of ulcers?
5. Why can Mr. F. not have caffeine?
6. Why is alcohol prohibited?
7. Why are cola drinks prohibited?
8. Write a day's menus for Mr. F. on his new regime.
9. Should Mr. F. eat at his desk when he gets back to work? Why?
10. What advice do you think a doctor might give Mr. F.?

Discussion Topics

1. Name the accessory organs in the gastrointestinal system and explain their roles in digestion and metabolism.
2. Discuss dyspepsia. Include its probable causes and the suggested diet therapy for it.
3. Describe the bland diet and name ten foods that would not be included in it. Discuss its uses. How does the bland diet differ from the regular diet? When is it prescribed? Is it nutritionally adequate? Do any of the students know anyone who has been on a bland diet? If so, have them describe their reaction to the diet.
4. Describe hiatus hernia. Name its symptoms and possible treatment.
5. Define ulcers. Where are they found in the gastrointestinal system and how are they treated? Why is the Sippy Diet seldom used? What substances should not be allowed an ulcer patient? Why?
6. Explain the difference between diverticulosis and diverticulitis. How are these conditions treated?
7. Discuss the high-fiber diet. For what conditions might it be used? Compare it to the low- and minimum-residue diets. Why is corn on the cob not allowed on the minimum-residue diet? Name other foods that are not allowed on the minimum-residue diet and tell why they would not be allowed.
8. Discuss ulcerative colitis. What is it? What causes it? How is it treated?

9. Explain the metabolic functions of the liver. How do cirrhosis and hepatitis affect it. Discuss the diet therapy for these conditions.
10. Discuss cholecystitis and cholelithiasis. What organ do they affect? What is the dietary treatment for these conditions?
11. What is pancreatitis and what is the diet therapy for it?

Suggested Activities

1. Hold a panel discussion on gastrointestinal disturbances and the dietary treatment of them.
2. Make a list of foods eaten yesterday. Circle the foods that would be allowed on a restricted-residue diet.
3. Find recipes for restricted-residue and minimum-residue diets and add them to the special diet recipe file.
4. Plan a day's menu for a restricted-residue diet, another for a minimum-residue diet, and another for a high-fiber diet. Evaluate the menus for nutritional value, using the Basic Four food groups as a guide. Exchange menu plans with a fellow student and evaluate each other's plans in terms of nutrient content, flavor, aroma, color, shape, appearance, texture, and satiety value.
5. Prepare at least one of the meals on each of the above menus. Evaluate each in terms of nutrient content, flavor, aroma, color, shape, appearance, texture, and satiety value.
6. Adapt the following menu to suit a patient on a minimum-residue diet:

Orange Juice
Fried Egg
Bacon
Whole Wheat Toast
with
Butter and Marmalade
Milk
Coffee

7. List 10 of your favorite foods. Circle those foods that would not be allowed in a bland diet.

Review

Multiple Choice. Select the letter that precedes the best answer.

1. Dyspepsia
   1. may be an indication of a serious gastrointestinal disturbance
   2. is usually psychological in origin
   3. may be overcome with improved eating habits
   4. is caused by high-fiber foods
      a) 1 & 2   b) 1, 2, & 3   c) 1 & 3   d) 2, 3, & 4

2. The bland diet
   1. is generally considered a very effective means of therapy for gastrointestinal disturbances
   2. contains mild but fibrous foods
   3. is intended to prevent irritation of the gastrointestinal tract
   4. is not always considered an effective therapeutic tool in the treatment of gastrointestinal disorders
      a) 1 & 2   b) 1, 2, & 3   c) 2 & 3   d) 3 & 4

3. The purpose of the bland diet is to reduce
   1. peristalsis
   2. the flow of gastric juices
   3. kcal intake
   4. iron absorption
      a) 1, 2 & 3   b) 2 & 3   c) 1 & 2   d) 3 & 4

4. The flavors of foods in the bland diet are generally
   1. spicy
   2. highly varied
   3. mild
   4. salty
      a) 1 & 2   b) 1, 2, & 3   c) 2 only   d) 3 only

5. The following foods would be allowed on a bland diet:
   1. peeled, fresh apple and oranges without membranes
   2. fried hamburger with catsup
   3. gingerale and 7-up
   4. hot chocolate with whipped cream
      a) 1 & 3   b) only 3   c) only 1   d) only 4

6. Hiatus hernia
   1. only occurs in the small intestine
   2. may cause regurgitation
   3. causes "heartburn"
   4. patients may be more comfortable with small, frequent meals
      a) 1 & 3   b) 2, 3, & 4   c) 2 & 4   d) 2 & 3

7. Peptic ulcers
   1. occur in the stomach or the duodenum
   2. may be partially caused by anxiety
   3. are always treated with the Sippy Diet
   4. are sometimes treated with a regular diet
      a) 1, 2 & 4   b) 1, 2, & 3   c) 1 & 2   d) 2 & 3

8. Protein foods may be somewhat restricted in cases of peptic ulcers because they
   1. contribute to uremia
   2. contain sodium
   3. provide amino acids
   4. stimulate gastric acid secretions
      a) 1 & 4   b) only 4   c) 2 & 3   d) only 3

9. The following should not be allowed an ulcer patient
   1. cola drinks
   2. milkshakes
   3. tea and coffee
   4. beer and wine
      a) 1, 3, & 4   b) 2, 3, & 4   c) 3 & 4   d) only 4

10. Diverticulitis
    1. is the inflammation of diverticula
    2. may be initially treated with a clear-liquid diet
    3. may be prevented with a high-fiber diet
    4. affects the intestines
       a) 1, 2 & 3   b) 2, 3, & 4   c) 1, 2, 3, & 4   d) 1, 3, & 4

11. Residue is that part of food that
    1. remains longest in the stomach
    2. is indigestible
    3. is left uneaten after the meal
    4. is inedible
       a) 1 & 2   b) 2 only   c) 3 only   d) 4 only

12. Food residue
    1. is ultimately evacuated in the feces
    2. never leaves the stomach
    3. never leaves the intestines
    4. results from incorrect cooking methods
       a) 1 only
       b) 2 & 3
       c) 3 & 4
       d) 4 only

13. Large amounts of food residue cause
   1. a decrease in fecal matter
   2. an increase in fecal matter
   3. weight gain
   4. diverticulosis
      a) 1 only (b) 2 only   c) 2 & 3   d) 3 & 4

14. The following foods would not be recommended for the high-fiber diet:
   1. pureed pears
   2. mashed potatoes
   3. rice pudding
   4. bran cereal
      (a) 1, 2, & 3   b) 2, 3, & 4   c) 3 & 4   d) only 4

15. The following foods would not be allowed on a low-residue diet:
   ·1. fresh oranges
   ·2. corn on the cob
   3. macaroni and cheese
   ·4. toast with butter
      a) 1, 2, & 3   b) 1 & 4   c) 1 & 2   d) only 4

16. The following foods would not be allowed on a minimum residue diet:
   1. corned beef and cabbage
   2. sliced, peeled apples
   3. peas and corn
   4. poached eggs on toast
      a) 1, 2, & 4   b) 1 & 2   c) 2 & 3   d) 1, 2, & 3

17. If the minimum-residue diet must be used for a period of time, the physician may
   1. alternate it weekly with the high-iron diet
   2. substitute the full liquid diet from time to time
   3. add fresh fruit juices before each meal
   4. prescribe a vitamin and mineral supplement
      a) 1 & 2   b) 1, 2, & 3   c) 2 & 3   (d) 4 only

18. Ulcerative colitis
   ·1. affects the colon
   2. always requires parenteral feedings
   ·3. may be treated with a low-residue diet that is also high in kcal and protein
   ·4. patients may be malnourished
      (a) 1, 3 & 4   b) 2, 3, & 4   c) 3 & 4   d) only 4

19. The following foods would be recommended for an ulcerative colitis patient; provided the patient tolerates <u>milk</u>:
    1. custard with whipped cream   3. eggnog
    2. chocolate milkshake   4. cream of tomato soup with crackers
       a) 1, 3, & 4   b) 1, 2, & 3   c) 2, 3, & 4   d) 1, 2, 3, & 4

20. The liver
    1. plays a major role in metabolism
    2. directs the distribution of amino acids
    3. converts glucose to glycogen
    4. stores iron and fat-soluble vitamins
       a) 1, 3, & 4   b) 1, 2, & 3   c) 2, 3, & 4   d) 1, 2, 3, & 4

21. Cirrhosis
    1. is a liver disease characterized by cell loss
    2. is always caused by alcoholism
    3. inevitably results in death
    4. affects the body's ability to tolerate fats
       a) 1 & 4   b) 1, 2, & 4   c) 1, 3, & 4   d) 1, 2, 3, & 4

22. Ascites
    1. is caused by cirrhosis
    2. is an accumulation of fluid in the abdomen
    3. may require the restriction of sodium and water
    4. is caused by a shortage of iron
       a) 1 & 4   b) 1, 2, & 3   c) 2 & 4   d) only 4

23. Hepatitis
    1. is an inflammation of the liver
    2. causes necrosis
    3. is always chronic
    4. may be caused by viruses or toxic agents
       a) 1 & 2   b) 1, 2, & 4   c) 2 & 3   d) 2, 3, &4

24. Gallbladder problems may require
    1. the dietary restriction of fat
    2. cholecystectomy
    3. loss of weight
    4. additional protein in the diet
       a) 1, 2, & 3   b) 1, 3, & 4   c) 1 & 3   d) 1 & 4

25. Inflammation of the pancreas
    1. is called pancreatitis
    2. may cause pain and nausea
    3. may require parenteral feeding
    4. always signifies cancer
       a) 1 & 2   b) 1 & 3   c) 2 & 3   d) 1, 2, & 3

References

Biology book of choice

Encyclopedia of choice

Bodinski, Lois H. 1982. *The Nurse's Guide to Diet Therapy*. New York: John Wiley & Sons.

Gray, Henry. 1977. *Gray's Anatomy*. New York: Bounty Books.

Krause, Marie, and Kathleen L. Mahan. 1979. *Food, Nutrition and Diet Therapy*, 6th ed. Philadelphia: W.B. Saunders Co.

U.S. Department of Agriculture. 1963, 1975. *Composition of Foods*.

University of Iowa Hospitals and Clinics. 1979. *Recent Advances in Therapeutic Diets*. Iowa City: Iowa State University Press.

Winick, Myron. 1980. *Nutrition in Health and Disease*. New York: John Wiley & Sons.

Chapter 29

DIETS FOR SURGICAL PATIENTS, AND PATIENTS WITH BURNS, FEVERS, AND INFECTIONS

VOCABULARY

antibodies	enterostomies	phlebitis
aspirated	fever	regurgitated
early dumping	hemorrhage	thrombosis
syndrome	hyperalimentation	TPN
elective surgery	hypermetabolic	traumas
endocrine system	nasogastric tube	
enteral feeding	parenteral feeding	

OBJECTIVES

After studying this chapter, you should be able to

- Describe the body's reaction to trauma and relate it to nutrition

- Explain the special dietary needs of surgical and burn patients

- Explain the special dietary needs of patients with fever and infection

---

The topics discussed in this chapter may be described as *traumas* (injuries). The body reacts to trauma by signaling the endocrine system, which activates a self-protective, hypermetabolic response. This includes the immediate provision of glucose and other substances necessary for energy, wound healing and tissue maintenance. The intensity of this response depends on the severity of the trauma.

Trauma causes protein and mineral losses. At the same time there is an increased need for them to rebuild tissue. When the trauma includes hemorrhage and vomiting, these losses are compounded. Energy output is increased during trauma and extra vitamins are needed for the increased metabolism and the rebuilding of tissue. Obviously, nutrition plays a major role in the treatment of trauma.

SURGERY

Pre-Surgery Dietary Care

Surgery is a trauma whether elective or emergency. If elective, the patient's nutritional status should be evaluated prior to surgery, and if improvement is needed, it should be undertaken. A good nutritional status prior to surgery enhances recovery. A diet history taken before surgery can help in this evaluation, and will be helpful to the dietician in providing foods that will be accepted by the patient after surgery when appetite is poor.

Improvement of nutritional status will usually mean providing extra protein, carbohydrates, vitamins, and minerals. The extra protein is needed for wound healing, tissue building, and blood regeneration. Extra carbohydrates will be converted to glycogen and stored, to help provide energy after surgery, when needs are high, and when patients may be unable to eat normally. The B vitamins are needed for the increased metabolism, vitamins A and C for wound healing, vitamin D for the absorption of calcium, and vitamin K for proper clotting of the blood. Iron is necessary for blood building, calcium and phosphorus for bones, and the other minerals for maintenance of acid-base, electrolyte, and fluid balance in the body.

In cases of overweight, improved nutritional status includes weight reduction prior to surgery. Excess fat is a surgical hazard because the extra tissue increases the chances of infection and fatty tissue tends to retain the anesthetic longer than other tissue.

Food usually is not allowed the patient after the evening meal on the day before surgery. This ensures that the stomach contains no food, which could be regurgitated and then *aspirated* (taken into the airway) during surgery. If there is to be gastrointestinal surgery, a low-residue diet may be ordered for a few days prior to surgery (see Chapter 28). This is intended to reduce intestinal residue.

Post-Surgery Dietary Care

The post-surgery diet is intended to provide kcal and nutrients in amounts suf-ficient to fulfill metabolic needs and to promote healing and subsequent recovery.

Immediately following surgery, most patients will be given intravenous solutions containing water and dextrose and sometimes, electrolytes and water-soluble vitamins. These solutions provide approximately 170 kcal per liter. Since no more than 2 1/2—3 liters can be given in a 24-hour period, the maximum number of kcal supplied by these solutions is about 500. The estimated kcal requirement for adults after trauma is estimated to be from 40—70 per kilogram of body weight. A 110-pound individual would require at least 2000 kcal per day. Obviously, until the patient can take food there will be a considerable kcal deficit each day. Body fat will be used to provide energy and to spare body protein, but the kcal intake must be increased to meet energy demands as soon as possible.

Because protein losses due to trauma can be significant, and because protein is especially needed after surgery to rebuild tissue, control edema, avoid shock, resist infection, and transport fats, a high protein diet of 100 grams or more each day may be recommended. (See Chap. 27 for High-Protein diet.) In addition, extra minerals and vitamins are needed. When peristalsis returns, oral feedings can begin. Peristalsis is evidenced by bowel sounds.

Normally, post-operative diets begin with the clear liquid diet and progress to the regular diet. Sometimes this is done directly, and sometimes by way of the full liquid, soft, or residue-restricted diets. It depends on the patient and the type of surgery. (See Chapter 23 for a review of hospital diets and Chapter 28 for residue-restricted diets).

The average patient will be able to take food within approximately four days after surgery. If the patient cannot take food then, parenteral or *enteral* (via a nasogastric tube or a tube directly into the stomach or small intestine) feeding may be required.

Sometimes following gastric surgery, *early dumping syndrome* occurs within 15—30 minutes after eating. This is characterized by dizziness, weakness, cramps, vomiting, and diarrhea. It is caused by food moving too quickly from the stomach into the small intestine. Reducing the amount of liquid given with meals seems to alleviate the problem as do meals somewhat restricted in carbohydrate because carbohydrates leave the stomach faster than proteins and fats. Sucrose is generally restricted in such situations. Complex carbohydrates, while restricted if this problem occurs, are gradually reintroduced. Also, the total daily food intake may be divided and served as several small meals rather than the usual three meals, in an attempt to avoid overloading the stomach. Some patients do not tolerate milk well after gastric surgery so its inclusion in the diet will depend upon the patient's tolerance.

The food habits of the post-operative patient should be closely observed because they will affect recovery. When the patient's appetite fails to improve, the physician and the dietician should be notified, and efforts made to offer nutritional foods that the patient will eat. The patient should be encouraged to eat and to eat slowly to avoid swallowing air, which can cause abdominal distension and pain.

PARENTERAL NUTRITION

Parenteral nutrition is the provision of nutrients via a vein. When such provision is only dextrose, water, vitamin, and electrolyte solutions, it can be done via a peripheral vein. However, in some cases, such as after burns or during coma, when the digestive tract must not be used or when the patient refuses to eat, it is necessary to provide the total nutritional requirements parenterally. This is called total parenteral nutrition (TPN) or hyperalimentation. A solution containing glucose, protein, vitamins, and minerals is given through a catheter inserted surgically in the superior vena cava. The vena cava is used because the blood flow is high; thus the nutrients are quickly diluted, reducing the possibility of *phlebitis* (inflammation of a vein), or *thrombosis* (blood clot). During a 24-hour period, 2500 to 3500 kcal can be given in this way.

TPN solutions are prepared under sterile conditions. When the TPN is to be discontinued, it must be done gradually. As the oral intake of food is gradually increased, the TPN should be gradually decreased.

ENTERAL NUTRITION

Enteral nutrition, or tube feeding, is sometimes used because of unconsciousness, surgery, stroke, severe malnutrition, extensive burns, emotional problems, or obstruction. These feedings are administered by a nasogastric tube (through the nose), or by various *enterostomies* (openings) directly into the esophagus, duodenum, jejunum, or stomach by means of a surgical incision. The nasogastric tube is inserted by a doctor or a registered nurse. The enterostomy tubes are inserted by the doctor during surgery. Patients who are tube fed require a great deal of patience and understanding. They have been deprived of a basic pleasure of life—eating. They may also be fearful and apprehensive about the tube itself. The condition requiring enteral nutrition may be temporary or permanent.

Diets for tube feeding must be liquid in consistency, nutritionally adequate, and free of contamination. Tube feedings are usually high in caloric value and often high in protein. Occasionally, a lactose-free feeding may be ordered. A food blender is very useful for converting some foods into liquid form. Baby foods may be used when diluted to liquid consistency. Feedings often must be strained to remove any lumps that may have formed from poor blending or preparation.

Commercially prepared tube feedings are available. These are nutritionally adequate and convenient because the unopened cans do not require refrigeration and no further preparation is necessary.

The first feedings are small and usually given every hour. If the patient has difficulty tolerating the feeding and regurgitates it, the person giving the feeding must be especially careful to prevent *aspiration* (breathing in) of the vomitus. First feedings are usually diluted to half strength with equal amounts of water to prevent diarrhea. Diarrhea causes the loss of essential nutrients and fluids, which weakens the patient. Diarrhea can also occur when feedings are too cold, given too rapidly or in too concentrated a form, or are contaminated by bacteria. As the patient tolerates the feedings, they may be gradually increased to full strength, larger feedings, and with a longer time span between feedings.

Tube feedings are a good medium for bacterial growth. At best, tube feeding is a clean procedure and not an absolutely sterile technique. However, precautions must be taken to prevent contamination.

1. Keep the tube clamped off between feedings.
2. Keep the end of the tube covered with sterile gauze between feedings.
3. Cover opened cans with clean plastic covers.
4. Keep opened cans covered tightly and stored in the refrigerator.
5. Flush the tube with water after every feeding.
6. Wash and dry the equipment between feedings.

ADMINISTERING THE TUBE FEEDING

A demonstration of the tube feeding procedure is first given by the instructor. The student must carefully observe and study the procedure before attempting it. The prescribed feeding must first be double-checked against the doctor's written order. It should be at room temperature before being administered. A feeding that is too cold may give the patient abdominal cramps or diarrhea.

There are two methods that may be used to administer nutrients to a patient who has had a nasogastric or enterostomy tube inserted for tube feeding purposes. The funnel method (figure 29-1) or the drip method (figure 29-2) may be used.

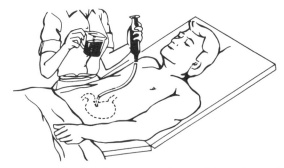

Figure 29-1 The funnel may be used to tube feed patients who have a gastrostomy tube or a nasogastric tube. The principles of nursing care are the same. This illustration shows tube feeding through a gastrostomy tube.

The Funnel Method

Supplies should be put on a tray and taken to the bedside:

- A large syringe (the barrel may be used as a funnel)
- Prescribed feeding at room temperature
- 60 ml (2 oz) of lukewarm water (to flush tubing)
- Glass of water (for checking position of tube)
- Sterile 2" × 2" gauze sponge
- Rubber band
- Emesis basin

The procedure should be described to the patient beforehand to reduce anxiety. Anyone who has a nasogastric tube inserted may be especially afraid of choking. If the patient has a nasogastric tube in place, she or he should be helped into a semi-Fowler's position. In this position, the patient lies on his back with the head and shoulders elevated to a 45° angle; the knees are slightly flexed and the heels are resting on the bed. This position helps the feeding to flow to the stomach using the force of gravity. If the patient has an enterostomy tube in place, the head of the bed should be raised to a semi-Fowler's position *only if the patient's condition permits it*. If the patient's condition does not permit a semi-sitting position, the feeding may be given while the patient is lying flat with his head on a pillow.

The doctor may order that the enterostomy tube be aspirated before the feeding is given. This is done to determine if the preceding feeding has passed into the small intestine. If the preceding feeding has not passed into the small intestine, the current feeding may need to be withheld. The doctor's order would indicate how to determine if a feeding is to be withheld.

It is essential that the nurse check that the tube is in the stomach before a tube feeding is given. (If the tube is in the lungs or trachea, the patient can aspirate the feeding causing choking, pneumonia, or death.) To check, the clamp on the tube should be opened or removed before testing:

- The open end of the tube should be placed in a glass of water. If there is bubbling each time the patient breathes, the tube may be in the lungs. If this occurs, the feeding must not be given and the doctor or the nurse in charge must be notified. If no bubbles can be seen in the water, the tube is probably in the stomach.
- To check if the tube is in the stomach, the nurse should aspirate the tube with a syringe and check for gastric content; an Asepto syringe may be used to gently suck out some of the stomach contents. The rubber bulb should be squeezed *before* it is inserted in the glass part of the Asepto syringe. If a greenish yellow fluid returns, the tube is in the stomach.

The funnel must be attached to the tubing. The tubing must be pinched off or clamped while the funnel is attached. This prevents excess air from entering the stomach. Excess air in the stomach causes gas pains and abdominal distention. Thirty milliliters (1 oz) of warm water should be poured into the funnel before the feeding. The water should be allowed to run in by gravity and not forced. If the water flows through the tube, it indicates the tube is open and the feeding may proceed. If the water does not run in, the nurse in charge should check the tube.

The prescribed feeding should be poured into the funnel and given in an unhurried manner. More of the solution should be added before the funnel has emptied. This prevents air from entering the stomach. When a feeding is given through a gastrostomy tube, the funnel should be held about two to three inches above the abdomen. The rate of the feeding can be controlled by raising or lowering the funnel, or by slightly pinching the tubing. A typical feeding takes about 20 minutes. An emesis basin should be available in case the patient regurgitates the feeding.

The patient should be carefully observed for signs of distress. **CAUTION:** If the patient with a nasogastric tube is coughing, choking, or becoming cyanotic (turning blue), he may be aspirating the fluid because the tube has become displaced. In such a case, the feeding must be stopped immediately and the nurse in charge notified.

After the feeding has been completed, about 30 ml (1 oz) of water should be poured into the tube to clear the tubing and prevent it from clogging. The tubing must be clamped just before the funnel empties. This prevents the feeding solution and gastric juices from escaping. After the funnel has been removed, the end of the tube should be covered with a sterile 2 × 2 inch gauze sponge and secured with a rubber band. This prevents bacteria from entering the tube.

The time, type, amount of feeding, and how well the patient tolerated it must be charted. Charting must be accurate, prompt, and complete. If an Intake and Output record is being kept for the patient, record the time, amount, and type of feeding on it also.

The patient's condition should be carefully monitored. A feeling of fullness or nausea after a meal may indicate that the patient is being fed too often or is receiving too much at each feeding. If the patient feels this way, the nurse in charge should be notified because the

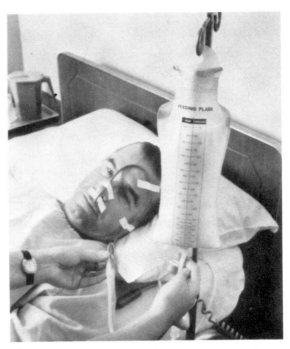

Figure 29-2 Continuous drip feeding

order for feeding may need to be changed.

The patient should rest for about 20 minutes after the feeding. She or he may remain in the semi-Fowler's position or be turned on the right side with the head elevated. An elevated position and relaxation aids digestion.

The Drip Method

Supplies should be collected and taken to the patient's bedside:

- Continuous drip feeding set with attached tubing
- IV stand
- Prescribed feeding at room temperature

The procedure should be clearly described to the patient before it is begun. The continuous drip set with the attached tubing should be hung on the IV stand. The tubing on the drip set must be clamped. The plastic bag with the prescribed solution should be filled. The tubing must be unclamped to allow the solution to run through and expel the air, which could cause uncomfortable gas pains for the patient. Then the tubing on the drip set must be reclamped.

The gastric tube should be temporarily unclamped to check if the tube is still in the patient's stomach. The drip set tubing must be attached to the gastric tube and the drip regulated according to the doctor's order. The drip set tubing is then unclamped and the procedure charted. This must be checked frequently to be sure the fluid is flowing properly. The tubing and bag should be changed at least every 8 hours. This is necessary to prevent the growth of bacteria.

DIET THERAPY FOR BURNS

The losses of protein, fluids and electrolytes caused by serious burns are extraordinary, and the tissue loss may continue for many days. These nutrient losses must, of course, be replaced. An enormous increase in energy is also needed for the healing process. Intravenous solutions and blood transfusions are initially used to replace lost fluids. A high protein, high kcal diet with largely increased amounts of vitamin C (to aid in healing) and B vitamins (for increased metabolic needs) is used.

TPN may be required due to facial burns and the *atony* (weakness) of the gastrointestinal tract which sometimes occurs in badly burned patients.

It is also essential that badly burned patients have sufficient fluids to help the kidneys hold the unusual load of wastes in solution. When food can be taken orally, meals should be small and frequent.

Burn patients need a great deal of encouragement. They may be in pain, worried about disfigurement and know they face a long, costly and painful hospital stay with the possibility of surgery.

DIET THERAPY DURING FEVERS AND INFECTIONS

Fever typically accompanies an infection. Fevers and infections may be acute or chronic. Fever is a hypermetabolic state in which each degree of fever on the Fahrenheit scale raises the metabolism rate 7 percent. If extra kcal are not provided during fever, the body first uses its supply of glycogen, then its stored fat and finally its own tissue for energy.

Protein intake should be increased during fever to one or two grams per kilogram of body weight. Protein is needed to replace body tissue and to produce antibodies to fight the infection. Extra kcal are needed for the increased metabolic rate. Extra vitamins are also necessary for the increased metabolic rate and to help fight the infection causing the fever.

Patients usually have very poor appetites with fever, but they will often accept ice water, fruit juice, and carbonated beverages. Some will accept boullion or consommé.

Usually, the diet during fever and infection progresses from the liquid to the regular diet with frequent, small meals recommended. It should be high protein, high kcal, and high vitamin. In some cases, parenteral or enteral feedings may be necessary.

SUMMARY

Surgery, burns, fevers, and infections are traumas that cause the body to react hyper-metabolically to promote healing. This creates the need for additional nutrients at the same time that the injury causes a loss of nutrients. Care must be taken to provide extra proteins, kcal, vitamins, minerals, and carbohydrates as needed in these stress situations. When surgery is elective, nutritional status should be improved prior to surgery, if necessary. When food cannot be taken orally, enteral or parenteral nutrition should be used.

Case Study—Surgery Patient

Anne was an extremely busy 46-year-old working wife and mother of two teenagers when she fell and broke her hip very badly. The surgeon pinned it and grafted bone, and instructed her to put no weight on it. During the surgery it was observed that Anne appeared to have early osteoporosis. The surgeon so advised her.

When Anne was in the hospital, the dietician took a careful diet history and learned that Anne had, in her young adult life, not eaten as she knew she should have. She admitted to having shorted herself on milk all of her adult life. She did eat cheese fairly often, however.

For several days after the surgery, Anne was unable to eat at all. She became extremely depressed. Vitamins were prescribed. As Anne did begin to eat a bit, she felt better and was less depressed. She was discharged after 2 1/2 weeks. When Anne returned home, she weighed 100 pounds and regained her strength very slowly. After 3 1/2 months, she went back to work on crutches.

After six months it became clear that the hip was not healing as the surgeon had hoped, and he advised Anne to have a hip replacement if she were to walk again without crutches. She agreed and a date was set. This time she prepared for surgery. The operation was a success. She suffered no depression, and she was discharged after two weeks. She is walking now without a cane.

Case Study Questions

1. What is osteoporosis and how might Anne have developed it? What can she do to prevent it from becoming worse? What relation is there between Anne's apparent liking for cheese and osteoporosis?
2. What might have contributed to Anne's depression after the first surgery?
3. Was Anne's first surgery elective or emergency? The second?
4. How might Anne have prepared for surgery the second time?
5. What might have contributed to Anne's lack of depression after the second operation?
6. What type of diet should Anne have been on after surgery?
7. What type of diet should Anne follow to limit any possible worsening of her osteoporosis? How long should she follow this diet?

8. What possible effect might the vitamins prescribed in the hospital have had on Anne's depression and feelings of weakness?
9. Although Anne had always done the family's housework and cooking as well as dog walking, she could do very few of these things after her fracture. How might these chores have been handled by her family?

Discussion Topics

1. Describe the body's reaction to trauma and how nutrition is related to it.
2. Why are extra nutrients needed during trauma?
3. When might surgery be elective?
4. In what ways might a diet history of a pre-surgical patient be helpful?
5. Explain why a trauma patient needs extra protein. What happens when the extra protein is not provided?
6. Why does a trauma patient need extra minerals?
7. Why must a patient's stomach be empty at the time of surgery?
8. Explain why the IV dextrose solutions are not sufficient to fulfill nutritional requirements after surgery.
9. Explain early dumping syndrome and tell how it may be alleviated.
10. Discuss enteral and parenteral nutrition. Explain the differences between them. Are they nutritionally adequate programs? When might each be used?
11. Could parenteral nutrition be used in the treatment of anorexia nervosa? Explain.

Suggested Activities

1. Ask a doctor or nurse to visit the class and discuss enterostomies, telling why and when they are used and problems associated with them.
2. Prepare a drawing of the body, featuring the endocrine system. Include a brief description of each gland and its function(s) in the body.
3. Ask if a class member has experienced a trauma as discussed in this chapter. If so, ask that person to describe it, her or his reactions to it, appetite and recovery.
4. Plan a day's menus for a 175-pound man who requires 100 grams of protein, and 70 kcal per kilogram of body weight.

5. Role-play a situation where a patient is 9 days post surgery, cannot eat, and the nurse is trying to convince her to eat.
6. Role-play a situation between a 10-year old child and a nurse. The child has rheumatic fever, a temperature of 100° F and refuses most food.

Review

Multiple Choice. Select the letter that precedes the best answer.

1. Trauma
   1. may be described as injury
   2. causes a hypermetabolic response in the body
   3. usually increases the body's need for protein
   4. has no relation to nutrition
      a) 1 & 2   b) 1, 2, 3   c) 2, 3, 4   d) 4 only

2. During trauma, there is usually
   1. reduced need for protein and minerals
   2. a hypermetabolic response in the body
   3. only minor changes in nutritional requirements
   4. an increased need for protein
      a) 1, 2   b) 1, 3   c) 2, 3   d) 2, 4

3. Wound healing, tissue building, and blood regeneration all require
   1. extra fat
   2. extra cholesterol
   3. reduced kcal intake
   4. protein
      a) only 4   b) only 3   c) 3, 4   d) 1, 2, 3

4. Intravenous solutions
   1. sometimes contain water-soluble vitamins
   2. sometimes contain fat-soluble vitamins
   3. are usually given immediately following surgery
   4. provide only about 170 kcal per gallon of solution
      a) 1, 2   b) 1, 3   c) 1, 4   d) 4 only

5. Protein is needed to
   1. build tissue
   2. resist infection
   3. control edema
   4. kill bacteria
      a) 1, 2   b) 2, 3   c) 1, 2, 3   d) 2, 3, 4

6. It would not be surprising for TPN to be used in the treatment of
   1. fractured hip
   2. third degree burns over a large part of the patient's body
   3. broken jaw
   4. appendicitis
      a) 1, 2   b) 2, 3   c) 3, 4   d) 4 only

7. Early dumping syndrome is characterized by
   1. migraine headache
   2. hypertension and tremors
   3. vomiting and diarrhea
   4. dizziness and cramps
      a) 1, 2   b) 1, 2, 3   c) 2, 3   d) 3, 4

8. TPN is given through
   1. a nasogastric tube
   2. a peripheral vein in the ankle
   3. the superior vena cava
   4. an enterostomy
      a) 1   b) 2   c) 3   d) 4

9. Severely burned patients will need
   1. to replace protein and fluids
   2. to replace electrolytes
   3. intravenous solutions and blood transfusions
   4. a high-protein, high-kcal diet
      a) 1, 2   b) 1, 2, 3   c) 2, 3, 4   d) 1, 2, 3, 4

10. Fever
    1. creates a need for extra kcal
    2. patients have enormous appetites
    3. patients require extra vitamins
    4. patients should be kept on a low-kcal diet
       a) 1, 2   b) 1, 4   c) 1, 3   d) 1, 2, 3, 4

11. Patients must occasionally be fed by tube because of
    1. accidents   3. surgery
    2. childbirth   4. unconsciousness
       a) 1, 2, 4   b) 1, 2, 3   c) 1, 3, 4   d) all

12. Tube feedings *must* be
    1. colorful   3. liquid
    2. nutritionally balanced meals   4. smooth
       a) 1, 2, 4   b) 1, 3, 4   c) 2, 3, 4   d) all

13. For tube feedings, one may use
    1. commercially prepared liquid diets
    2. baby foods
    3. regular diets blended to a liquid consistency
    4. high-calorie diets blended to a liquid consistency
        a) 1, 2, 3   b) 2, 3, 4   c) 1, 3, 4   d) all
14. To prevent diarrhea during tube feedings, one should
    1. add iron to the feeding
    2. give feeding very slowly
    3. give feeding very quickly
    4. give feeding at room temperature
        a) 1, 3   b) 2, 4   c) 3   d) all
15. The first tube feedings are usually
    1. small   3. diluted to half strength
    2. given hourly   4. given slowly
        a) 1, 3   b) 2, 4   c) 1, 3, 4   d) all

References

Bodinski, Lois H. 1982. *The Nurse's Guide to Diet Therapy*. New York: John Wiley & Sons.

Robinson, Corinne H. 1980. *Basic Nutrition and Diet Therapy*, 4th ed. New York: Macmillan Publishing Company.

U.S. Department of Agriculture. *Composition of Foods*. 1963, 1975.

Williams, Sue Rodwell. 1982. *Essentials of Nutrition and Diet Therapy*, 3rd ed., St. Louis: C.V. Mosby Co.

Chapter 30

DIET THERAPY FOR CANCER PATIENTS

OBJECTIVES

After studying this chapter, you should be able to

- State the effects of cancer on the nutritional status of the host

- Describe nutritional problems resulting from the medical treatment of cancer

- Describe nutritional therapy for cancer patients

THE NATURE OF CANCER

Cancer is a disease characterized by abnormal cell growth, and can occur in any organ. In some way the genes lose control of cell growth and reproduction becomes unstructured and excessive. The developing mass caused by the abnormal growth is called a tumor or *neoplasm* (new growth). Cancer is also called *neoplasia*. Cancerous tumors are *malignant* (life threatening), affect the structure, and consequently the function of organs. When cancer cells break away from their original site, move through the blood, and spread to a new site, they are said to *metastasize*. Cancer is the second leading cause of death in the United States. However, it must

be noted that cancer does not always cause death. When it is found early in its development, prompt treatment can irradicate it.

THE CAUSES OF CANCER

The precise etiology (cause) of cancer is not known, but it is thought that heredity, viruses, and environmental *carcinogens* (cancer causing substances) contribute to its development. Cancer is *not inherited*, but some families appear to have a *genetic predisposition* (inherited *tendency*) toward it. When such seems to be the case, environmental carcinogens should be carefully avoided and medical checkups made regularly. Environmental carcinogens include radiation (whether from X-rays, sun, or atomic wastes); certain chemicals ingested in food or water; certain chemicals that touch the skin regularly; and certain substances that are breathed in such as tobacco smoke, and asbestos.

Carcinogens are not known to cause cancer from one or even a few exposures, but after prolonged exposure. For example, skin cancer does not develop after one sunburn. Certain substances in foods are thought to be carcinogenic. As research continues, more information will become available. Until it is, the suspect food need not be eliminated from the diet, but its use might be limited. In general, it seems wise for people to limit their exposure to suspected carcinogens whenever possible. Some foods or food substances are thought to prevent or even cure cancer. While there may be some prophylactic (preventive) qualities in some foods, as yet there is no known cure from them and the promotion of such cures is deceptive quackery.

Stress is thought by some to be a contributing cause. An immune system that has been damaged—possibly through malnutrition—may also be a contributing factor toward cancer. Protein, for example, is essential for the maintenance of a healthy immune system.

THE EFFECTS OF CANCER

One of the first indications of cancer may be unexplained weight loss. This is because the tumor cells use for their own metabolism and development the nutrients the host has taken in. The host may suffer from weakness, and anorexia may occur, which compounds the weight loss. The weight loss includes the loss of muscle tissue and *hypoalbuminemia* (low albumin [protein] content of the blood),

and anemia may develop. The sense of taste and of smell may become abnormal in cancer patients. This may be because of nutrient deficiency. A zinc deficiency, for example, affects the sense of taste. Foods may taste less sweet and more bitter than they would to healthy people. Cancer patients become satiated earlier than normal, possibly due to decreased digestive secretions. Insulin production may be abnormal and *hyperglycemia* (high levels of blood sugar) can delay the stomach's emptying and dull the appetite. Some cancers cause hypercalcemia. If this is chronic, kidney stones and impaired kidney function can occur.

The location of a tumor can affect the host. For example, an esophageal or intestinal tumor can cause blockage in the gastrointestinal tract, causing malabsorption as well. If the cancer is untreated, the continued anorexia and weight loss will create a state of malnutrition, which in turn can lead to *cachexia* (severe wasting) and ultimately, death.

THE TREATMENT OF CANCER

Medical treatment of cancer may include surgical removal, radiation, *chemotherapy* (drug), or a combination of these methods. These very treatments, unfortunately, have side effects that may further undermine the nutritional status of the patient. The nutritional effects of surgery in general were discussed in Chapter 29 and may be reviewed at this time. Cancer surgery, however, may have some additional effects. Surgery on the mouth, for example, might well affect the ability to chew or swallow. Gastric or intestinal *resection* (partial removal) can affect absorption and result in nutritional deficiencies. The removal of the pancreas will result in diabetes mellitus.

Radiation can change the senses of taste and smell, particularly if it is done for cancer of the head or neck. It may also cause a decrease in salivary secretions, which will cause dry mouth (xerostomia) and difficulty in swallowing. This reduction in saliva also causes tooth decay and sometimes the loss of teeth. Radiation reduces the amount of absorptive tissue in the small intestine. In addition, it can cause bowel obstruction or diarrhea.

Chemotherapy reduces the ability of the small intestine to regenerate absorptive cells and it can cause hemorrhagic colitis. Both radiation and chemotherapy depress appetite. They may cause nausea, vomiting, and diarrhea that can lead to fluid and electrolyte imbalances. If therapy is given near meal times and the patient is subsequently ill from the therapy, she or he may relate the illness to the food, and later refuse those foods.

However, when the therapy is completed and the patient is able to return to a well-balanced diet, these problems may disappear.

IMPROVING THE NUTRITIONAL STATUS OF THE CANCER PATIENT _____

The goal of improving the cancer patient's nutritional status includes the prevention of further weight loss. This is not easily attained. The anorexia of cancer is particularly difficult to combat because cancer patients tend to develop strong food aversions that are thought to be caused by chemotherapy. Patients receiving chemotherapy near mealtime associate the foods at that meal with the nausea experienced from the chemother-

apy, and often form aversions to those particular foods. These aversions result in very limited acceptance of food and contribute further to the patient's malnutrition. It is preferable that chemotherapy be withheld from two to three hours before and after meals. The appetite and absorption usually improve after chemotherapy so the patient can improve nutritional status between chemotherapy treatments.

Diet plans for cancer patients require an individual approach. The patient's diet history should be taken at the outset of hospitalization. Kcal and nutrient needs must be determined by the diet counselor, but the patient's diet guidelines should be made in consultation with the patient. It is essential that favorite foods, prepared in familiar ways and served attractively be included. Nutritious food beautifully served is useless if the patient refuses it.

If chewing is a problem, a soft diet may be helpful. (See Chapter 23 for a review of the soft diet.) If diarrhea is a problem, a residue-restricted diet may help. (See Chapter 28 for a review of residue-restricted diets.) Patients should be evaluated continuously, but inconspicuously.

If the patient is scheduled to undergo radiation or chemotherapy, these factors must be included in the diet planning.

It is important that the diet counselor establishes a good relationship with the patient and that constant reminders to eat be avoided. The patient usually understands the situation and such reminders are in fact only depressing reminders of the cancer. Energy demands are high because of the hypermetabolic state caused by the cancer. Kcal needs will vary from patient to patient. Carbohydrates and fat will be needed to provide this energy and spare protein for tissue building and the immune system. Patients with good nutritional status will need from 80—100 grams of protein a day. Malnourished patients may need from 100—200 grams of protein a day. Vitamins and minerals are essential for metabolism, tissue maintenance, and appetite, and they may be supplied in supplemental form. Fluids are important to help the kidneys eliminate the metabolic wastes and the toxins from drugs.

The patient's food habits may require change if the patient has scrupulously avoided desserts and high kcal foods to maintain normal weight previous to the cancer.

Sometimes patients may be willing to eat foods that are brought from home. Some may find cold foods more appealing than hot foods. Meats may taste bitter so milk, cheese, eggs, and fish may be more appealing. If foods taste less sweet to the cancer patient than to the well person, sugar may be added to juices and fruits. This may please the patient and adds kcal to the diet.

Supplementation with high kcal, high protein, liquid foods between meals may be useful but not if their consumption reduces the patient's appetite at meals.

If the patient suffers from dry mouth, salad dressings, gravies, sauces, and syrups appropriately served on foods will be helpful. Several small meals may be better tolerated than three large meals. It is preferable to serve the nutritionally richer meals early in the day because the patient is less tired and may have a better appetite at that time. If nausea or pain are a continuous problem, drugs to control them, particularly at mealtimes, may be helpful. While oral feedings are definitely preferred, enteral or parenteral feedings may become necessary if cachexia is extreme. Sometimes an oral diet may be used in conjunction with an enteral feeding plan. (See Chapter 29 for a review of enteral and parenteral nutrition.) As the patient improves, kcal and nutritional content of the diet should be gradually increased.

SUMMARY

Cancer is a disease characterized by abnormal cell growth. It can strike any body tissue. Energy needs increase because of the hypermetabolic state and the tumor's needs for energy nutrients at the same time anorexia occurs in the patient. Its cause is not known. It causes severe wasting, blockages, anemia, and various metabolic problems. Treatment of cancer includes surgery, radiation, and chemotherapy. Improving the patient's nutritional state is difficult because of the illness and anorexia. Parenteral or enteral nutrition may be necessary.

Case Study—Cancer Patient

The doctor found a tumor in Betty G.'s left breast at Betty's annual exam. She scheduled Betty for a biopsy the next day and admitted her to the hospital the same day as the exam. The doctor explained that if the tumor were malignant, a radical mastectomy may be necessary.

When Betty awoke from anesthesia 24 hours after the discovery of her tumor, she had only one breast. She was depressed, but not as depressed as some women in this situation. The doctor told her that she believed the entire mass had been eradicated.

Betty was offered broth later on the day of surgery, but declined. The next day she was served a clear liquid diet, but could swallow only a bit of gingerale. On the second day, she was served a full liquid diet and on the third day, a soft diet. Betty ate nothing and her depression increased.

Betty's husband, son, daughter-in-law, and friends were very supportive and visited often, frequently bringing home-made cookies, fruit juice, and candy, but Betty could not eat. When her doctor asked her about her appetite, she said she was not eating much. She was being supported with IV solution, but had taken only about 200 kcal of gingerale orally. After one week, the doctor asked the dietitian to consult with Betty. She did and afterward Betty began to eat a bit. At the end of two weeks, Betty was discharged. She had lost ten pounds.

Case Study Questions

1. Why was Betty's biopsy and possible surgery scheduled so quickly?
2. What are some reasons Betty's depression increased with time?
3. What are some possible reasons for Betty's inability to eat?
4. Why did Betty lose weight?
5. What things would the dietitian probably have asked Betty during their consultation?
6. What are some possible reasons for Betty's improved appetite after the consultation with the dietitian?
7. What type of nutritional support might Betty need after her discharge? (Her husband is an executive with a local company.)
8. Do you think Betty's depression will leave her after she returns home? Explain.
9. What type of support—in addition to nutritional—might Betty require after she returns home? Explain.
10. Betty will not be able to fully use her left arm for some time. What activities can she undertake once she is home and feeling better?

Discussion Topics

1. Discuss cancer, telling what it is and how it affects body functions and nutritional status.
2. Discuss the etiology of cancer. Include any current news items that relate.
3. Explain how lung cancer moves to the brain or breast cancer to the bones.

4. Explain why cancer patients lose weight.
5. Discuss current medical treatment of cancer. How does it affect nutritional status?
6. Why is the anorexia of cancer patients especially difficult to combat? What causes it? Are there any ways it can be prevented?
7. How does one attempt to improve the nutritional status of a cancer patient?
8. Are supplemental feedings of liquid foods useful in the nutritional rehabilitation of a cancer patient? Explain.
9. Discuss enteral and parenteral nutrition in relation to cancer patients.

Suggested Activities

1. Invite an oncologist (physician specializing in cancer) to speak to the class.
2. Role-play a situation where a nurse is attempting to help a cancer patient with lunch. The patient had chemotherapy an hour after yesterday's lunch and was quite ill.
3. Write an essay giving your feelings if you had just been told that you had a malignant breast tumor.
4. Assume you are Chief Dietitian in the local hospital. Write your instructions for your assistant who will be making diet plans for a new patient with throat cancer. The patient is seriously malnourished, has xerostomia, and is hospitalized for chemotherapy.
5. Plan a day's menus for a cancer patient who will eat only the following foods:

sweetened orange juice	soda crackers
bananas	milkshakes
applesauce	eggnog
cooked pears	cottage cheese
puffed rice cereal	cream of chicken soup
rice pudding	poached eggs
white toast with current jelly	boullion

Review

Matching

K _____ 1. cachexia 339
F _____ 2. carcinogen 338
O _____ 3. chemotherapy 339
N _____ 4. genetic predisposition
C _____ 5. hyperglycemia 339
M _____ 6. hypoalbuminemia 339
J _____ 7. malignant 338
D _____ 8. metastasize 338
A _____ 9. neoplasia 338
I _____ 10. neoplasm 338
L _____ 11. resection 339
P _____ 12. xerostomia 340
B _____ 13. host 339
H _____ 14. malabsorption 339
E _____ 15. bowel obstruction 340

a. cancer
b. supports the parasite
c. high level of blood sugar
d. to move from one organ to another
e. blockage
f. cancer-causing substance
g. etiology
h. poor absorption
i. tumor
j. life-threatening
k. severe wasting
l. partial removal
m. reduced amounts of protein in the blood
n. inherited tendency
o. treatment of cancer with drugs
p. dry mouth
q. not inherited

Multiple Choice. Select the letter that precedes the best answer.

1. Cancer
   1. is characterized by abnormal cell growth 338
   2. tumor may also be called neoplasm 338
   3. inevitably causes death 338
   4. can metastasize 338
       a) 1, 2   b) 1, 2, 3   c) 1, 2, 4   d) Only 4

2. Carcinogens include
   1. viruses
   2. smoke 339
   3. X-rays 339
   4. salmonella
       a) 1, 2, 3   b) 2, 3, 4   c) 3, 4   d) only 4

3. Carcinogens
   1. cause cancer after only limited exposure 339
   2. include some chemical substances 339
   3. are never found in food or water 339
   4. should be avoided whenever possible 338
      a) 1, 2   b) 1, 3   c) 2, 4   d) 3, 4
4. Cancer patients
   1. tend to lose weight 339
   2. may experience a change in their senses of taste and smell 339
   3. seldom suffer from anorexia 339
   4. may suffer from cachexia 339
      a) 1, 2   b) 1, 2, 3   c) 2, 3   d) 1, 2, 4
5. Radiation and chemotherapy
   1. seldom affect cancer patients' nutritional status 339
   2. may depress appetite 340
   3. may cause nausea
   4. may create food aversions
      a) 1, 2   b) 1, 2, 3   c) 2, 3   d) 2, 3, 4

References

Howard, Roseanne B., and Nancie H. Herbold. 1982. *Nutrition in Clinical Care*, 2nd ed. New York: McGraw Hill Book Company.

Hui, Y.H. 1983. *Human Nutrition and Diet Therapy*. Monterey, Calif.: Wadsworth Health Sciences Division of Wadsworth Inc.

Krause, Marie V., and Kathleen L. Mahan. 1979. *Food, Nutrition and Diet Therapy*, 6th ed. Philadelphia: W.B. Saunders Co.

Robinson, Corinne H., and Marilyn R. Lawler. 1982. *Normal and Therapeutic Nutrition*, 16th ed. New York: MacMillan Publishing Company.

Suitor, Carol W., and Merrily F. Crowley. 1984. *Nutrition Principles and Application in Health Promotion*. Philadelphia: J.B. Lippincott Company.

Chapter 31

DIETS FOR PATIENTS WITH FOOD ALLERGIES, BLOOD AND METABOLIC DISORDERS

OBJECTIVES

After studying this chapter, you should be able to

- Describe allergy diets and their uses

- Identify foods appropriate for patients with blood disorders

- Explain given metabolic disorders and identify foods appropriate for them

ALLERGIES

An *allergy* is an altered reaction of the tissues of certain individuals who are exposed to substances which, in similar amounts, are harmless to other persons. The substances causing this *hypersensitivity* (abnormal adverse reaction) are called *allergens*. Allergic individuals seem most prone to allergic reactions during periods of stress. People may be allergic to various things such as pollen, dust, certain drugs, cosmetics, and foods. The discussion in this chapter will be limited to allergic reactions to foods.

Types of Allergic Reactions

Some of the typical symptoms of food allergies include "hay fever," asthma, gastro-

intestinal disturbances, *urticaria* (hives), edema, headache, and dermatitis. Because allergies are uncomfortable and can be detrimental to health, they should be treated to relieve the symptoms. The simplest treatment is to remove the item that causes the allergic reaction. Finding the cause or causes of an allergy, however, is the most difficult part of treatment. This is because allergic reactions to the same food may differ in two individuals. For example, the fact that someone gets hives from eating strawberries does not mean that an allergic reaction to strawberries will appear as hives in another member of the family. Allergic reactions may even differ from time to time with the same individual. People do not *inherit* allergies; they inherit the tendency to them.

Although children frequently outgrow their sensitivities, it is wise to delay the introduction of known food allergens to young children if their parents suffer from allergies.

Treatment of Allergies

When someone suspects food allergies, it is wise to keep a food diary and record all food, drink, and allergic reactions.

Skin tests (application of a common allergen to a small area of skin) are frequently used to detect allergies. Because food allergies are rather difficult to determine from skin tests, elimination diets are often prescribed to find the food or foods that cause the allergic reaction. *Elimination diets* are diets composed of very few, specific foods that are not common allergens.

The elimination diet identifies specific foods as allergens by their individual and gradual addition to a basic diet composed of relatively nonallergenic foods. Doctors specializing in allergies have found that some of the most common food allergens are: milk, wheat, eggs, oranges, chocolate, fish, tomatoes, and strawberries. It is common for other foods in the same class as the allergens to cause allergic reactions as well. Cooking, however, alters the foods and may eliminate allergic reactions. Diets are planned that eliminate common food allergens and include only those foods that seldom cause trouble, such as rice, lamb, sugar, and canned pears.

Four elimination diets are given in table 31-1. The patient is kept on one of these diets for a week. If allergic reactions continue, another elimination diet is tried for a week, and so on. If the reactions continue even during the fourth diet, then it may be assumed that the allergy is due to something other than food and other treatment is sought.

When and if relief is found from the allergic symptoms while on one of the recommended diets, the patient is continued on it for a second week and then, very gradually, other foods are introduced to the diet. Those foods most likely to produce allergic reactions are added last until an allergic reaction occurs. The allergy can then be traced to one or two foods, and these can be eliminated from the diet. Knowing the cause of the allergy enables the patient to lead a healthy, normal life, provided that eliminating these foods does not affect her or his nutrition.

If the elimination of the allergen results in a diet deficient in certain nutrients, suitable substitutes for these nutrients must be found. For example, if a patient is allergic to citrus fruits, other foods rich in vitamin C to which the patient is not allergic must be found. If the allergy is to milk, soybean milk may be substituted. When the patient is allergic to foods for which it is extremely difficult to find substitutes, concentrated forms of their essential nutrients may be prescribed.

Sometimes, however, the allergies require such a restriction of foods that the diet does become nutritionally inadequate. As in all cases of allergy, and particularly in such cases, it is hoped that the patient can become *desensitized* (made less sensitive) to the allergens so that a nutritionally balanced diet can be restored. To desensitize the patient, a minute amount of food allergen is given after a period of complete *abstinence* (avoidance) from it. The amount of the allergen is gradually increased until the patient can tolerate it.

The patient must be taught the food sources of the nutrient or nutrients lacking so that other foods may be substituted that are nutritionally equal to those causing the allergy. It is essential that the patient be taught to read

Table 31-1 Elimination Diets

Diet 1	Diet 2	Diet 3	Diet 4
Rice	Corn	Tapioca	Milk†
Tapioca	Rye	White potato	Tapioca
Rice biscuit	Corn pone	Breads made of any	Cane
Rice bread	Corn-rye muffins	combination of	Sugar
	Rye bread	soy, Lima, potato	
	Ry-Krisp	starch and tapioca	
		flours	
Lettuce	Beets	Tomato	
Chard	Squash	Carrot	
Spinach	Asparagus	Lima beans	
Carrot	Artichoke	String beans	
Sweet potato		Peas	
or yam			
Lamb	Chicken (no hens)	Beef	
	Bacon	Bacon	
Lemon	Pineapple	Lemon	
Grapefruit	Peach	Grapefruit	
Pears	Apricot	Peach	
	Prune	Apricot	
Cane sugar	Cane or beet sugar	Cane sugar	
Sesame oil	Mazola	Sesame oil	
Olive oil*	Sesame oil	Soybean oil	
Salt	Salt	Gelatin, plain or	
Gelatin, plain or	Gelatin, plain or	flavored with	
flavored with	flavored with	lime or lemon	
lime or lemon	pineapple	Salt	
Maple syrup or	Karo corn syrup	Maple syrup or	
syrup made	White vinegar	syrup made	
with cane sugar	Royal baking	with cane sugar	
flavored with	powder	flavored with	
maple	Baking soda	maple	
Royal baking	Cream of tartar	Royal baking	
powder	Vanilla extract	powder	
Baking soda		Baking soda	
Cream of tartar		Cream of tartar	
Vanilla extract		Vanilla extract	
Lemon extract		Lemon extract	

*Allergy to it may occur with or without allergy to olive pollen. Mazola may be used if corn allergy is not present.

†Milk should be taken up to 2 or 3 quarts a day. Plain cottage cheese and cream may be used. Tapioca cooked with milk and milk sugar may be taken.

Source: Rowe, A. H. *Elimination Diets and the Patient's Allergies* ed. 2, Philadelphia: Lee & Febiger, 1944

the labels on commercially prepared foods, and to check the ingredients of restaurant foods carefully. Baked products, mixes, meat-loaf, or pancakes may contain egg, milk, or wheat that may be responsible for the allergic reaction.

METABOLIC DISORDERS

Congenital disabilities preventing the normal metabolism of specific nutrients are inborn errors of metabolism. They are caused by *mutations* (changes) in the genes. There is great variation in the seriousness of the conditions caused by these defects. Some cause death at an early age and some can be minimized so that life can be supported by adjustments in the normal diet. Among children born with these defects, there is, however, the common danger of damage to the central nervous system because of their abnormal body chemistry. This results in mental retardation and sometimes retarded growth. Early diagnosis of these inborn errors combined with diet therapy increases the chances of preventing retardation. Hospitals test newborns for some of these disorders as a matter of course. Where there is a family history of a certain genetic disorder, genetic screening can be done. In addition, some of these abnormalities can be discovered by *amniocentesis* (testing of the baby in utero).

Galactosemia

Galactosemia is a condition in which there is a lack of the liver enzyme, *transferase*. Transferase normally converts galactose to glucose. Galactose is the simple sugar resulting from the digestion of lactose, the sugar found in milk (which was discussed in Chapter 3). When transferase is missing, and the infant ingests anything containing galactose, the amount of galactose in the blood becomes so excessive that it is toxic. When this happens to a newborn, she or he suffers diarrhea, vomiting, edema, and the child's liver does not function normally. Cataracts may develop, *galactosuria* (galactose in the urine) occurs, and mental retardation ensues.

Diet Therapy

Diet therapy for galactosemia is the exclusion of anything containing milk from any mammal. During infancy, the treatment is simple because parents can feed the baby lactose-free, commercially-prepared formula and provide supplemental minerals and vitamins. As the child grows, and moves on to adult foods, parents must be extremely careful to avoid any food, beverage, or medicine that contains lactose. Nutritional supplements of calcium, vitamin D, and riboflavin must be given so that the diet is nutritionally adequate. This restricted diet may be necessary throughout life, but some physicians allow a somewhat liberalized diet as the child reaches school age. This may mean only small amounts of baked or processed foods that contain small amounts of milk. Even this must be accompanied by careful and regular monitoring for galactosuria.

Phenylketonuria (PKU)

In phenylketonuria, infants lack the liver enzyme, *phenylalanine hydroxylase*, which is necessary for the metabolism of the amino acid, *phenylalanine*. Infants seem to be normal at birth, but if the disease is not treated, most of them become hyperactive, suffer seizures between 6 and 18 months, and become mentally retarded. Most hospitals today test newborns for phenylketonuria. PKU babies typically have light-colored skin and hair.

Diet Therapy

There is a special, nutritionally-adequate, commercial infant formula available for PKU babies. It provides just enough phenylalanine for basic needs, but no excess. The specific amount depends on the infant's size and growth rate. Regular blood tests determine the adequacy of the amounts. Diets are carefully monitored for kcal and nutrient intake, and adjusted frequently as needs change. Except for fats and sugars, there is some protein in all foods. Some of that protein is phenylalanine, so diets for the growing child eating normal food must be carefully planned. There is a synthetic milk for older children that can be used as a beverage or in puddings and baked products. Diets should be monitored throughout life to avoid mental retardation.

Maple Syrup Urine Disease (MSUD)

Maple Syrup Urine Disease is a congenital defect resulting in the inability to metabolize three amino acids—*leucine, isoleucine,* and *valine.* It is named for the odor of the urine of these patients. When the infant ingests food protein, there are increased blood levels of these amino acids. Hypoglycemia, apathy, and convulsions occur very early. If the disease is not treated promptly, the child will die.

Diet Therapy

The diet must provide sufficient kcal and nutrients, but with extremely restricted amounts of leucine, isoleucine, and valine. A special formula and low-protein foods are used. Diet therapy appears to be necessary throughout life.

Gout

Gout is a metabolic disorder in which the joints of the fingers and toes become very painful. It is caused by an inborn error of purine metabolism that upsets uric acid production (See Chapter 27 for discussion of purines). Normally, uric acid is excreted via the kidneys, but in gout, some of it is deposited in the joints of the fingers and toes, causing pain.

It is rare among women and children, appearing most often in men over 30. It has been associated with obesity and excessive use of alcohol. Chronic gout can cause degenerative changes in the affected joints.

Treatment

The treatment of gout is with drugs that inhibit the metabolic production of uric acid and improve excretion of it. Physicians vary in their inclusion of diet therapy in the treatment. Some prescribe a purine-restricted diet and some simply restrict the use of high-purine foods such as organ meats, anchovies, sardines, meat extracts, and soups. Fasting or weight reduction should not be undertaken during an attack of gout and, if persons with this disorder want to lose weight, it must be done gradually since fasting or rapid weight loss increase the blood level of uric acid.

Hyperthyroidism

Metabolism is regulated by the thyroid gland. When this gland secretes too much thyroxine, the metabolism rate is increased, and the patient experiences excessive hunger and in most cases weight loss. The daily kcal requirement may reach 4,000—5,000 to prevent weight loss. Medical treatment or surgery may be necessary to improve the condition. The use of coffee, tea, and alcohol is usually restricted.

Hypothyroidism

In this condition, the thyroid gland secretes too little thyroxine and metabolic activity is slowed. Patients have a tendency to gain weight and to feel the cold more readily than normal. Treatment may include medication and a diet reduced in kcal.

ANEMIAS

Anemias are diseases of the red blood cells (*erythrocytes*).

Iron Deficiency Anemia

Iron deficiency anemia is the most common nutritional deficiency in the United States. It is found in all age groups and all economic classes. It is a condition in which the number of red blood cells or the amount of hemoglobin each contains is less than normal. It may be due to an inadequate diet (*nutritional anemia*), inadequate absorption, hemorrhage from accident, or diseases causing chronic hemorrhage, reduced red blood cell production, or reduced life span of the cells.

Treatment

If the iron deficiency anemia is caused by disease, this disease must be treated. If the anemia is due to inadequate diet, an iron-, vitamin C-, and protein-rich diet in combination with supplemental iron is used (See Chapter 5). Vitamin C is an iron enhancer. (It improves iron absorption and should be included in some form with each meal.)

Pernicious Anemia

Pernicious anemia is a severe and chronic deficiency of vitamin B_{12}. It is caused by the body's inability to absorb vitamin B_{12} because of the lack of a certain gastric secretion called *intrinsic factor*. Vitamin B_{12} attaches to the intrinsic factor and is then transported to the ileum, where it is absorbed. Pernicious anemia can also occur after a long period of the strict

Table 31-2 Suggested Menus for Iron Deficiency Anemia

Breakfast	Lunch	Dinner
Orange Juice	Pineapple Juice	Melon Slice
Poached Egg	Macaroni and Cheese	Braised Liver
Whole Wheat Toast	Spinach-Mushroom-Bacon Salad	Boiled Potato with Parsley
Milk	Corn Muffins	Green Peas
Coffee	Prune Whip	Tomato Salad
	Milk	Cracked Wheat Bread with Butter
		Vanilla Ice Cream
Snacks		Milk
Dried fruits		
Oatmeal-raisin cookies		

use of a vegetarian diet because such a diet provides no vitamin B_{12}. In this condition, the activity of the bone marrow is slowed and the resulting red blood cells are fewer in number, larger than normal, and not completely mature. Patients experience poor appetite and disturbances of the gastrointestinal and nervous systems. Coordination and mental processes may be affected.

Treatment

The treatment of pernicious anemia includes regular and frequent intramuscular injections of vitamin B_{12} throughout the patient's lifetime, and a diet that is rich in animal protein, iron, and vitamins.

Sickle Cell Anemia

Sickle Cell Anemia is a hereditary condition that primarily affects the Black community. Red blood cells become "sickle" shaped. The odd shape limits the amount of oxygen a cell carries because its perimeter is reduced, and it can cause *occlusions* (blockages) of blood vessels, causing severe pain. Liver and kidney function are adversely affected. A low-iron diet may be prescribed because of the excess iron stored from the abnormal destruction of red blood cells. Children five years and younger are at greatest risk from this disease.

SUMMARY

Food allergies can cause many different and unpleasant symptoms. To determine their causes, elimination diets are used. Some of the most common food allergens have been found to be milk, chocolate, oranges, tomatoes, fish, strawberries, and wheat.

Inborn errors of metabolism cause various problems, some more serious than others. In these conditions, diet therapy is the primary tool in maintaining the patient's health.

Anemias are diseases of the red blood cells and stem from varying factors. Diet therapy plays an important role in their treatment.

Case Study—Food Allergy

At the age of 35, Carrie T. began to suffer severe and frequent headaches. After seeing several doctors, she was advised that her headaches were common migraine. After much urging, she visited an allergist. Skin tests were made and she was found to be allergic to several environmental substances, but no food allergies were discovered. The doctor gave her a list of foods (chocolate, tomatoes, oranges, red wine, fish, strawberries), however, to which many people are allergic. She ignored it, saying she did not "believe in" allergies. She had heard too often about her parents' allergies and considered them to be "just a state of mind".

Finally, after an extremely severe and long-lasting headache, she began to wonder if she were wrong about allergies and if there were certain foods to which she was allergic. She considered the foods she had eaten the day before this last headache. She had orange juice and eggs at breakfast, chocolate cake and milk in the afternoon, and wine and shrimp at dinner. All of these foods were common allergens. Although she remained somewhat skeptical, she did begin to record her diet. The following day she had another slice of chocolate cake. The day after that, she suffered another headache. The next time she suffered a headache, she realized she had had red wine the previous evening. There were as yet no headaches after she had eaten tomatoes, oranges, or fish. However, after a period of family stress during which Carrie had 2 and 3 migraines a week, she began to suspect fish, certain ice creams, and some raw fruits, as well as chocolate. When the family situation was resolved and the stress was relieved, the frequency of Carrie's headaches was reduced. Except for chocolate, eating foods she had begun to suspect as allergens did not always result in headache.

Now, since Carrie has learned to cope more comfortably with stressful situations and to avoid known food allergens, the frequency of her headaches has been greatly reduced.

Case Study Questions

1. Was it surprising that the allergist did not discover Carrie's food allergies with the skin tests? Explain.
2. Carrie's parents both suffer from allergies that affect their nasal passages. Is it not rather strange that Carrie's allergies were from foods? Explain.
3. Why did the headaches increase in frequency during periods of stress?
4. Why did Carrie begin to keep a food diary? How can that be useful in a situation such as Carrie's?
5. Carrie discovered that she could not eat raw apples, but that she could eat applesauce. Explain.
6. Would Carrie be apt to suffer migraine from eating a meal of lamb, rice, and canned pears? Explain.
7. Later on, Carrie did develop an allergy to oranges. Do you think she would be wise to eat grapefruit instead? Why?
8. Carrie's husband suffers from asthma. Do you think Carrie's daughter may develop allergies? Explain.
9. Carrie is expecting a second child soon. How would you advise her regarding the introduction of solid foods to the baby?
10. Carrie has discovered that she cannot eat chocolate, fish, oranges, raw apples, nuts, and coconut. Is she likely to develop nutritional deficiencies because of her allergies? Why?

Discussion Topics

1. What are *allergies*? What may cause them?
2. What are some common allergic reactions to food? How can they be avoided?

3. Do people inherit allergies? Explain.
4. Of what use is a food diary in relation to allergies? What are elimination diets and when are they used?
5. What is the most difficult part of treating food allergies?
6. How may an allergic patient be desensitized?
7. Is an allergy diet always nutritious? Explain.
8. Explain how eggs, wheat, or milk may be hidden in each of the following foods: mayonnaise, bread, rye crackers, potato salad, gravy, meatloaf, breaded veal cutlet, bologna, malted milk.
9. What is meant by inborn errors of metabolism? What causes them? How may they affect people?
10. What is galactosemia? How is it acquired? How does it affect the body? Is it serious? How is it treated?
11. Discuss PKU. Include its cause, symptoms, effects, and treatment.
12. Discuss MSUD. Include its cause, reason for its name, symptoms, treatment, and prognosis if it is not treated.
13. What is *gout*? Who is most apt to be afflicted with it? How is it treated?
14. Compare hyperthyroidism and hypothyroidism, and their treatments.
15. What is anemia? What may cause anemia? How can nutritional anemia be treated?

Suggested Activities

1. Organize a panel discussion on metabolic disorders. Assign individual students to individual disorders. Use outside sources.
2. Ask someone with food allergies to speak to the class. Follow this talk with questions from the audience.
3. Ask an endocrinologist to speak to the class on thyroid disorders.
4. Role-play a situation where the doctor must explain PKU to the parents of a PKU baby. Include cause, symptoms, effects, and treatment.
5. Visit a supermarket and make a list of high-purine foods available.
6. Write a day's menus that include your favorite foods. Adapt it for a patient with nutritional anemia.
7. Adapt the following menu for someone who is allergic to milk.

Cream Soup	Baker's Bread
Roast Beef	Butter
Mashed Potatoes	Ice Cream
Buttered Peas	Black Coffee

8. Visit a local supermarket and look for the ingredients wheat, eggs, and milk in frozen prepared meals, baked products and baking mixes.
9. Find recipes that are suitable for diets in which eggs, wheat, or milk must be eliminated.
10. Plan a luncheon for a patient who is allergic to wheat.
11. Ask a doctor or registered nurse to explain skin tests to the class. Discuss these tests after the lecture.
12. Write the menus of the meals eaten yesterday. Adapt one meal to a wheat-free diet. Adapt another to an egg-free diet. Adapt a third meal to a milk-free diet.

Review

A. Multiple Choice. Select the *letter* that precedes the best answer.

1. An adverse physical reaction to a food is called a food
   a. refusal
   b. allergy
   c. symptom
   d. allergen

2. Substances that cause altered physical reactions are called
   a. symptoms
   b. allergies
   c. allergens
   d. abstinence

3. One of the typical symptoms of food allergies is
   a. diabetes mellitus
   b. colitis
   c. hives
   d. atherosclerosis

4. The simplest treatment for a food allergy is
   a. a skin test
   b. the clear-liquid diet
   c. elimination of the allergen
   d. the use of penicillin

5. In cases of food allergy, an elimination diet may be prescribed to
   a. desensitize the patient
   b. avoid medication
   c. avoid surgery
   d. find the allergen

6. Some foods that frequently cause an allergic reaction are
   a. milk, eggs, and wheat
   b. lamb, rice, and sugar
   c. canned pears and tapioca
   d. rice and pears

7. If a person is found to be allergic to milk,
   a. milk of any kind must be eliminated
   b. ordinary cheese may be substituted
   c. soy milk may be substituted
   d. dry milk may be substituted

8. The person on an egg-free diet may not have
   a. cow's milk
   b. ordinary bakery cake
   c. fresh fruits
   d. olives

9. Foods that seldom cause food allergies are
   a. rice, canned pears, and lamb
   b. milk, eggs, and wheat
   c. chocolate, oranges, and tomatoes
   d. strawberries and fish

10. A congenital disease preventing normal metabolism
    a. occurs only in men over 30
    b. is called in inborn error of metabolism
    c. occurs only in the thyroid gland
    d. is also called the basal metabolic state

11. In galactosemia, the body
    a. lacks transferase
    b. needs large amounts of lactose
    c. cannot metabolize any protein
    d. is unable to digest sugar

12. If untreated, inborn errors of metabolism may cause
    a. cancer
    b. mental retardation
    c. vitamin C deficiency
    d. premature births

13. Maple Syrup Urine Disease is
    a. a form of diabetes
    b. a form of anemia
    c. an inborn error of metabolism
    d. never fatal

14. Gout
    a. causes mental retardation
    b. occurs only in men under 30
    c. is another name for PKU
    d. is an error in purine metabolism

15. Anemias
    a. occur in the endocrine glands only
    b. are usually caused by inborn errors of metabolism
    c. are extremely uncommon
    d. affect the blood

References

American Dietetic Association. 1981. *Handbook of Clinical Dietetics*. New Haven: Yale University.

U.S. Department of Agriculture. *Composition of Foods*. 1963, 1975.

Massachusetts General Hospital Dietary Department. 1976. *Diet Manual*. Boston: Little, Brown & Co.

Howard, Roseanne B., and Nancie H. Herbold. 1982. *Nutrition in Clinical Care*, 2nd ed. New York: McGraw Hill Book Company.

Iowa Dietetic Association. 1984. *Simplified Diet Manual with Meal Patterns*, 5th ed. Ames: Iowa State University Press.

Kerschner, Velma L. 1983. *Nutrition and Diet Therapy*. Philadelphia: F.A. Davis Co.

University of Iowa Hospitals and Clinics. 1979. *Recent Advances in Therapeutic Diets*. Iowa City: State University Press.

Appendix

Table A-1 Recommended Daily Dietary Allowances,[a]—Revised 1980

	Age (years)	Weight (kg)	Weight (lb)	Height (cm)	Height (in)	Protein (g)	Vitamin A (μg RE)[b]	Vitamin D (μg)[c]	Vitamin E (mg α-TE)[d]
Infants	0.0–0.5	6	13	60	24	kg × 2.2	420	10	3
	0.5–1.0	9	20	71	28	kg × 2.0	400	10	4
Children	1–3	13	29	90	35	23	400	10	5
	4–6	20	44	112	44	30	500	10	6
	7–10	28	62	132	52	34	700	10	7
Males	11–14	45	99	157	62	45	1000	10	8
	15–18	66	145	176	69	56	1000	10	10
	19–22	70	154	177	70	56	1000	7.5	10
	23–50	70	154	178	70	56	1000	5	10
	51+	70	154	178	70	56	1000	5	10
Females	11–14	46	101	157	62	46	800	10	8
	15–18	55	120	163	64	46	800	10	8
	19–22	55	120	163	64	44	800	7.5	8
	23–50	55	120	163	64	44	800	5	8
	51+	55	120	163	64	44	800	5	8
Pregnant						+30	+200	+5	+2
Lactating						+20	+400	+5	+3

[a]The allowances are intended to provide for individual variations among most normal persons as they live in the United States under usual environmental stresses. Diets should be based on a variety of common foods in order to provide other nutrients for which human requirements have been less well defined.

[b]Retinol equivalents. 1 retinol equivalent = 1 μg retinol or 6 μg β carotene.

[c]As cholecalciferol. 10 μg cholecalciferol = 400 IU of vitamin D.

[d]α-tocopherol equivalents. 1 mg d-α tocopherol = 1 α-TE.

[e]1 NE (niacin equivalent) is equal to 1 mg of niacin or 60 mg of dietary tryptophan.

Table A-1 (*Continued*)

Water-Soluble Vitamins							Minerals					
Vita-min C (mg)	Thia-min (mg)	Ribo-flavin (mg)	Niacin (mg NE)[e]	Vita-min B-6 (mg)	Fola-cin[f] (μg)	Vitamin B-12 (μg)	Cal-cium (mg)	Phos-phorus (mg)	Mag-nesium (mg)	Iron (mg)	Zinc (mg)	Iodine (μg)
35	0.3	0.4	6	0.3	30	0.5[g]	360	240	50	10	3	40
35	0.5	0.6	8	0.6	45	1.5	540	360	70	15	5	50
45	0.7	0.8	9	0.9	100	2.0	800	800	150	15	10	70
45	0.9	1.0	11	1.3	200	2.5	800	800	200	10	10	90
45	1.2	1.4	16	1.6	300	3.0	800	800	250	10	10	120
50	1.4	1.6	18	1.8	400	3.0	1200	1200	350	18	15	150
60	1.4	1.7	18	2.0	400	3.0	1200	1200	400	18	15	150
60	1.5	1.7	19	2.2	400	3.0	800	800	350	10	15	150
60	1.4	1.6	18	2.2	400	3.0	800	800	350	10	15	150
60	1.2	1.4	16	2.2	400	3.0	800	800	350	10	15	150
50	1.1	1.3	15	1.8	400	3.0	1200	1200	300	18	15	150
60	1.1	1.3	14	2.0	400	3.0	1200	1200	300	18	15	150
60	1.1	1.3	14	2.0	400	3.0	800	800	300	18	15	150
60	1.0	1.2	13	2.0	400	3.0	800	800	300	18	15	150
60	1.0	1.2	13	2.0	400	3.0	800	800	300	10	15	150
+20	+0.4	+0.3	+2	+0.6	+400	+1.0	+400	+400	+150	h	+5	+25
+40	+0.5	+0.5	+5	+0.5	+100	+1.0	+400	+400	+150	h	+10	+50

[f]The folacin allowances refer to dietary sources as determined by *Lactobacillus casei* assay after treatment with enzymes (conjugases) to make polyglutamyl forms of the vitamin available to the test organism.

[g]The recommended dietary allowance for vitamin B-12 in infants is based on average concentration of the vitamin in human milk. The allowances after weaning are based on energy intake (as recommended by the American Academy of Pediatrics) and consideration of other factors, such as intestinal absorption.

[h]The increased requirement during pregnancy cannot be met by the iron content of habitual American diets nor by the existing iron stores of many women; therefore the use of 30–60 mg of supplemental iron is recommended. Iron needs during lactation are not substantially different from those of nonpregnant women, but continued supplementation of the mother for 2–3 months after parturition is advisable in order to replenish stores depleted by pregnancy.

Source: Food and Nutrition Board, National Academy of Sciences—National Research Council.

Table A-2 1983 Metropolitan Height and Weight Tables. Weights at ages 25–29 based on lowest mortality. Weight in pounds according to frame (in indoor clothing weighing 5 lbs. for men and 3 lbs. for women; shoes with 1″ heels).

Men					Women				
Height		Small Frame	Medium Frame	Large Frame	Height		Small Frame	Medium Frame	Large Frame
Feet	Inches				Feet	Inches			
5	2	128–134	131–141	138–150	4	10	102–111	109–121	118–131
5	3	130–136	133–143	140–153	4	11	103–113	111–123	120–134
5	4	132–138	135–145	142–156	5	0	104–115	113–126	122–137
5	5	134–140	137–148	144–160	5	1	106–118	115–129	125–140
5	6	136–142	139–151	146–164	5	2	108–121	118–132	128–143
5	7	138–145	142–154	149–168	5	3	111–124	121–135	131–147
5	8	140–148	145–157	152–172	5	4	114–127	124–138	134–151
5	9	142–151	148–160	155–176	5	5	117–130	127–141	137–155
5	10	144–154	151–163	158–180	5	6	120–133	130–144	140–159
5	11	146–157	154–166	161–184	5	7	123–136	133–147	143–163
6	0	149–160	157–170	164–188	5	8	126–139	136–150	146–167
6	1	152–164	160–174	168–192	5	9	129–142	139–153	149–170
6	2	155–168	164–178	172–197	5	10	132–145	142–156	152–173
·6	3	158–172	167–182	176–202	5	11	135–148	145–159	155–176
6	4	162–176	171–187	181–207	6	0	138–151	148–162	158–179

Source: *Metropolitan Life Insurance Company* Source of basic data 1979 Build Study Society of Actuaries and Association of Life Insurance Medical Directors of America 1980.

Table A-3 Mild Sodium-Restricted Diet Plans (Based on Daily Number of Calories Allowed)

Food List	1200-Calorie Diet	1800-Calorie Diet	Unrestricted-Calorie Diet
1	Not applicable	2	2 or more
1A	2	Not applicable	Not applicable
2	At least one each from groups A, B, C	At least one each from groups A, B, C	At least one each from groups A, B, C
3	4	4	2 or more
4	5	7	4 or more
5	5	5	5 or more
6	None	4	As desired
7	1	2	As desired

Source: Adapted from "Your Mild Sodium-Restricted Diet" (Revised), American Heart Association

Table A-4 Food Lists for the Mild Sodium-Restricted Diet*

LIST 1: MILK

Note: Each unit contains about 170 calories, 8 grams protein, 10 grams fat, and 12 grams carbohydrate. Two units from List 5, Meat, may be substituted for not more than one milk unit a day, or 6 ounces of plain yogurt (3/4 cup)

CAUTION: Do not use any commercial foods made of milk such as ice cream, sherbet, milkshakes, chocolate milk, malted milk, milk mixes, and condensed milk.

Evaporated whole milk, reconstituted	1 cup
Nonfat buttermilk.	2 fat units and 1 cup
Nonfat dry milk, powdered	2 fat units and 3 tablespoons (Use amount specified on package for making one cup of milk.)
Nonfat dry milk, reconstituted or skim milk	2 fat units and 1 cup
Whole milk.	1 cup
Whole milk buttermilk	1 cup

LIST 1A: MILK FOR 1200-CALORIE DIET PLAN

Note: Each unit contains about 85 calories, 8 grams protein, negligible fat, and 12 grams carbohydrate. One unit from List 5, Meat may be substituted for not more than one milk unit a day.

Caution: When milk is used in cooking be sure to count it as part of the day's allowance. Do not use whole milk or any commercial foods made of milk such as ice cream, sherbet, milkshakes, chocolate milk, malted milk, milk mixes, and condensed milk.

Evaporated skim milk, reconstituted	1 cup
Nonfat buttermilk.	1 cup
Nonfat dry milk, powdered	3 tablespoons (Use amount specified on package for making one cup of milk.)
Nonfat dry milk, reconstituted or skim milk	1 cup

LIST 2: VEGETABLES

Use fresh, frozen, or canned. Frozen peas and lima beans usually contain a small amount of salt, and often this is enough to season them adequately for the mild sodium-restricted diet. Do not use sauerkraut, pickles, or other vegetables prepared with brine or salted.

Group A

Note: Each unit contains negligible calories, protein, fat and carbohydrate. Each unit is a 1/2-cup serving.

Artichoke	Cucumber	Okra
Asparagus	Dandelion greens	Peppers, green or red
Beet greens	Eggplant	Radishes

*It is important to keep in touch with your physician while on any sodium-restricted diet.

Table A-4 *(Continued)*

Group A

Broccoli	Endive	Spinach
Brussels sprouts	Escarole	Squash, summer (yellow, zucchini)
Cabbage	Green beans	Tomato juice
Cauliflower	Kale	Tomatoes
Celery	Lettuce	Turnip greens
Chard, Swiss	Mushrooms	Wax beans
Chicory	Mustard greens	

Group B

Note: Each unit contains about 35 calories, 2 grams protein, negligible fat, and 7 grams carbohydrate. Each unit is a 1/2-cup serving. Two units from Group A may be substituted for one unit from Group B.

Beets	Peas	Squash, winter (acorn, Hubbard)
Carrots	Pumpkin	Turnip, white
Onions	Rutabaga (yellow turnip)	

Group C

Note: Each unit contains about 70 calories, 2 grams protein, negligible fat, and 15 grams carbohydrate. One unit from List 4, Breads, Cereals, and Cereal Products, may be substituted for one unit from Group C.

Beans, lima or navy, fresh, frozen, or dried. . . .	1/2 cup, cooked	Parsnips.	2/3 cup
Beans, baked (no pork). . .	1/4 cup	Peas, dried (split green or yellow, cowpeas).	1/2 cup, cooked
Corn.	1/3 cup or 1/2 small ear	Potato, white	1 small
Hominy.	1/2 cup	Potatoes, mashed.	1/2 cup
Lentils, dried	1/2 cup, cooked	Sweet potato	1/4 cup, or 1/2 small

LIST 3: FRUIT

Use frozen, fresh, canned, or dried. Fresh lemons and limes and their juice, unsweetened cranberries and cranberry juice, and unsweetened rhubarb may be used as desired.

Note: Each unit contains about 40 calories, negligible protein and fat, and 10 grams carbohydrate.

CAUTION: If following the 1200- or 1800-calorie diet plan do not use crystallized or glazed fruit, sweetened fruit, or fruit canned or frozen in sugar syrup.

Apple	1 small	Grape juice.	1/4 cup
Apple juice or apple cider .	1/3 cup	Honeydew melon	1/8 medium
Applesauce.	1/2 cup	Mango.	1/2 small
Apricots, dried	4 halves	Orange	1 small
Apricots, fresh	2 medium	Orange juice	1/2 cup

Table A-4 *(Continued)*

LIST 3: FRUIT

Apricot nectar	1/4 cup	Papaya	1/3 medium
Banana	1/2 small	Peach	1 medium
Blackberries	1 cup	Pear	1 small
Blueberries	2/3 cup	Pineapple	1/2 cup diced or 2 small slices
Cantaloupe	1/4 small		
Cherries	10 large	Pineapple juice	1/3 cup
Cranberries, sweetened	1 tablespoon	Plums	2 medium
Cranberry juice, sweetened	1/3 cup	Prunes	2 medium
Dates	2	Prune juice	1/4 cup
Fig	1 medium	Raisins	2 tablespoons
Fruit cup or mixed fruits	1/2 cup	Raspberries	1 cup
Grapefruit	1/2 small	Rhubarb, sweetened	2 tablespoons
Grapefruit juice	1/2 cup	Strawberries	1 cup
Grapes	12	Tangerine	1 large
		Tangerine juice	1/2 cup
		Watermelon	1 cup

LIST 4: BREADS, CEREALS, AND CEREAL PRODUCTS

Note: Each unit contains about 70 calories, 2 grams protein, negligible fat, and 15 grams carbohydrates. One unit from List 2, Vegetables, Group C, may be substituted for one bread unit.

CAUTION: Do not use breads and rolls with salt toppings, potato chips, pretzels, regular salted popcorn, and other heavily salted snack foods. If following the 1200- or 1800-calorie diet plan, do not use sugar-coated cereals.

Breads and Rolls

Bread	1 slice
Melba toast	4 pieces (3 1/2″ x 1 1/2″ x 1/8″)
Roll	1 medium
Biscuit	1 medium
Cornbread	1 cube (1 1/2″)
Griddle cakes	two 3-inch
Muffin	1 medium

Cooked Cereals, Lightly Salted: Each unit is a 1/2-cup serving.

Farina	Rolled wheat
Grits	Wheat meal
Oatmeal	

Table A-4 *(Continued)*

LIST 4: BREADS, CEREALS, AND CEREAL PRODUCTS

Dry Cereals

Shredded wheat	2/3 biscuit
Other dry cereal	3/4 cup

Cereal Products

Barley	1 1/2 tablespoons, uncooked
Cornmeal	2 tablespoons
Cornstarch	2 1/2 tablespoons
Crackers, preferably with unsalted tops	five 2-inch square
Flour	2 1/2 tablespoons
Graham crackers	2
Macaroni	1/2 cup cooked
Matzo	one 5-inch square
Noodles	1/2 cup, cooked
Popcorn, lightly salted	1 1/2 cups
Rice, brown or white	1/2 cup, cooked
Spaghetti	1/2 cup, cooked
Tapioca	2 tablespoons, uncooked
Waffle	one 3-inch square section

LIST 5: MEAT, POULTRY, FISH, EGGS, CHEESE, AND LOW-SODIUM PEANUT BUTTER

Note: Units allowed per day average about 75 calories, 7 grams protein, 5 grams fat, and negligible carbohydrate.

Meat or Poultry, Fresh, Frozen, or Canned

CAUTION: Do not use salty or smoked meat such as bacon, bologna, chipped or corned beef, frankfurters, ham, meats koshered by salting, luncheon meats, salt pork, sausage, and smoked tongue.

One ounce, cooked, of any of the following is one unit.

Beef	Pork
Brain	Quail
Chicken	Rabbit
Duck	Tongue
Kidney	Turkey
Lamb	Veal
Liver (beef, calf, chicken, pork)	

Table A-4 *(Continued)*

LIST 5: MEAT, POULTRY, FISH, EGGS, CHEESE, AND LOW-SODIUM PEANUT BUTTER

Fish or Fish Fillets (Fresh, Frozen, or Canned)

CAUTION: Do not use salty or smoked fish such as anchovies, caviar, salted and dried cod, herring, and sardines.

One ounce, cooked, of any of the following is one unit.

Bass	Clams	Eels	Lobster	Salmon	Sole
Bluefish	Cod	Flounder	Oyster	Scallops	Trout
Catfish	Crab	Halibut	Rockfish	Shrimp	Tuna

Eggs, Cheese, and Peanut Butter

CAUTION: Do not use processed cheese or cheese spreads unless they are low-sodium dietetic. Do not use any cheese such as Roquefort, Camembert, or Gorgonzola.

American cheddar or Swiss cheese	1 ounce
Cottage cheese (lightly salted)	1/4 cup
Egg	1
Low-sodium dietetic peanut butter	2 tablespoons

LIST 6: FAT

Note: Each unit contains about 45 calories and 5 grams fat.

CAUTION: Do not use salted nuts, olives, bacon and bacon fat, salt pork, and heavily salted snack foods such as potato chips and sticks, and crackers.

Avocado	1/8 of 4-inch fruit
Butter	1 teaspoon (1 small pat)
Cream, heavy (sweet or sour)	1 tablespoon
Cream, light (sweet or sour)	2 tablespoons
Fat or oil for cooking	1 teaspoon
French dressing	1 tablespoon
Margarine	1 teaspoon
Mayonnaise	1 teaspoon
Nuts, unsalted	6 small

Table A-4 *(Continued)*

LIST 7: FREE CHOICE

Note: Each free choice unit contains about 75 calories. One free choice unit daily is allowed on the 1200-calorie diet, and two free choice units daily are allowed on the 1800-calorie diet. If calories are not restricted, patient may have as many free choice units as desired. The free choice unit may be divided. For example, the patient may have one unit from the fruit list and two teaspoons of sugar as the free choice unit.

```
List 6, fat. . . . . . . . . . . . . . . . . . . . . . . . . . . . .  2 units
List 3, fruit . . . . . . . . . . . . . . . . . . . . . . . . . . .  2 units
Sugar, white or brown . . . . . . . . . . . . . . . . . . .  4 teaspoons
Syrup, honey, jelly, jam, or marmalade . . . . . . . . . . .  4 teaspoons
List 2, vegetables, Group C . . . . . . . . . . . . . . . . .  1 unit
List 4, Breads . . . . . . . . . . . . . . . . . . . . . . . . .  1 unit
*Candy made without salted nuts. . . . . . . . . . . . . . . . .75 calories
```
*The following amounts of candy furnish approximately 75 calories:

1 piece (1″ x 1″ x 3/4″) fondant or fudge 24 pieces to a pound)
2 large, or 16 small, gum drops (2/3 ounce)
4 pieces (1″ x 1″ x 1/2″), or 7 - 8 pieces, hard candy (2/3 ounce)
3 marshmallows (2/3 ounce)
10 jelly beans (1 ounce)

SEASONINGS: FLAVORING EXTRACTS; HERBS, SPICES, AND AROMATIC SEEDS

The following seasonings may be used:

Allspice	Mint
Almond extract	Mustard, dry, or mustard seed
Anise seed	Nutmeg
Basil	Onion, onion juice, or onion powder
Bay leaf	Orange extract
Bouillon cube, low-sodium dietetic	Oregano
Caraway seed	Paprika
Cardamom	Parsley or parsley flakes
Catsup, dietetic	Pepper, fresh green or red
Celery leaves, dried or fresh	Pepper, black, red, or white
Celery seed	Peppermint extract
Chili powder	Pimiento peppers
Chives	Poppy seed
Cinnamon	Poultry seasoning
Cloves	Purslane
Cocoa	Rosemary

Table A-4 *(Continued)*

SEASONINGS: FLAVORING EXTRACTS; HERBS, SPICES, AND AROMATIC SEEDS

Coconut
Cumin
Curry
Dill
Fennel
Garlic, garlic juice, or garlic powder
Ginger
Horseradish
Juniper
Lemon juice or extract
Mace
Maple extract
Marjoram
Meat extract, low-sodium dietetic
Meat tenderizers, low-sodium dietetic

Saffron
Sage
Salt, used lightly in cooking
Salt substitutes, if recommended by the physician
Savory
Sesame seeds
Sorrel
Sugar
Tarragon
Thyme
Turmeric
Vanilla extract
Vinegar
Wine, if allowed
Walnut extract

The following may not be used:

Artificial sweeteners unless recommended by the
   physician
Commercial bouillon in any form
Catsup
Celery salt, except when used as allowed
   seasoning
Chili sauce
Garlic salt except when used as allowed seasoning
Meat extracts, sauces, and tenderizers if not low-
   sodium dietetic

Mustard, prepared
Olives
Onion salt, except when used as allowed seasoning
Pickles
Relishes
Salt substitutes unless recommended by the
   physician
Saccharin, unless recommended by the physician
Cooking wine (salt has been added)
Worcestershire sauce

MISCELLANEOUS FOODS

The following may be used:
Beverages

Alcoholic beverages, if allowed by the physician
Cocoa made with milk from diet
Coffee, instant or regular
Coffee substitute
Fruit juices (must be counted as fruit units)
Lemonade, using sugar allowance from diet
Milk as allowed on Milk List 1 or 1A
Tea

Table A-4 *(Continued)*

MISCELLANEOUS FOODS

Candy

If calories are restricted, candy may be used as a 75-calorie free choice

Cornstarch

Gelatin

Leavening Agents

Baking powder
Baking soda (for baking only)
Cream of tartar
Potassium bicarbonate
Yeast

Rennet Tablets

Use milk and sugar from the day's allowance

Tapioca

For thickening fruit, or milk tapioca pudding (Be sure to count the tapioca, fruit, milk, and egg from the day's allowance.)

The following may be used unless the patient is on the 1200- or 1800-calorie diet plan:

Baking chocolate
Instant cocoa mixes
Prepared beverage mixes, including fruit-flavored powders
Malted milk and other milk preparations
Fountain beverages
Sugar-sweetened carbonated beverages
Candies, except as free choice
Sugar-sweetened gelatin desserts
Prepared pudding mixes, including rennet powder desserts
Molasses, honey, syrups

Source: "Your Mild Sodium-Restricted Diet (revised)," American Heart Association

°F	°C	°F	°C	°F	°C	°F	°C
70	21.1	117	47.2	160	71.1	197.6	92
71	21.7	118	47.8	161	71.7	198	92.2
72	22.2	119	48.3	161.6	72	199	92.8
73	22.8	120	48.9	162	72.2	199.4	93
74	23.3	121	49.4	163	72.8	200	93.3
75	23.9	122	50	163.4	73	201	93.9
76	24.4	123	50.6	164	73.3	201.2	94
77	25	124	51.1	165	73.9	202	94.4
78	25.6	125	51.7	165.2	74	203	95
79	26.1	126	52.2	166	74.4	204	95.6
80	26.7	127	52.8	167	75	204.8	96
81	27.2	128	53.3	168	75.6	205	96.1
82	27.8	129	53.9	168.8	76	206	96.7
83	28.3	129.2	54	169	76.1	206.6	97
84	28.9	130	54.4	170	76.7	207	97.2
85	29.4	131	55	170.6	77	208	97.8
86	30	132	55.6	171	77.2	208.4	98
87	30.6	132.8	56	172	77.8	209	98.3
88	31.1	133	56.1	172.4	78	210	98.9
89	31.7	134	56.7	173	78.3	211	99.4
90	32.2	135	57.2	174	78.9	212	100
91	32.8	136	57.8	174.2	79	213	100.6
92	33.3	136.4	58	175	79.4	214	101.1
93	33.9	137	58.3	176	80	215	101.7
94	34.4	138	58.9	177	80.6	215.6	102
95	35	139	59.4	177.8	81	216	102.2
96	35.6	140	60	178	81.1	217	102.8
96.8	36	141	60.6	179	81.7	218	103.3
97	36.1	141.8	61	179.6	82	219	103.9
98	36.7	142	61.1	180	82.2	219.2	104
98.6	37	143	61.7	181	82.8	220	104.4
99	37.2	144	62.2	181.4	83	221	105
100	37.8	145	62.8	182	83.3	225	107.2
100.4	38	145.4	63	183.2	84	230	110
101	38.3	146	63.3	184	84.4	235	112.8
102	38.9	147	63.9	185	85	239	115
102.2	39	147.2	64	186	85.6	240	115.6
103	39.4	148	64.4	186.8	86	245	118.3
104	40	149	65	187	86.1	248	120
105	40.6	150	65.6	188	86.7	250	121.1
105.8	41	150.8	66	188.6	87	255	123.9
106	41.1	151	66.1	189	87.2	257	125
107	41.7	152	66.7	190	87.8	260	126.7
107.6	42	152.6	67	190.4	88	265	129.4
108	42.2	153	67.2	191	88.3	266	130
109	42.8	154	67.8	192	88.9	270	132.2
110	43.3	154.4	68	192.2	89	275	135
111	43.9	155	68.3	193	89.4	280	137.8
112	44.4	156	68.9	194	90	284	140
113	45	156.2	69	195	90.6	285	140.6
114	45.6	157	69.4	195.8	91	290	143.3
115	46.1	158	70	196	91.1	295	146.1
116	46.7	159	70.6	197	91.7	300	148.9
116.6	47	159.8	71				

Table A-6 Exchange Lists for Meal Planning

LIST 1. Milk Exchanges (Includes Non-Fat Low-Fat and Whole Milk)

This list shows the kinds and amounts of milk or milk products to use for one milk exchange. Those which appear in **bold type** are **non-fat**. Low-fat and whole milk contain saturated fat. One exchange of milk contains 12 grams of carbohydrate, 8 grams of protein, a trace of fat and 80 calories.

Non-Fat Fortified Milk
Skim or non-fat milk	1 cup
Powdered (non-fat dry, before adding liquid)	1/3 cup
Canned, evaporated—skim milk	1/2 cup
Buttermilk made from skim milk	1 cup
Yogurt made from skim milk (plain, unflavored)	1 cup

Low-Fat Fortified Milk
1% fat fortified milk	1 cup
(omit 1/2 Fat Exchange)	
2% fat fortified milk	1 cup
(omit 1 Fat Exchange)	
Yogurt made from 2% fortified milk (plain, unflavored)	1 cup
(omit 1 Fat Exchange)	

Whole Milk (Omit 2 Fat Exchanges)
Whole milk	1 cup
Canned evaporated whole milk	1/2 cup
Buttermilk made from whole milk	1 cup
Yogurt made from whole milk (plain, unflavored)	1 cup

LIST 2. Vegetable Exchanges

This list shows the kinds of **vegetables** to use for one vegetable exchange. One exchange is ½ cup. One exchange of vegetables contains about 5 grams of carbohydrate, 2 grams of protein and 25 calories.

Asparagus
Bean Sprouts
Beets
Broccoli
Brussels Sprouts
Cabbage
Carrots
Cauliflower
Celery
Eggplant

Greens:
  Mustard
  Spinach
  Turnip
Mushrooms
Okra
Onions
Rhubarb
Rutabaga
Sauerkraut

Table A-6 *(Continued)*

LIST 2. Vegetable Exchanges

Green Pepper	String Beans, green or yellow
Greens:	Summer Squash
Beet	Tomatoes
Chards	Tomato Juice
Collards	Turnips
Dandelion	Vegetable Juice Cocktail
Kale	Zucchini

The following **raw vegetables** may be used as desired:

Chicory	Lettuce
Chinese Cabbage	Parsley
Cucumbers	Pickles, Dill
Endive	Radishes
Escarole	Watercress

Starchy Vegetables are found in the Bread Exchange List.

LIST 3. Fruit Exchanges

This list shows the kinds and amounts of **fruits** to use for one fruit exchange. One exchange of fruit contains 10 grams of carbohydrate and 40 calories.

Apple	1 small	Mango	1/2 small
Apple Juice	1/3 cup	Melon	
Applesauce (unsweetened)	1/2 cup	Cantaloupe	1/4 small
Apricots, fresh	2 medium	Honeydew	1/8 medium
Apricots, dried	4 halves	Watermelon	1 cup
Banana	1/2 small	Nectarine	1 small
Berries		Orange	1 small
Blackberries	1/2 cup	Orange Juice	1/2 cup
Blueberries	1/2 cup	Papaya	3/4 cup
Raspberries	1/2 cup	Peach	1 medium
Strawberries	3/4 cup	Pear	1 small
Cherries	10 large	Persimmon, native	1 medium
Cider	1/3 cup	Pineapple	1/2 cup
Dates	2	Pineapple Juice	1/3 cup
Figs, fresh	1	Plums	2 medium
Figs, dried	1	Prunes	2 medium
Grapefruit	1/2	Prune Juice	1/4 cup
Grapefruit Juice	1/2 cup	Raisins	2 tablespoons
Grapes	12	Tangerine	1 medium
Grape Juice	1/4 cup		

Cranberries may be used as desired if no sugar is added.

Table A-6 *(Continued)*

LIST 4. Bread Exchanges (Includes **Bread, Cereal** and **Starchy Vegetables**)

This list shows the kinds and amounts of **breads, cereals, starchy vegetables** and Prepared Foods to use for one Bread Exchange. Those which appear in **bold type** are **low-fat**. One exchange of bread contains 15 grams of carbohydrate, 2 grams of protein and 70 calories.

Bread

White (including French and Italian)	1 slice
Whole Wheat	1 slice
Rye or Pumpernickel	1 slice
Raisin	1 slice
Bagel, small	1/2
English Muffin, small	1/2
Plain Roll, bread	1
Frankfurter Roll	1/2
Hamburger Bun	1/2
Dried Bread Crumbs	3 Tbs.
Tortilla, 6″	1

Cereal

Bran Flakes	1/2 cup
Other ready-to-eat unsweetened Cereal	3/4 cup
Puffed Cereal (unfrosted)	1 cup
Cereal (cooked)	1/2 cup
Grits (cooked)	1/2 cup
Rice or Barley (cooked)	1/2 cup
Pasta (cooked), Spaghetti, Noodles, Macaroni	1/2 cup
Popcorn (popped, no fat added, large kernel)	3 cups
Cornmeal (dry)	2Tbs.
Flour	2-1/2Tbs.
Wheat Germ	1/4 cup

Crackers

Arrowroot	3
Graham, 2-1/2″ sq.	2
Matzoth, 4″ × 6″	1/2
Oyster	20
Pretzels, 3-1/8″ long × 1/8″ dia.	25
Rye Wafers, 2″ × 3-1/2″	3
Saltines	6
Soda, 2-1/2″ sq.	4

Dried Beans, Peas and Lentils

Beans, Peas, Lentils (dried and cooked)	1/2 cup
Baked Beans, no pork (canned)	1/4 cup

Starchy Vegetables

Corn	1/3 cup
Corn on Cob	1 small
Lima Beans	1/2 cup
Parsnips	2/3 cup
Peas, Green (canned or frozen)	1/2 cup
Potato, White	1 small
Potato (mashed)	1/2 cup
Pumpkin	3/4 cup
Winter Squash, Acorn or Butternut	1/2 cup
Yam or Sweet Potato	1/4 cup

Prepared Foods

Biscuit 2″ dia. (omit 1 Fat Exchange)	1
Corn bread, 2″ × 2″ × 1″ (omit 1 Fat Exchange)	1
Corn Muffin, 2″ dia. (omit 1 Fat Exchange)	1
Crackers, round butter type (omit 1 Fat Exchange)	5
Muffin, plain small (omit 1 Fat Exchange)	1
Potatoes, French Fried, length 2″ to 3-1/2″ (omit 1 Fat Exchange)	8
Potato or Corn chips (omit 2 Fat Exchanges)	15
Pancake, 5″ × 1/2″ (omit 1 Fat Exchange)	1
Waffle, 5″ × 1/2″ (omit 1 Fat Exchange)	1

Table A-6 *(Continued)*

LIST 5. Meat Exchanges Lean Meat

The list shows the kinds and amounts of *lean meat* and other protein-rich foods to use for one low-fat meat exchange. **Trim off all visible fat.** One exchange of lean meat (1 oz.) contains 7 grams of protein, 3 grams of fat and 55 calories.

Beef:	**Baby Beef (very lean), Chipped Beef, Chuck, Flank Steak, Tenderloin, Plate Ribs, Plate Skirt Steak, Round (bottom, top), All cuts Rump, Spare Ribs, Tripe**	1 oz.
Lamb:	**Leg, Rib, Sirloin, Loin (roast and chops), Shank, Shoulder**	1 oz.
Pork:	**Leg (Whole Rump, Center Shank), Ham, Smoked (center slices)**	1 oz.
Veal:	**Leg, Loin, Rib, Shank, Shoulder, Cutlets**	1 oz.
Poultry:	**Meat *without skin* of Chicken, Turkey, Cornish Hen, Guinea Hen, Pheasant**	1 oz.
Fish:	**Any fresh or frozen**	1 oz.
	Canned Salmon, Tuna, Mackerel, Crab and Lobster,	1/4 cup
	Clams, Oysters, Scallops, Shrimp,	5 or 1 oz.
	Sardines, drained	3
Cheeses containing less than 5% butterfat		1 oz.
Cottage Cheese, Dry and 2% butterfat		1/4 cup
Dried Beans and Peas (omit 1 Bread Exchange)		1/2 cup

LIST 5. Meat Exchanges Medium-Fat Meat

This list shows the kinds and amounts of medium-fat meat and other protein-rich foods to use for one medium-fat meat exchange. **Trim off all visible fat.** One exchange of medium-fat meat (1 oz.) contains 7 grams of protein, 5 grams of fat and 75 calories.

Beef:	Ground (15% fat), Corned Beef (canned), Rib Eye, Round (ground commercial)	1 oz.
Pork:	Loin (all cuts Tenderloin), Shoulder Arm (picnic), Shoulder Blade, Boston Butt, Canadian Bacon, Boiled Ham	1 oz.
Liver, Heart, Kidney and Sweetbreads (these are high in cholesterol)		1 oz.
Cottage Cheese, creamed		1/4 cup
Cheese: Mozzarella, Ricotta, Farmer's cheese, Neufchatel,		1 oz.
Parmesan		3 tbs.
Egg (high in cholesterol)		1
Peanut Butter (omit 2 additional Fat Exchanges)		2 tbs.

LIST 5. Meat Exchanges High-Fat Meat

This list shows the kinds and amounts of high-fat meat and other protein-rich foods to use for one high-fat meat exchange. **Trim off all visible fat.** One exchange of high-fat meat (1 oz.) contains 7 grams of protein, 8 grams of fat and 100 calories.

Beef:	Brisket, Corned Beef (Brisket), Ground Beef (more than 20% fat), Hamburger (commercial), Chuck (ground commercial), Roasts (Rib), Steaks (Club and Rib)	1 oz.
Lamb:	Breast	1 oz.
Pork:	Spare Ribs, Loin (Back Ribs), Pork (ground), Country style Ham, Deviled Ham	1 oz.
Veal:	Breast	1 oz.

Table A-6 *(Continued)*

LIST 5. **Meat Exchanges** High-Fat Meat

Poultry: Capon, Duck (domestic), Goose	1 oz.
Cheese: Cheddar Types	1 oz.
Cold Cuts	4-1/2″ × 1/8″ slice
Frankfurter	1 small

LIST 6. Fat Exchanges

This list shows the kinds and amounts of fat-containing foods to use for one fat exchange. To plan a diet low in saturated fat select only those exchanges which appear in **bold type**. They are **polyunsaturated**. One exchange of fat contains 5 grams of fat and 45 calories.

Margarine, soft, tub or stick*	1 teaspoon
Avocado (4″ in diameter)**	1/8
Oil, Corn, Cottonseed, Safflower, Soy, Sunflower	1 teaspoon
Oil, Olive**	1 teaspoon
Oil, Peanut**	1 teaspoon
Olives**	5 small
Almonds**	10 whole
Pecans**	2 large whole
Peanuts**	
Spanish	20 whole
Virginia	10 whole
Walnuts	6 small
Nuts, other**	6 small
Margarine, regular stick	1 teaspoon
Butter	1 teaspoon
Bacon fat	1 teaspoon
Bacon, crisp	1 strip
Cream, light	2 tablespoons
Cream, sour	2 tablespoons
Cream, heavy	1 tablespoon
Cream Cheese	1 tablespoon
French dressing***	1 tablespoon
Italian dressing***	1 tablespoon
Lard	1 teaspoon
Mayonnaise***	1 teaspoon
Salad dressing, mayonnaise type***	2 teaspoons
Salt pork	3/4 inch cube

  *Made with corn, cottonseed, safflower, soy or sunflower oil only
  **Fat content is primarily monounsaturated
***If made with corn, cottonseed, safflower, soy or sunflower oil can be used on fat modified diet

    The exchange lists are based on material in the *Exchange Lists for Meal Planning* prepared by Committees of the American Diabetes Association, Inc. and the American Dietetic Association in cooperation with the National Institute of Arthritis, Metabolism and Digestive Diseases and the National Heart and Lung Institutes of Health, Public Health Service, U.S. Department of Health and Human Services.

Table A-7 Nutritive Values of the Edible Part of Foods (Courtesy of the United States Department of Agriculture)

DAIRY PRODUCTS (CHEESE, CREAM, IMITATION CREAM, MILK; RELATED PRODUCTS)

Butter. See Fats, oils; related products, items 103-108.

								Fatty Acids												
									Unsaturated											
Item No. (A)	Foods, approximate measures, units, and weight (edible part unless footnotes indicate otherwise) (B)	Grams	Water (C) Per cent	Food energy (D) Calories	Protein (E) Grams	Fat (F) Grams	Saturated (total) (G) Grams	Oleic (H) Grams	Linoleic (I) Grams	Carbohydrate (J) Grams	Calcium (K) Milligrams	Phosphorus (L) Milligrams	Iron (M) Milligrams	Potassium (N) Milligrams	Vitamin A value (O) International units	Thiamin (P) Milligrams	Riboflavin (Q) Milligrams	Niacin (R) Milligrams	Ascorbic acid (S) Milligrams
	Cheese:																		
	Natural:																		
1	Blue----- 1 oz-----	28	42	100	6	8	5.3	1.9	0.2	1	150	110	0.1	73	200	0.01	0.11	0.3	0
2	Camembert (3 wedges per 4-oz container). 1 wedge	38	52	115	8	9	5.8	2.2	.2	Trace	147	132	.1	71	350	.01	.19	.2	0
	Cheddar:																		
3	Cut pieces----- 1 oz-----	28	37	115	7	9	6.1	2.1	.2	Trace	204	145	.2	28	300	.01	.11	Trace	0
4	----- 1 cu in-----	17.2	37	70	4	6	3.7	1.3	.1	Trace	124	88	.1	17	180	Trace	.06	Trace	0
5	Shredded----- 1 cup-----	113	37	455	28	37	24.2	8.5	.7	1	815	579	.8	111	1,200	.03	.42	.1	0
	Cottage (curd not pressed down):																		
	Creamed (cottage cheese, 4% fat):																		
6	Large curd----- 1 cup-----	225	79	235	28	10	6.4	2.4	.2	6	135	297	.3	190	370	.05	.37	.3	Trace
7	Small curd----- 1 cup-----	210	79	220	26	9	6.0	2.2	.2	6	126	277	.3	177	340	.04	.34	.3	Trace
8	Low fat (2%)----- 1 cup-----	226	79	205	31	4	2.8	1.0	.1	8	155	340	.4	217	160	.05	.42	.3	Trace
9	Low fat (1%)----- 1 cup-----	226	82	165	28	2	1.5	.5	.1	6	138	302	.3	193	80	.05	.37	.3	Trace
10	Uncreamed (cottage cheese dry curd, less than 1/2% fat)----- 1 cup-----	145	80	125	25	1	.4	.1	Trace	3	46	151	.3	47	40	.04	.21	.2	0
11	Cream----- 1 oz-----	28	54	100	2	10	6.2	2.4	.2	1	23	30	.3	34	400	Trace	.06	Trace	0
	Mozzarella, made with—																		
12	Whole milk----- 1 oz-----	28	48	90	6	7	4.4	1.7	.2	1	163	117	.1	21	260	Trace	.08	Trace	0
13	Part skim milk----- 1 oz-----	28	49	80	8	5	3.1	1.2	.1	1	207	149	.1	27	180	.01	.10	Trace	0
	Parmesan, grated:																		
14	Cup, not pressed down----- 1 cup-----	100	18	455	42	30	19.1	7.7	.3	4	1,376	807	1.0	107	700	.05	.39	.3	0
15	Tablespoon----- 1 tbsp-----	5	18	25	2	2	1.0	.4	Trace	Trace	69	40	Trace	5	40	Trace	.02	Trace	0
16	Ounce----- 1 oz-----	28	18	130	12	9	5.4	2.2	.1	1	390	229	.3	30	200	.01	.11	.1	0
17	Provolone----- 1 oz-----	28	41	100	7	8	4.8	1.7	.1	1	214	141	.1	39	230	.01	.09	Trace	0
	Ricotta, made with—																		
18	Whole milk----- 1 cup-----	246	72	428	28	32	20.4	7.1	.7	7	509	389	.9	257	1,210	.03	.48	.3	0
19	Part skim milk----- 1 cup-----	246	74	340	28	19	12.1	4.7	.5	13	669	449	1.1	308	1,060	.05	.46	.2	0
20	Romano----- 1 oz-----	28	31	110	9	8				1	302	215			160		.11	Trace	0
21	Swiss----- 1 oz-----	28	37	105	8	8	5.0	1.7	.2	1	272	171	Trace	31	240	.01	.10	Trace	0
	Pasteurized process cheese:																		
22	American----- 1 oz-----	28	39	105	6	9	5.6	2.1	.2	Trace	174	211	.1	46	340	.01	.10	Trace	0
23	Swiss----- 1 oz-----	28	42	95	7	7	4.5	1.7	.1	1	219	216	.2	61	230	Trace	.08	Trace	0
24	Pasteurized process cheese food, American----- 1 oz-----	28	43	95	6	7	4.4	1.7	.1	2	163	130	.2	79	260	.01	.13	Trace	0
25	Pasteurized process cheese spread, American.----- 1 oz-----	28	48	82	5	6	3.8	1.5	.1	2	159	202	.1	69	220	.01	.12	Trace	0
	Cream, sweet:																		
26	Half-and-half (cream and milk)----- 1 cup-----	242	81	315	7	28	17.3	7.0	.6	10	254	230	.2	314	260	.08	.36	.2	2
27	----- 1 tbsp-----	15	81	20	Trace	2	1.1	.4	Trace	1	16	14	Trace	19	20	.01	.02	Trace	Trace
28	Light, coffee, or table----- 1 cup-----	240	74	470	6	46	28.8	11.7	1.0	9	231	192	.1	292	1,730	.08	.36	.1	2
29	----- 1 tbsp-----	15	74	30	Trace	3	1.8	.7	.1	1	14	12	Trace	18	110	Trace	.02	Trace	Trace

NUTRIENTS IN INDICATED QUANTITY

TABLE A-7
NUTRITIVE VALUES OF THE EDIBLE PART OF FOODS - Continued

(Dashes (—) denote lack of reliable data for a constituent believed to be present in measurable amount)

NUTRIENTS IN INDICATED QUANTITY

Item No. (A)	Foods, approximate measures, units, and weight (edible part unless footnotes indicate otherwise) (B)	Water (C)	Food energy (D)	Protein (E)	Fat (F)	Fatty Acids — Saturated (total) (G)	Fatty Acids — Unsaturated Oleic (H)	Fatty Acids — Linoleic (I)	Carbohydrate (J)	Calcium (K)	Phosphorus (L)	Iron (M)	Potassium (N)	Vitamin A Value (O)	Thiamin (P)	Riboflavin (Q)	Niacin (R)	Ascorbic acid (S)
	Whipping, unwhipped (volume about double when whipped):																	
30	Light ---- cup (239)	64	700	5	74	46.2	18.3	1.5	7	166	146	0.1	231	2,690	0.06	0.30	0.1	1
31	---- tbsp (15)	64	45	Trace	5	2.9	1.1	.1	Trace	10	9	Trace	15	170	Trace	.02	Trace	1
32	Heavy ---- cup (238)	58	820	5	88	54.8	22.2	2.0	7	154	149	.1	179	3,500	.05	.26	.1	1
33	---- tbsp (15)	58	80	Trace	6	3.5	1.4	.1	Trace	10	9	Trace	11	220	Trace	.02	Trace	Trace
34	Whipped topping, (pressurized) ---- cup (60)	61	155	2	13	8.3	3.4	.3	7	61	54	Trace	88	550	.02	.04	Trace	0
35	---- tbsp (3)	61	10	Trace	1	.4	.2	Trace	Trace	3	3	Trace	4	30	Trace	Trace	Trace	0
36	Cream, sour ---- cup (230)	71	495	7	48	30.0	12.1	1.1	10	268	195	.1	331	1,820	.08	.34	.2	2
37	---- tbsp (12)	71	25	Trace	3	1.6	.6	.1	1	14	10	Trace	17	90	Trace	.02	Trace	Trace
	Cream products, imitation (made with vegetable fat):																	
	Sweet:																	
	Creamers:																	
38	Liquid (frozen) ---- cup (245)	77	335	2	24	22.8	Trace	Trace	28	23	157	.1	467	¹220	0	0	0	0
39	---- tbsp (15)	77	20	Trace	2	1.4	Trace	0	2	1	10	Trace	29	¹10	0	0	0	0
40	Powdered ---- cup (94)	2	515	5	33	30.6	.9	0	52	21	397	Trace	763	¹190	0	.16	0	0
41	---- tsp (2)	2	10	Trace	1	.7	Trace	0	1	Trace	8	Trace	16	¹Trace	0	¹Trace	0	0
	Whipped topping:																	
42	Frozen ---- cup (75)	50	240	1	19	16.3	1.0	.2	17	5	6	.1	14	¹650	0	0	0	0
43	---- tbsp (4)	50	15	Trace	1	.9	.1	Trace	1	Trace	Trace	Trace	1	¹30	0	0	0	0
44	Powdered, made with whole milk. ---- cup (80)	67	150	3	10	8.5	.6	.1	13	72	69	Trace	121	¹290	.02	.09	Trace	1
45	---- tbsp (4)	67	10	Trace	Trace	.4	Trace	Trace	1	4	3	Trace	6	¹10	Trace	Trace	Trace	Trace
46	Pressurized ---- cup (70)	60	185	1	16	13.2	1.4	.2	11	4	13	Trace	13	¹330	0	0	0	0
47	---- tbsp (4)	60	10	Trace	1	.8	.1	Trace	1	Trace	Trace	Trace	1	¹20	0	0	0	0
48	Sour dressing (imitation sour cream) made with nonfat dry milk. ---- cup (235)	75	415	8	39	31.2	4.4	1.1	11	266	205	.1	380	¹20	.09	.38	.2	2
49	Ice cream. See Milk desserts, frozen (items 75–80). ---- tbsp (12)	75	20	Trace	2	1.6	.2	.1	1	14	10	Trace	19	¹Trace	.01	.02	Trace	Trace
	Ice milk. See Milk desserts, frozen (items 81–83).																	
	Milk:																	
	Fluid:																	
50	Whole (3.3% fat) ---- 1 cup (244)	88	150	8	8	5.1	2.1	.2	11	291	228	.1	370	²310	.09	.40	.2	2
	Lowfat (2%):																	
51	No milk solids added ---- 1 cup (244)	89	120	8	5	2.9	1.2	.1	12	297	232	.1	377	500	.10	.40	.2	2
	Milk solids added:																	
52	Label claim less than 10 g of protein per cup. ---- 1 cup (245)	89	125	9	5	2.9	1.2	.1	12	313	245	.1	397	500	.10	.42	.2	2
53	Label claim 10 or more grams of protein per cup (protein fortified). ---- 1 cup (246)	88	135	10	5	3.0	1.2	.1	14	352	276	.1	447	500	.11	.48	.2	3
	Lowfat (1%):																	
54	No milk solids added ---- 1 cup (244)	90	100	8	3	1.6	.7	.1	12	300	235	.1	381	500	.10	.41	.2	2
	Milk solids added:																	
55	Label claim less than 10 g of protein per cup. ---- 1 cup (245)	90	105	9	2	1.5	.6	.1	12	313	245	.1	397	500	.10	.42	.2	2
56	Label claim 10 or more grams of protein per cup (protein fortified). ---- 1 cup (246)	89	120	10	3	1.8	.7	.1	14	349	273	.1	444	500	.11	.47	.2	3
	Nonfat (skim):																	
57	No milk solids added ---- 1 cup (245)	91	85	8	Trace	.3	.1	Trace	12	302	247	.1	406	500	.09	.37	.2	2

¹Vitamin A value is largely from beta-carotene used for coloring. Riboflavin value for items 40–41 apply to products with added riboflavin.
²Applies to product without added vitamin A. With added vitamin A, value is 500 International Units (I.U.).

DAIRY PRODUCTS (CHEESE, CREAM, IMITATION CREAM, MILK; RELATED PRODUCTS)—Con.

(A)	(B)	Grams	(C) Per-cent	(D) Cal-ories	(E) Grams	(F) Grams	(G) Grams	(H) Grams	(I) Grams	(J) Grams	(K) Milli-grams	(L) Milli-grams	(M) Milli-grams	(N) Milli-grams	(O) Inter-national units	(P) Milli-grams	(Q) Milli-grams	(R) Milli-grams	(S) Milli-grams
	Milk—Continued																		
	Fluid—Continued																		
	Nonfat (skim)—Continued																		
	Milk solids added:																		
58	Label claim less than 10 g of protein per cup. 1 cup	245	90	90	9	1	0.4	0.1	Trace	12	316	255	0.1	416	500	0.10	0.43	0.2	2
59	Label claim 10 or more grams of protein per cup (protein fortified). 1 cup	246	89	100	10	1	.4	.1	Trace	14	352	275	.1	446	500	.11	.48	.2	3
	Buttermilk—																		
60	1 cup	245	90	100	8	2	1.3	.5	Trace	12	285	219	.1	371	380	.08	.38	.1	2
	Canned:																		
	Evaporated, unsweetened:																		
61	Whole milk 1 cup	252	74	340	17	19	11.6	5.3	0.4	25	657	510	.5	764	[3]610	.12	.80	.5	5
62	Skim milk 1 cup	255	79	200	19	1	.3	.1	Trace	29	738	497	.7	845	[4]1,000	.11	.79	.4	3
63	Sweetened, condensed 1 cup	306	27	980	24	27	16.8	6.7	.7	166	868	775	.6	1,136	[3]1,000	.28	1.27	.6	8
	Dried:																		
	Buttermilk:																		
64	1 cup	120	3	465	41	7	4.3	1.7	.2	59	1,421	1,119	.4	1,910	[3]260	.47	1.90	1.1	7
	Nonfat instant:																		
65	Envelope, net wt., 3.2 oz[5] 1 envelope	91	4	325	32	1	.4	.1	Trace	47	1,120	896	.3	1,552	[6]2,160	.38	1.59	.8	5
66	Cup[7] 1 cup	68	4	245	24	Trace	.3	.1	Trace	35	837	670	.2	1,160	[6]1,610	.28	1.19	.6	4
	Milk beverages:																		
	Chocolate milk (commercial):																		
67	Regular 1 cup	250	82	210	8	8	5.3	2.2	.2	26	280	251	.6	417	[3]300	.09	.41	.3	2
68	Lowfat (2%) 1 cup	250	84	180	8	5	3.1	1.3	.1	26	284	254	.6	422	500	.10	.42	.3	2
69	Lowfat (1%) 1 cup	250	85	160	8	3	1.5	.7	.1	26	287	257	.6	426	500	.10	.40	.2	2
70	Eggnog (commercial) 1 cup	254	74	340	10	19	11.3	5.0	.6	34	330	278	.5	420	890	.09	.48	.3	4
	Malted milk, home-prepared with 1 cup of whole milk and 2 to 3 heaping tsp of malted milk powder (about 3/4 oz):																		
71	Chocolate 1 cup of milk plus 3/4 oz of powder.	265	81	235	9	9	5.5	—	—	29	304	265	.5	500	330	.14	.43	.7	2
72	Natural 1 cup of milk plus 3/4 oz of powder.	265	81	235	11	10	6.0	—	—	27	347	307	.3	529	380	.20	.54	1.3	2
	Shakes, thick:[8]																		
73	Chocolate, container, net wt., 10.6 oz. 1 container	300	72	355	9	8	5.0	2.0	.2	63	396	378	.9	672	260	.14	.67	.4	0
74	Vanilla, container, net wt., 11 oz. 1 container	313	74	350	12	9	5.9	2.4	.2	56	457	361	.3	572	360	.09	.61	.5	0
	Milk desserts, frozen:																		
	Ice cream:																		
	Regular (about 11% fat):																		
75	Hardened 1/2 gal	1,064	61	2,155	38	115	71.3	28.8	2.6	254	1,406	1,075	1.0	2,052	4,340	.42	2.63	1.1	6
76	1 cup	133	61	270	5	14	8.9	3.6	.3	32	176	134	.1	257	540	.05	.33	.1	1
77	3-fl oz container	50	61	100	2	5	3.4	1.4	.1	12	66	51	Trace	96	200	.02	.12	.1	Trace
78	Soft serve (frozen custard) 1 cup	173	60	375	7	23	13.5	5.9	.6	38	236	199	.4	338	790	.08	.45	.2	1
79	Rich (about 16% fat), hardened. 1/2 gal	1,188	59	2,805	33	190	118.3	47.8	4.3	256	1,213	927	.8	1,771	7,200	.36	2.27	.9	5
80	1 cup	148	59	350	4	24	14.7	6.0	.5	32	151	115	.1	221	900	.04	.28	.1	1
	Ice milk:																		
81	Hardened (about 4.3% fat) 1/2 gal	1,048	69	1,470	41	45	28.1	11.3	1.0	232	1,409	1,035	1.5	2,117	1,710	.61	2.78	.9	6
82	1 cup	131	69	185	5	6	3.5	1.4	.1	29	176	129	.1	265	210	.08	.35	.1	1

TABLE A-7
NUTRITIVE VALUES OF THE EDIBLE PART OF FOODS - Continued

(Dashes (—) denote lack of reliable data for a constituent believed to be present in measurable amount)

Item No. (A)	Foods, approximate measures, units, and weight (edible part unless footnotes indicate otherwise) (B)		Water (C)	Food energy (D)	Protein (E)	Fat (F)	Fatty Acids Saturated (total) (G)	Unsaturated Oleic (H)	Unsaturated Linoleic (I)	Carbohydrate (J)	Calcium (K)	Phosphorus (L)	Iron (M)	Potassium (N)	Vitamin A value (O)	Thiamin (P)	Riboflavin (Q)	Niacin (R)	Ascorbic acid (S)
83	Soft serve (about 2.6% fat)	1 cup 175	70	225	8	5	2.9	1.2	0.1	38	274	202	0.3	412	180	0.12	0.54	0.2	1
84	Sherbet (about 2% fat)	1/2 gal 1,542	66	2,160	17	31	19.0	7.7	.7	469	827	594	2.5	1,585	1,480	.26	.71	1.0	31
85		1 cup 193	66	270	2	4	2.4	1.0	.1	59	103	74	.3	198	190	.03	.09	.1	4
	Milk desserts, other:																		
86	Custard, baked	1 cup 265	77	305	14	15	6.8	5.4	.7	29	297	310	1.1	387	930	.11	.50	.3	1
	Puddings: From home recipe: Starch base:																		
87	Chocolate	1 cup 260	66	385	8	12	7.6	3.3	.3	67	250	255	1.3	445	390	.05	.36	.3	1
88	Vanilla (blancmange)	1 cup 255	76	285	9	10	6.2	2.5	.2	41	298	232	Trace	352	410	.08	.41	.3	2
89	Tapioca cream	1 cup 165	72	220	8	8	4.1	2.5	.5	28	173	180	.7	223	480	.07	.30	.2	2
	From mix (chocolate) and milk:																		
90	Regular (cooked)	1 cup 260	70	320	9	8	4.3	2.6	.2	59	265	247	.8	354	340	.05	.39	.3	2
91	Instant	1 cup 260	69	325	8	7	3.6	2.2	.3	63	374	237	1.3	335	340	.08	.39	.3	2
	Yogurt: With added milk solids: Made with lowfat milk:																		
92	Fruit-flavored[9]	container, net wt, 8 oz 227	75	230	10	3	1.8	.6	.1	42	343	269	.2	439	[10]120	.08	.40	.2	1
93	Plain	container, net wt, 8 oz 227	85	145	12	4	2.3	.8	.1	16	415	326	.2	531	[10]150	.10	.49	.3	2
94	Made with nonfat milk	container, net wt, 8 oz 227	85	125	13	Trace	.3	.1	Trace	17	452	355	.2	579	[10]20	.11	.53	.3	2
	Without added milk solids:																		
95	Made with whole milk	container, net wt, 8 oz 227	88	140	8	7	4.8	1.7	.1	11	274	215	.1	351	280	.07	.32	.2	1
	EGGS																		
	Eggs, large (24 oz per dozen): Raw:																		
96	Whole, without shell	1 egg 50	75	80	6	6	1.7	2.0	.6	1	28	90	1.0	65	260	.04	.15	Trace	0
97	White	1 white 33	88	15	3	Trace	0	0	0	Trace	4	4	Trace	45	0	Trace	.09	Trace	0
98	Yolk	1 yolk 17	49	65	3	6	1.7	2.1	.6	Trace	26	86	.9	15	310	.04	.07	Trace	0
	Cooked:																		
99	Fried in butter	1 egg 46	72	85	5	6	2.4	2.2	.6	1	26	80	1.0	58	290	.03	.13	Trace	0
100	Hard-cooked, shell removed	1 egg 50	74	80	6	6	1.7	2.0	.6	1	28	90	1.0	65	260	.04	.14	Trace	0
101	Poached	1 egg 50	74	80	6	6	1.7	2.0	.6	1	28	90	1.0	65	260	.04	.13	Trace	0
102	Scrambled (milk added) in butter. Also omelet.	1 egg 64	76	95	6	7	2.8	2.3	.6	1	47	97	.9	85	310	.04	.16	Trace	0
	FATS, OILS; RELATED PRODUCTS																		
	Butter: Regular (1 brick or 4 sticks per lb):																		
103	Stick (1/2 cup)	1 stick 113	16	815	1	92	57.3	23.1	2.1	Trace	27	26	.2	29	[11]3,470	.01	.04	Trace	0
104	Tablespoon (about 1/8 stick)	1 tbsp 14	16	100	Trace	12	7.2	2.9	.3	Trace	3	3	Trace	4	[11]430	Trace	Trace	Trace	0
105	Pat (1 in square, 1/3 in high; 90 per lb)	1 pat 5	16	35	Trace	4	2.5	1.0	.1	Trace	1	1	Trace	1	[11]150	Trace	Trace	Trace	0
	Whipped (6 sticks or two 8-oz containers per lb).																		
106	Stick (1/2 cup)	1 stick 76	16	540	1	61	38.2	15.4	1.4	Trace	18	17	.1	20	[11]2,310	Trace	.03	Trace	0
107	Tablespoon (about 1/8 stick)	1 tbsp 9	16	65	Trace	8	4.7	1.9	.2	Trace	2	2	Trace	2	[11]290	Trace	Trace	Trace	0
108	Pat (1 1/4 in square, 1/3 in high; 120 per lb)	1 pat 4	16	25	Trace	3	1.9	.8	.1	Trace	1	1	Trace	1	[11]120	0	Trace	Trace	0

3 Applies to product without vitamin A added.
4 Applies to product with added vitamin A. Without added vitamin A, value is 20 International Units (I.U.).
5 Yields 1 qt of fluid milk when reconstituted according to package directions.
6 Applies to product with added vitamin A.
7 Weight applies to product with label claim of 1 1/3 cups equal 3.2 oz.
8 Applies to product with label claim of 1 1/3 cups equal 3.2 oz.
9 Content of fat, vitamin A, and carbohydrate varies. Consult the label when precise values are needed for special diets.
10 Applies to products made from thick shake mixes and that do not contain added ice cream. Products made from milk shake mixes are higher in fat and usually contain added ice cream.
11 Applies to product made with milk containing no added vitamin A.
11 Based on year-round average.

FATS, OILS; RELATED PRODUCTS—Con.

(A)	(B)		(C)	(D)	(E)	(F)	(G)	(H)	(I)	(J)	(K)	(L)	(M)	(N)	(O)	(P)	(Q)	(R)	(S)
		Grams	Per-cent	Cal-ories	Grams	Grams	Grams	Grams	Grams	Grams	Milli-grams	Milli-grams	Milli-grams	Milli-grams	Inter-national units	Milli-grams	Milli-grams	Milli-grams	Milli-grams
109	Fats, cooking (vegetable shortenings). 1 cup	200	0	1,770	0	200	48.8	88.2	48.4	0	0	0	0	0	—	0	0	0	0
110	Lard 1 tbsp	13	0	110	0	13	3.2	5.7	3.1	0	0	0	0	0	0	0	0	0	0
111	1 cup	205	0	1,850	0	205	81.0	83.8	20.5	0	0	0	0	0	0	0	0	0	0
112	1 tbsp	13	0	115	0	13	5.1	5.3	1.3	0	0	0	0	0	0	0	0	0	0
	Margarine:																		
	Regular (1 brick or 4 sticks per lb):																		
113	Stick (1/2 cup)	113	16	815	1	92	16.7	42.9	24.9	Trace	27	26	.2	29	[12]3,750	.01	.04	Trace	0
114	Tablespoon (about 1/8 stick)	14	16	100	Trace	12	2.1	5.3	3.1	Trace	3	3	Trace	4	[12]470	Trace	Trace	Trace	0
115	Pat (1 in square, 1/3 in high; 90 per lb).	5	16	35	Trace	4	.7	1.9	1.1	Trace	1	1	Trace	1	[12]170	Trace	Trace	Trace	0
116	Soft, two 8-oz containers per lb. 1 container	227	16	1,635	1	184	32.5	71.5	65.4	Trace	53	52	.4	59	[12]7,500	.01	.08	.1	0
117	1 tbsp	14	16	100	Trace	12	2.0	4.5	4.1	Trace	3	3	Trace	4	[12]470	Trace	Trace	Trace	0
	Whipped (6 sticks per lb):																		
118	Stick (1/2 cup)	76	16	545	Trace	61	11.2	28.7	16.7	Trace	18	17	.1	20	[12]2,500	Trace	.03	Trace	0
119	Tablespoon (about 1/8 stick)	9	16	70	Trace	8	1.4	3.6	2.1	Trace	2	2	Trace	2	[12]310	Trace	Trace	Trace	0
	Oils, salad or cooking:																		
120	Corn 1 cup	218	0	1,925	0	218	27.7	53.6	125.1	0	0	0	0	0	—	0	0	0	0
121	1 tbsp	14	0	120	0	14	1.7	3.3	7.8	0	0	0	0	0	—	0	0	0	0
122	Olive 1 cup	216	0	1,910	0	216	30.7	154.4	17.7	0	0	0	0	0	—	0	0	0	0
123	1 tbsp	14	0	120	0	14	1.9	9.7	1.1	0	0	0	0	0	—	0	0	0	0
124	Peanut 1 cup	216	0	1,910	0	216	37.4	98.5	67.0	0	0	0	0	0	—	0	0	0	0
125	1 tbsp	14	0	120	0	14	2.3	6.2	4.2	0	0	0	0	0	—	0	0	0	0
126	Safflower 1 cup	218	0	1,925	0	218	20.5	25.9	159.8	0	0	0	0	0	—	0	0	0	0
127	1 tbsp	14	0	120	0	14	1.3	1.6	10.0	0	0	0	0	0	—	0	0	0	0
128	Soybean oil, hydrogenated (partially hardened). 1 cup	218	0	1,925	0	218	31.8	93.1	75.6	0	0	0	0	0	—	0	0	0	0
129	1 tbsp	14	0	120	0	14	2.0	5.8	4.7	0	0	0	0	0	—	0	0	0	0
130	Soybean-cottonseed oil blend, hydrogenated. 1 cup	218	0	1,925	0	218	38.2	63.0	99.6	0	0	0	0	0	—	0	0	0	0
131	1 tbsp	14	0	120	0	14	2.4	3.9	6.2	0	0	0	0	0	—	0	0	0	0
	Salad dressings:																		
	Commercial:																		
	Blue cheese:																		
132	Regular 1 tbsp	15	32	75	1	8	1.6	1.7	3.8	1	12	11	Trace	6	30	Trace	.02	Trace	Trace
133	Low calorie (5 Cal per tsp) 1 tbsp	16	84	10	Trace	1	.5	.3	Trace	1	10	8	Trace	5	30	Trace	.01	Trace	Trace
	French:																		
134	Regular 1 tbsp	16	39	65	Trace	6	1.1	1.3	3.2	3	2	2	.1	13	—	Trace	Trace	Trace	—
135	Low calorie (5 Cal per tsp) 1 tbsp	16	77	15	Trace	1	.1	.1	.4	2	2	2	.1	13	—	Trace	Trace	Trace	—
	Italian:																		
136	Regular 1 tbsp	15	28	85	Trace	9	1.6	1.9	4.7	1	2	1	Trace	2	Trace	Trace	Trace	Trace	—
137	Low calorie (2 Cal per tsp) 1 tbsp	15	90	10	Trace	1	.1	.1	.4	Trace	Trace	1	Trace	2	Trace	Trace	Trace	Trace	—
138	Mayonnaise 1 tbsp	14	15	100	Trace	11	2.0	2.4	5.6	Trace	3	4	.1	5	40	Trace	.01	Trace	—
	Mayonnaise type:																		
139	Regular 1 tbsp	15	41	65	Trace	6	1.1	1.4	3.2	2	2	4	Trace	1	30	Trace	Trace	Trace	Trace
140	Low calorie (8 Cal per tsp) 1 tbsp	16	81	20	Trace	2	.4	.4	1.0	2	3	4	Trace	1	40	Trace	Trace	Trace	Trace
141	Tartar sauce, regular 1 tbsp	14	34	75	Trace	8	1.5	1.8	4.1	1	3	4	.1	11	30	Trace	Trace	Trace	Trace
	Thousand Island:																		
142	Regular 1 tbsp	16	32	80	Trace	8	1.4	1.7	4.0	2	2	3	.1	18	50	Trace	Trace	Trace	Trace
143	Low calorie (10 Cal per tsp) 1 tbsp	15	68	25	Trace	2	.4	.4	1.0	2	2	3	.1	17	50	Trace	Trace	Trace	Trace
144	From home recipe: Cooked type[3] 1 tbsp	16	68	25	1	2	.5	.6	.3	2	14	15	.1	19	80	.01	.03	Trace	Trace

TABLE A-7
NUTRITIVE VALUES OF THE EDIBLE PART OF FOODS · Continued
(Dashes (—) denote lack of reliable data for a constituent believed to be present in measurable amount)

NUTRIENTS IN INDICATED QUANTITY

Item No. (A)	Foods, approximate measures, units, and weight (edible part unless footnotes indicate otherwise) (B)	Grams	Water (C)	Food energy (D)	Pro-tein (E)	Fat (F)	Satu-rated (total) (G)	Unsat. Oleic (H)	Linoleic (I)	Carbo-hydrate	Calcium (K)	Phos-phorus (L)	Iron (M)	Potas-sium (N)	Vitamin A value (O)	Thiamin (P)	Ribo-flavin (Q)	Niacin (R)	Ascorbic acid (S)
	FISH, SHELLFISH, MEAT, POULTRY: RELATED PRODUCTS																		
	Fish and shellfish:																		
145	Bluefish, baked with butter or margarine. 3 oz	85	68	135	22	4	—	—	—	0	25	244	0.6	—	40	0.09	0.08	1.6	—
	Clams:																		
146	Raw, meat only. 3 oz	85	82	65	11	1	—	—	—	2	59	138	5.2	154	90	.08	.15	1.1	—
147	Canned, solids and liquid. 3 oz	85	86	45	7	1	0.2	Trace	Trace	2	47	116	3.5	119	—	.01	.09	.9	8
148	Crabmeat (white or king), canned, not pressed down. 1 cup	135	77	135	24	3	.6	0.4	0.1	1	61	246	1.1	149	—	.11	.11	2.6	—
149	Fish sticks, breaded, cooked, frozen (stick, 4 by 1 by 1/2 in). 1 fish stick or 1 oz	28	66	50	5	3	—	—	—	2	3	47	.1	—	0	.01	.02	.5	—
150	Haddock, breaded, fried[14]. 3 oz	85	66	140	17	5	1.4	2.2	1.2	5	34	210	1.0	296	—	.03	.06	2.7	—
151	Ocean perch, breaded, fried[14]. 1 fillet	85	59	195	16	11	2.7	4.4	2.3	6	28	192	1.1	242	—	.10	.10	1.6	2
152	Oysters, raw, meat only (13–19 medium Selects). 1 cup	240	85	160	20	4	1.3	.8	.1	8	226	343	13.2	290	740	.34	.43	6.0	—
153	Salmon, pink, canned, solids and liquid. 3 oz	85	71	120	17	5	.9	.8	.1	0	[15]167	243	.7	307	60	.03	.16	6.8	—
154	Sardines, Atlantic, canned in oil, drained solids. 3 oz	85	62	175	20	9	3.0	2.5	.5	0	372	424	2.5	502	190	.02	.17	4.6	—
155	Scallops, frozen, breaded, fried, reheated. 6 scallops	90	60	175	16	8	—	—	—	9	—	—	—	—	—	—	—	—	—
156	Shad, baked with butter or margarine, bacon. 3 oz	85	64	170	20	10	—	—	—	0	20	266	.5	320	30	.11	.22	7.3	—
	Shrimp:																		
157	Canned meat[16]. 3 oz	85	70	100	21	1	.1	.1	Trace	1	98	224	2.6	104	50	.01	.03	1.5	—
158	French fried[16]. 3 oz	85	57	190	17	9	2.3	3.7	2.0	9	61	162	1.7	195	—	.03	.07	2.3	—
159	Tuna, canned in oil, drained solids. 3 oz	85	61	170	24	7	1.7	1.7	.7	0	7	199	1.6	—	70	.04	.10	10.1	—
160	Tuna salad[17]. 1 cup	205	70	350	30	22	4.3	6.3	6.7	7	41	291	2.7	—	590	.08	.23	10.3	2
	Meat and meat products:																		
161	Bacon, (20 slices per lb, raw), broiled or fried, crisp. 2 slices	15	8	85	4	8	2.5	3.7	.7	Trace	2	34	.5	35	0	.08	.05	.8	—
	Beef,[18] cooked: Cuts braised, simmered or pot roasted:																		
162	Lean and fat (piece, 2 1/2 by 2 1/2 by 3/4 in). 3 oz	85	53	245	23	16	6.8	6.5	.4	0	10	114	2.9	184	30	.04	.18	3.6	—
163	Lean only from item 162. 2.5 oz	72	62	140	22	5	2.1	1.8	.2	0	10	108	2.7	176	10	.04	.17	3.3	—
	Ground beef, broiled:																		
164	Lean with 10% fat. 3 oz or patty 3 by 5/8 in	85	60	185	23	10	4.0	3.9	.3	0	10	196	3.0	261	20	.08	.20	5.1	—
165	Lean with 21% fat. 2.9 oz or patty 3 by 5/8 in	82	54	235	20	17	7.0	6.7	.4	0	9	159	2.6	221	30	.07	.17	4.4	—
	Roast, oven cooked, no liquid added: Relatively fat, such as rib:																		
166	Lean and fat (2 pieces, 4 1/8 by 2 1/4 by 1/4 in). 3 oz	85	40	375	17	33	14.0	13.6	.8	0	8	158	2.2	189	70	.05	.13	3.1	—
167	Lean only from item 166. 1.8 oz	51	57	125	14	7	3.0	2.5	.3	0	6	131	1.8	161	10	.04	.11	2.6	—
	Relatively lean, such as heel of round:																		
168	Lean and fat (2 pieces, 4 1/8 by 2 1/4 by 1/4 in). 3 oz	85	62	165	25	7	2.8	2.7	.2	0	11	208	3.2	279	10	.06	.19	4.5	—

[12] Based on average vitamin A content of fortified margarine. Federal specifications for fortified margarine require a minimum of 15,000 International Units (I.U.) of vitamin A per pound.
[13] Fatty acid values apply to product made with regular-type margarine.
[14] Dipped in egg, milk or water, and breadcrumbs; fried in vegetable shortening.
[15] If bones are discarded, value for calcium will be greatly reduced.
[16] Dipped in egg, breadcrumbs, and flour or batter.
[17] Prepared with tuna, celery, salad dressing (mayonnaise type), pickle, onion, and egg.
[18] Outer layer of fat on the cut was removed to within approximately 1/2 in of the lean. Deposits of fat within the cut were not removed.

(A)	(B)	Grams	(C) Percent	(D) Calories	(E) Grams	(F) Grams	(G) Grams	(H) Grams	(I) Grams	(J) Grams	(K) Milligrams	(L) Milligrams	(M) Milligrams	(N) Milligrams	(O) International units	(P) Milligrams	(Q) Milligrams	(R) Milligrams	(S) Milligrams
	Meat and meat products—Continued																		
	Beef,[18] cooked—Continued																		
	Roast, oven cooked, no liquid added—Continued																		
	Relatively lean such as heel of round—Continued																		
169	Lean only from item 168--- 2.8 oz---	78	65	125	24	3	1.2	1.0	0.1	0	10	199	3.0	268	Trace	0.06	0.18	4.3	—
	Steak:																		
	Relatively fat—sirloin, broiled:																		
170	Lean and fat (piece, 2 1/2 by 2 1/2 by 3/4 in) --- 3 oz---	85	44	330	20	27	11.3	11.1	.6	0	9	162	2.5	220	50	.05	.15	4.0	—
171	Lean only from item 170--- 2.0 oz---	56	59	115	18	4	1.8	1.6	.2	0	7	146	2.2	202	10	.05	.14	3.6	—
	Relatively lean—round, braised:																		
172	Lean and fat (piece, 4 1/8 by 2 1/4 by 1/2 in) --- 3 oz---	85	55	220	24	13	5.5	5.2	.4	0	10	213	3.0	272	20	.07	.19	4.8	—
173	Lean only from item 172--- 2.4 oz---	68	61	130	21	4	1.7	1.5	.2	0	9	182	2.5	238	10	.05	.16	4.1	—
	Beef, canned:																		
174	Corned beef--- 3 oz---	85	59	185	22	10	4.9	4.5	.2	0	17	90	3.7	—	—	.01	.20	2.9	—
175	Corned beef hash--- 1 cup---	220	67	400	19	25	11.9	10.9	.5	24	29	147	4.4	440	—	.02	.20	4.6	—
176	Beef, dried, chipped--- 2 1/2-oz jar---	71	48	145	24	4	2.1	2.0	.1	0	14	287	3.6	142	—	.05	.23	2.7	0
177	Beef and vegetable stew--- 1 cup---	245	82	220	16	11	4.9	4.5	.2	15	29	184	2.9	613	2,400	.15	.17	4.7	17
178	Beef potpie (home recipe), baked[19] (piece, 1/3 of 9-in diam. pie)--- 1 piece---	210	55	515	21	30	7.9	12.8	6.7	39	29	149	3.8	334	1,720	.30	.30	5.5	6
179	Chili con carne with beans, canned--- 1 cup---	255	72	340	19	16	7.5	6.8	.3	31	82	321	4.3	594	150	.08	.18	3.3	33
180	Chop suey with beef and pork (home recipe)--- 1 cup---	250	75	300	26	17	8.5	6.2	.7	13	60	248	4.8	425	600	.28	.38	5.0	1
181	Heart, beef, lean, braised--- 3 oz---	85	61	160	27	5	1.5	1.1	.6	1	5	154	5.0	197	20	.21	1.04	6.5	1
	Lamb, cooked:																		
	Chop, rib (cut 3 per lb with bone), broiled:																		
182	Lean and fat--- 3.1 oz---	89	43	360	18	32	14.8	12.1	1.2	0	8	139	1.0	200	—	.11	.19	4.1	—
183	Lean only from item 182--- 2 oz---	57	60	120	16	6	2.5	2.1	.2	0	6	121	1.1	174	—	.09	.15	3.4	—
	Leg, roasted:																		
184	Lean and fat (2 pieces, 4 1/8 by 2 1/4 by 1/4 in).--- 3 oz---	85	54	235	22	16	7.3	6.0	.6	0	9	177	1.4	241	—	.13	.23	4.7	—
185	Lean only from item 184--- 2.5 oz---	71	62	130	20	5	2.1	1.8	.2	0	9	169	1.4	227	—	.12	.21	4.4	—
	Shoulder, roasted:																		
186	Lean and fat (3 pieces, 2 1/2 by 2 1/2 by 1/4 in).--- 3 oz---	85	50	285	18	23	10.8	8.8	.9	0	9	146	1.0	206	—	.11	.20	4.0	—
187	Lean only from item 186--- 2.3 oz---	64	61	130	17	6	3.6	2.3	.2	0	8	140	1.0	193	—	.10	.18	3.7	—
188	Liver, beef, fried[20] (slice, 6 1/2 by 2 3/8 by 3/8 in).--- 3 oz---	85	56	195	22	9	2.5	3.5	.9	5	9	405	7.5	323	[21]45,390	.22	3.56	14.0	23
189	Pork, cured, cooked: Ham, light cure, lean and fat, roasted (2 pieces, 4 1/8 by 2 1/4 by 1/4 in).[22]--- 3 oz---	85	54	245	18	19	6.8	7.9	1.7	0	8	146	2.2	199	0	.40	.15	3.1	—
	Luncheon meat:																		
190	Boiled ham, slice (8 per 8-oz pkg.).--- 1 oz---	28	59	65	5	5	1.7	2.0	.4	0	3	47	.8	—	0	.12	.04	.7	—
191	Canned, spiced or unspiced: Slice, approx. 3 by 2 by 1/2 in.--- 1 slice---	60	55	175	9	15	5.4	6.7	1.0	1	5	65	1.3	133	0	.19	.13	1.8	—

TABLE A-7

NUTRITIVE VALUES OF THE EDIBLE PART OF FOODS · Continued

(Dashes (—) denote lack of reliable data for a constituent believed to be present in measurable amount)

Item No.	Foods, approximate measures, units, and weight (edible part unless footnotes indicate otherwise)	Weight	Water	Food energy	Protein	Fat	Saturated (total)	Unsaturated Oleic	Unsaturated Linoleic	Carbohydrate	Calcium	Phosphorus	Iron	Potassium	Vitamin A value	Thiamin	Riboflavin	Niacin	Ascorbic acid
(A)	(B)		(C)	(D)	(E)	(F)	(G)	(H)	(I)	(J)	(K)	(L)	(M)	(N)	(O)	(P)	(Q)	(R)	(S)
	Pork, fresh,[18] cooked: Chop, loin (cut 3 per lb with bone), broiled:																		
192	Lean and fat ---- 2.7 oz	78	42	305	19	25	8.9	10.4	2.2	0	9	209	2.7	216	0	0.75	0.22	4.5	—
193	Lean only from item 192 ---- 2 oz	56	53	150	17	9	3.1	3.6	.8	0	7	181	2.2	192	0	.63	.18	3.8	—
	Roast, oven cooked, no liquid added:																		
194	Lean and fat (piece, 2 1/2 by 2 1/2 by 3/4 in.), 3 oz	85	46	310	21	24	8.7	10.2	2.2	0	9	218	2.7	233	0	.78	.22	4.8	—
195	Lean only from item 194, 2.4 oz	68	55	175	20	10	3.5	4.1	.8	0	9	211	2.6	224	0	.73	.21	4.4	—
	Shoulder cut, simmered:																		
196	Lean and fat (3 pieces, 2 1/2 by 2 1/2 by 1/4 in.), 3 oz	85	46	320	20	26	9.3	10.9	2.3	0	9	118	2.6	158	0	.46	.21	4.1	—
197	Lean only from item 196 ---- 2.2 oz	63	60	135	18	6	2.2	2.6	.6	0	8	111	2.3	146	0	.42	.19	3.7	—
	Sausages (see also Luncheon meat (items 190-191)):																		
198	Bologna, slice (8 per 8-oz pkg.), 1 slice	28	56	85	3	8	3.0	3.4	.5	Trace	2	36	.5	65	—	.05	.06	.7	—
199	Braunschweiger, slice (6 per 6-oz pkg.), 1 slice	28	53	90	4	8	2.6	3.4	.8	1	3	69	1.7	—	1,850	.05	.41	2.3	—
200	Brown and serve (10-11 per 8-oz pkg.), browned, 1 link	17	40	70	3	6	2.3	2.8	.7	Trace	—	—	—	—	—	—	—	—	—
201	Deviled ham, canned ---- 1 tbsp	13	51	45	2	4	1.5	1.8	.4	0	1	12	.3	—	0	.02	.01	.2	—
202	Frankfurter (8 per 1-lb pkg.), cooked (reheated), 1 frankfurter	56	57	170	7	15	5.6	6.5	1.2	1	3	57	.8	—	—	.08	.11	1.4	—
203	Meat, potted (beef, chicken, turkey), canned, 1 tbsp	13	61	30	2	2	—	—	—	0	—	—	—	35	—	Trace	.03	.2	—
204	Pork link (16 per 1-lb pkg.), cooked, 1 link	13	35	60	2	6	2.1	2.4	.5	Trace	1	21	.3	—	0	.10	.04	.5	—
	Salami:																		
205	Dry type, slice (12 per 4-oz pkg.), 1 slice	10	30	45	2	4	1.6	1.6	.1	Trace	1	28	.4	—	—	.04	.03	.5	—
206	Cooked type, slice (8 per 8-oz pkg.), 1 slice	28	51	90	5	7	3.1	3.0	.2	Trace	3	57	.7	—	—	.07	.07	1.2	—
207	Vienna sausage (7 per 4-oz can), 1 sausage	16	63	40	2	3	1.2	1.4	.2	Trace	1	24	.3	—	—	.01	.02	.4	—
	Veal, medium fat, cooked, bone removed:																		
208	Cutlet (4 1/8 by 2 1/4 by 1/2 in.), braised or broiled, 3 oz	85	60	185	23	9	4.0	3.4	.1	0	9	196	2.7	258	—	.06	.21	4.6	—
209	Rib (2 pieces, 4 1/8 by 2 1/4 by 1/4 in.), roasted, 3 oz	85	55	230	23	14	6.1	5.1	.6	0	10	211	2.9	259	—	.11	.26	6.6	—
	Poultry and poultry products: Chicken, cooked:																		
210	Breast, fried,[23] bones removed, 1/2 breast (3.3 oz with bones), 2.8 oz	79	58	160	26	5	1.4	1.8	1.1	1	9	218	1.3	—	70	.04	.17	11.6	—
211	Drumstick, fried,[23] bones removed (2 oz with bones), 1.3 oz	38	55	90	12	4	1.1	1.3	.9	Trace	6	89	.9	—	50	.03	.15	2.7	—
212	Half broiler, broiled, bones removed (10.4 oz with bones), 6.2 oz	176	71	240	42	7	2.2	2.5	1.3	0	16	355	3.0	483	160	.09	.34	15.5	—
213	Chicken, canned, boneless ---- 3 oz	85	65	170	18	10	3.2	3.8	2.0	0	18	210	1.3	117	200	.03	.11	3.7	3
214	Chicken a la king, cooked (home recipe), 1 cup	245	68	470	27	34	12.7	14.3	3.3	12	127	358	2.5	404	1,130	.10	.42	5.4	12
215	Chicken and noodles, cooked (home recipe), 1 cup	240	71	365	22	18	5.9	7.1	3.5	26	26	247	2.2	149	430	.05	.17	4.3	Trace

[18] Outer layer of fat on the cut was removed to within approximately 1/2 in. of the lean. Deposits of fat within the cut were not removed.
[19] Crust made with vegetable shortening and enriched flour.
[20] Regular-type margarine used.
[21] Value varies widely.
[22] About one-fourth of the outer layer of fat on the cut was removed. Deposits of fat within the cut were not removed.
[23] Vegetable shortening used.

(A)	(B)		(C)	(D)	(E)	(F)	(G)	(H)	(I)	(J)	(K)	(L)	(M)	(N)	(O)	(P)	(Q)	(R)	(S)
		Grams	Percent	Calories	Grams	Grams	Grams	Grams	Grams	Grams	Milligrams	Milligrams	Milligrams	Milligrams	International units	Milligrams	Milligrams	Milligrams	Milligrams
	FISH, SHELLFISH, MEAT, POULTRY; RELATED PRODUCTS—Con.																		
	Poultry and poultry products—Continued																		
	Chicken chow mein:																		
216	Canned-- 1 cup	250	89	95	7	Trace	—	—	—	18	45	35	1.3	418	150	0.05	0.10	1.0	13
217	From home recipe-- 1 cup	250	78	255	31	10	2.4	3.4	3.1	10	58	293	2.5	473	280	.08	.23	4.3	10
218	Chicken potpie (home recipe), baked, [19] piece (1/3 or 9-in diam. pie). 1 piece	232	57	545	23	31	11.3	10.9	5.6	42	70	232	3.0	343	3,090	.34	.31	5.5	5
	Turkey, roasted, flesh without skin:																		
219	Dark meat, piece, 2 1/2 by 1 5/8 by 1/4 in. 4 pieces	85	61	175	26	7	2.1	1.5	1.5	0	—	—	2.0	338	—	.03	.20	3.6	—
220	Light meat, piece, 4 by 2 by 1/4 in. 2 pieces	85	62	150	28	3	.9	.6	.7	0	—	—	1.0	349	—	.04	.12	9.4	—
	Light and dark meat:																		
221	Chopped or diced-- 1 cup	140	61	265	44	9	2.5	1.7	1.8	0	11	351	2.5	514	—	.07	.25	10.8	[2]52
222	Pieces (1 slice white meat, 4 by 2 by 1/4 in with 2 slices dark meat, 2 1/2 by 1 5/8 by 1/4 in). 3 pieces	85	61	160	27	5	1.5	1.0	1.1	0	7	213	1.5	312	—	.04	.15	6.5	[2]52
	FRUITS AND FRUIT PRODUCTS																		
	Apples, raw, unpeeled, without cores:																		
223	2 3/4-in diam. (about 3 per lb with cores). 1 apple	138	84	80	Trace	1	—	—	—	20	10	14	.4	152	120	.04	.03	.1	6
224	3 1/4-in diam. (about 2 per lb with cores). 1 apple	212	84	125	Trace	1	—	—	—	31	15	21	.6	233	190	.06	.04	.2	8
225	Applejuice, bottled or canned[24]-- 1 cup	248	88	120	Trace	Trace	—	—	—	30	15	22	1.5	250	—	.02	.05	.2	[2]52
	Applesauce, canned:																		
226	Sweetened-- 1 cup	255	76	230	1	Trace	—	—	—	61	10	13	1.3	166	100	.05	.03	.1	[2]53
227	Unsweetened-- 1 cup	244	89	100	Trace	Trace	—	—	—	26	10	12	1.2	190	100	.05	.02	.1	[2]52
	Apricots:																		
228	Raw, without pits (about 12 per lb with pits). 3 apricots	107	85	55	1	Trace	—	—	—	14	18	25	.5	301	2,890	.03	.04	.6	11
229	Canned in heavy sirup (halves and sirup). 1 cup	258	77	220	2	Trace	—	—	—	57	28	39	.8	604	4,490	.05	.05	1.0	10
	Dried:																		
230	Uncooked (28 large or 37 medium halves per cup). 1 cup	130	25	340	7	1	—	—	—	86	87	140	7.2	1,273	14,170	.01	.21	4.3	16
231	Cooked, unsweetened, fruit and liquid. 1 cup	250	76	215	4	1	—	—	—	54	55	88	4.5	795	7,500	.01	.13	2.5	8
232	Apricot nectar, canned-- 1 cup	251	85	145	1	Trace	—	—	—	37	23	30	.5	379	2,380	.03	.03	.5	[2]36
	Avocados, raw, whole, without skins and seeds:																		
233	California, mid- and late-winter (with skin and seed, 3 1/8-in diam.; wt. 10 oz). 1 avocado	216	74	370	5	37	5.5	22.0	3.7	13	22	91	1.3	1,303	630	.24	.43	3.5	30
234	Florida, late summer and fall (with skin and seed, 3 5/8-in diam.; wt., 1 lb). 1 avocado	304	78	390	4	33	6.7	15.7	5.3	27	30	128	1.8	1,836	880	.33	.61	4.9	43
235	Banana without peel (about 2.6 per lb with peel). 1 banana	119	76	100	1	Trace	—	—	—	26	10	31	.8	440	230	.06	.07	.8	12
236	Banana flakes-- 1 tbsp	6	3	20	Trace	Trace	—	—	—	5	2	6	.2	92	50	.01	.01	.2	Trace

TABLE A-7

NUTRITIVE VALUES OF THE EDIBLE PART OF FOODS - Continued

(Dashes (—) denote lack of reliable data for a constituent believed to be present in measurable amount)

Item No. (A)	Foods, approximate measures, units, and weight (edible part unless footnotes indicate otherwise) (B)	Weight (g)	Water % (C)	Food energy (D)	Pro-tein (E)	Fat (F)	Satu-rated (total) (G)	Oleic (H)	Lino-leic (I)	Carbo-hydrate (J)	Calcium (K)	Phos-phorus (L)	Iron (M)	Potas-sium (N)	Vitamin A value (O)	Thiamin (P)	Ribo-flavin (Q)	Niacin (R)	Ascorbic acid (S)
237	Blackberries, raw --- 1 cup	144	85	85	2	1	—	—	—	19	46	27	1.3	245	290	0.04	0.06	0.6	30
238	Blueberries, raw --- 1 cup	145	83	90	1	1	—	—	—	22	22	19	1.5	117	150	.04	.09	.7	20
	Cantaloup. See Muskmelons (item 271).																		
	Cherries:																		
239	Sour (tart), red, pitted, canned, water pack --- 1 cup	244	88	105	2	Trace	—	—	—	26	37	32	.7	317	1,660	.07	.05	.5	12
240	Sweet, raw, without pits and stems --- 10 cherries	68	80	45	1	Trace	—	—	—	12	15	13	.3	129	70	.03	.04	.3	7
241	Cranberry juice cocktail, bottled, sweetened --- 1 cup	253	83	165	Trace	Trace	—	—	—	42	13	8	.8	25	Trace	.03	.03	.1	[27]81
242	Cranberry sauce, sweetened, canned, strained --- 1 cup	277	62	405	Trace	1	—	—	—	104	17	11	.6	83	60	.03	.03	.1	6
	Dates:																		
243	Whole, without pits --- 10 dates	80	23	220	2	Trace	—	—	—	58	47	50	2.4	518	40	.07	.08	1.8	0
244	Chopped --- 1 cup	178	23	490	4	1	—	—	—	130	105	112	5.3	1,153	90	.16	.18	3.9	0
245	Fruit cocktail, canned, in heavy sirup --- 1 cup	255	80	195	1	Trace	—	—	—	50	23	31	1.0	411	360	.05	.03	1.0	5
	Grapefruit: Raw, medium, 3 3/4-in diam. (about 1 lb 1 oz):																		
246	Pink or red --- 1/2 grapefruit with peel[28]	241	89	50	1	Trace	—	—	—	13	20	20	.5	166	540	.05	.02	.2	44
247	White --- 1/2 grapefruit with peel[28]	241	89	45	1	Trace	—	—	—	12	19	19	.5	159	10	.05	.02	.2	44
248	Canned, sections with sirup --- 1 cup	254	81	180	2	Trace	—	—	—	45	33	36	.8	343	30	.08	.05	.5	76
	Grapefruit juice:																		
249	Raw, pink, red, or white --- 1 cup	246	90	95	1	Trace	—	—	—	23	22	37	.5	399	(29)	.10	.05	.5	93
	Canned, white:																		
250	Unsweetened --- 1 cup	247	89	100	1	Trace	—	—	—	24	20	35	1.0	400	20	.07	.05	.5	84
251	Sweetened --- 1 cup	250	86	135	1	Trace	—	—	—	32	20	35	1.0	405	30	.08	.05	.5	73
	Frozen, concentrate, unsweetened:																		
252	Undiluted, 6-fl oz can --- 1 can	207	62	300	4	1	—	—	—	72	70	124	.8	1,250	60	.29	.12	1.4	286
253	Diluted with 3 parts water by volume --- 1 cup	247	89	100	1	Trace	—	—	—	24	25	42	.2	420	20	.10	.04	.5	96
254	Dehydrated crystals, prepared with water (1 lb yields about 1 gal) --- 1 cup	247	90	100	1	Trace	—	—	—	24	22	40	.2	412	20	.10	.05	.5	91
	Grapes, European type (adherent skin), raw:																		
255	Thompson Seedless --- 10 grapes	50	81	35	Trace	Trace	—	—	—	9	6	10	.2	87	50	.03	.02	.2	2
256	Tokay and Emperor, seeded types --- 10 grapes[30]	60	81	40	Trace	Trace	—	—	—	10	7	11	.2	99	60	.03	.02	.2	2
	Grapejuice:																		
257	Canned or bottled --- 1 cup	253	83	165	1	Trace	—	—	—	42	28	30	.8	293	—	.10	.05	.5	[25]Trace
	Frozen concentrate, sweetened:																		
258	Undiluted, 6-fl oz can --- 1 can	216	53	395	1	Trace	—	—	—	100	22	32	.9	255	40	.13	.22	1.5	[31]32
259	Diluted with 3 parts water by volume --- 1 cup	250	86	135	1	Trace	—	—	—	33	8	10	.3	85	10	.05	.08	.5	[31]10
260	Grape drink, canned --- 1 cup	250	86	135	Trace	Trace	—	—	—	35	8	10	.3	88	—	[32].03	.03	.3	[32]
261	Lemon, raw, size 165, without peel and seeds (about 4 per lb with peels and seeds) --- 1 lemon	74	90	20	1	Trace	—	—	—	6	19	12	.4	102	10	.03	.01	.1	39
	Lemon juice:																		
262	Raw --- 1 cup	244	91	60	1	Trace	—	—	—	20	17	24	.5	344	50	.07	.02	.2	112
263	Canned, or bottled, unsweetened --- 1 cup	244	92	55	1	Trace	—	—	—	19	17	24	.5	344	50	.07	.02	.2	102
264	Frozen, single strength, unsweetened, 6-fl oz can --- 1 can	183	92	40	1	Trace	—	—	—	13	13	16	.5	258	40	.05	.02	.2	81
	Lemonade concentrate, frozen:																		
265	Undiluted, 6-fl oz can --- 1 can	219	49	425	Trace	Trace	—	—	—	112	9	13	.4	153	40	.05	.06	.7	66
266	Diluted with 4 1/3 parts water by volume --- 1 cup	248	89	105	Trace	Trace	—	—	—	28	3	3	.1	40	10	.01	.02	.2	17

19 Crust made with vegetable shortening and enriched flour.
24 Also applies to pasteurized apple cider.
25 Applies to product without added ascorbic acid. For value of product with added ascorbic acid, refer to label.
26 Based on product with label claim of 45% of U.S. RDA in 6 fl oz.
27 Based on product with label claim of 100% of U.S. RDA in 6 fl oz.
28 Weight includes peel and membranes between sections. Without these parts, the weight of the edible portion is 123 g for item 246 and 118 g for item 247.
29 For white-fleshed varieties, value is about 20 International Units (I.U.) per cup; for red-fleshed varieties, 1,080 I.U.
30 Weight includes seeds. Without seeds, weight of the edible portion is 57 g.
31 Applies to product without added ascorbic acid. With added ascorbic acid, based on claim that 6 fl oz of reconstituted juice contain 45% or 50% of the U.S. RDA, value in milligrams is 108 or 120 for a 6-fl oz can (item 258), 36, or 40 for 1 cup of diluted juice (item 259).
32 For products with added thiamin and riboflavin but without added ascorbic acid, values in milligrams would be 0.60 for thiamin, 0.80 for riboflavin, and trace for ascorbic acid. For products with only ascorbic acid added, value varies with the brand. Consult the label.

FRUITS AND FRUIT PRODUCTS—Con.

(A)	(B)		grams	(C) Per-cent	(D) Cal-ories	(E) Grams	(F) Grams	(G) Grams	(H) Grams	(I) Grams	(J) Grams	(K) Milli-grams	(L) Milli-grams	(M) Milli-grams	(N) Milli-grams	(O) Inter-national units	(P) Milli-grams	(Q) Milli-grams	(R) Milli-grams	(S) Milli-grams
	Limeade concentrate, frozen:																			
267	Undiluted, 6-fl oz can	1 can	218	50	410	Trace	Trace	---	---	---	108	11	13	0.2	129	Trace	0.02	0.02	0.2	26
268	Diluted with 4 1/3 parts water by volume.	1 cup	247	89	100	Trace	Trace	---	---	---	27	3	3	Trace	32	Trace	Trace	Trace	Trace	6
	Limejuice:																			
269	Raw	1 cup	246	90	65	Trace	Trace	---	---	---	22	22	27	.5	256	20	.05	.02	.2	79
270	Canned, unsweetened	1 cup	246	90	65	Trace	Trace	---	---	---	22	22	27	.5	256	20	.05	.02	.2	52
	Muskmelons, raw, with rind, without seed cavity:																			
271	Cantaloup, orange-fleshed (with rind and seed cavity, 5-in diam., 2 1/3 lb).	1/2 melon with rind[33]	477	91	80	2	Trace	---	---	---	20	38	44	1.1	682	9,240	.11	.08	1.6	90
272	Honeydew (with rind and seed cavity, 6 1/2-in diam., 5 1/4 lb).	1/10 melon with rind[33]	226	91	50	1	Trace	---	---	---	11	21	24	.6	374	60	.06	.04	.9	34
	Oranges, all commercial varieties, raw:																			
273	Whole, 2 5/8-in diam., without peel and seeds (about 2 1/2 per lb with peel and seeds).	1 orange	131	86	65	1	Trace	---	---	---	16	54	26	.5	263	260	.13	.05	.5	66
274	Sections without membranes	1 cup	180	86	90	2	Trace	---	---	---	22	74	36	.7	360	360	.18	.07	.7	90
	Orange juice:																			
275	Raw, all varieties	1 cup	248	88	110	2	Trace	---	---	---	26	27	42	.5	496	500	.22	.07	1.0	124
276	Canned, unsweetened	1 cup	249	87	120	2	Trace	---	---	---	28	25	45	1.0	496	500	.17	.05	.7	100
	Frozen concentrate:																			
277	Undiluted, 6-fl oz can	1 can	213	55	360	5	Trace	---	---	---	87	75	126	.9	1,500	1,620	.68	.11	2.8	360
278	Diluted with 3 parts water by volume.	1 cup	249	87	120	2	Trace	---	---	---	29	25	42	.2	503	540	.23	.03	.9	120
279	Dehydrated crystals, prepared with water (1 lb yields about 1 gal).	1 cup	248	88	115	1	Trace	---	---	---	27	25	40	.5	518	500	.20	.07	1.0	109
	Orange and grapefruit juice: Frozen concentrate:																			
280	Undiluted, 6-fl oz can	1 can	210	59	330	4	1	---	---	---	78	61	99	.8	1,308	800	.48	.06	2.3	302
281	Diluted with 3 parts water by volume.	1 cup	248	88	110	1	Trace	---	---	---	26	20	32	.2	439	270	.15	.02	.7	102
282	Papayas, raw, 1/2-in cubes	1 cup	140	89	55	1	Trace	---	---	---	14	28	22	.4	328	2,450	.06	.06	.4	78
	Peaches: Raw:																			
283	Whole, 2 1/2-in diam., peeled, pitted (about 4 per lb with peels and pits).	1 peach	100	89	40	1	Trace	---	---	---	10	9	19	.5	202	[3]1,330	.02	.05	1.0	7
284	Sliced	1 cup	170	89	65	1	Trace	---	---	---	16	15	32	.9	343	[3]2,260	.03	.09	1.7	12
	Canned, yellow-fleshed, solids and liquid (halves or slices):																			
285	Sirup pack	1 cup	256	79	200	1	Trace	---	---	---	51	10	31	.8	333	1,100	.03	.05	1.5	8
286	Water pack	1 cup	244	91	75	1	Trace	---	---	---	20	10	32	.7	334	1,100	.02	.07	1.5	7
	Dried:																			
287	Uncooked	1 cup	160	25	420	5	1	---	---	---	109	77	187	9.6	1,520	6,240	.02	.30	8.5	29
288	Cooked, unsweetened, halves and juice.	1 cup	250	77	205	3	1	---	---	---	54	38	93	4.8	743	3,050	.01	.15	3.8	5

TABLE A-7

NUTRITIVE VALUES OF THE EDIBLE PART OF FOODS - Continued

(Dashes (—) denote lack of reliable data for a constituent believed to be present in measurable amount)

Item No. (A)	Foods, approximate measures, units, and weight (edible part unless footnotes indicate otherwise) (B)	Water (C)	Food energy (D)	Protein (E)	Fat (F)	Saturated (total) (G)	Unsaturated Oleic (H)	Linoleic (I)	Carbohydrate (J)	Calcium (K)	Phosphorus (L)	Iron (M)	Potassium (N)	Vitamin A value (O)	Thiamin (P)	Riboflavin (Q)	Niacin (R)	Ascorbic acid (S)
	Frozen, sliced, sweetened:																	
289	10-oz container——— 1 container———	284	250	1	Trace	—	—	—	64	11	37	1.4	352	1,850	0.03	0.11	2.0	[35]116
290	1 cup———	250	220	1	Trace	—	—	—	57	10	33	1.3	310	1,630	.03	.10	1.8	[35]103
	Pears:																	
	Raw, with skin, cored:																	
291	Bartlett, 2 1/2-in diam. (about 2 1/2 per lb with cores and stems). 1 pear———	164	100	1	1	—	—	—	25	13	18	.5	213	30	.03	.07	.2	7
292	Bosc, 2 1/2-in diam. (about 3 per lb with cores and stems). 1 pear———	141	85	1	1	—	—	—	22	11	16	.4	83	30	.03	.06	.1	6
293	D'Anjou, 3-in diam. (about 2 per lb with cores and stems). 1 pear———	200	120	1	1	—	—	—	31	16	22	.6	260	40	.04	.08	.2	8
294	Canned, solids and liquid, sirup pack, heavy (halves or slices). 1 cup———	255	195	1	1	—	—	—	50	13	18	.5	214	10	.03	.05	.3	3
	Pineapple:																	
295	Raw, diced——— 1 cup———	155	80	1	Trace	—	—	—	21	26	12	.8	226	110	.14	.05	.3	26
	Canned, heavy sirup pack, solids and liquid:																	
296	Crushed, chunks, tidbits——— 1 cup———	255	190	1	Trace	—	—	—	49	28	13	.8	245	130	.20	.05	.5	18
	Slices and liquid:																	
297	Large——— 1 slice; 2 1/4 tbsp liquid.	105	80	Trace	Trace	—	—	—	20	12	5	.3	101	50	.08	.02	.2	7
298	Medium——— 1 slice; 1 1/4 tbsp liquid.	58	45	Trace	Trace	—	—	—	11	6	3	.2	56	30	.05	.01	.1	4
299	Pineapple juice, unsweetened, canned. 1 cup———	250	140	1	Trace	—	—	—	34	38	23	.8	373	130	.13	.05	.5	[27]80
	Plums:																	
	Raw, without pits:																	
300	Japanese and hybrid (2 1/8-in diam., about 6 1/2 per lb with pits). 1 plum———	66	30	Trace	Trace	—	—	—	8	8	12	.3	112	160	.02	.02	.3	4
301	Prune-type (1 1/2-in diam., about 15 per lb with pits). 1 plum———	28	20	Trace	Trace	—	—	—	6	3	5	.1	48	80	.01	.01	.1	1
	Canned, heavy sirup pack (Italian prunes), with pits and liquid:																	
302	Cup——— 1 cup[36]	272	215	1	Trace	—	—	—	56	23	26	2.3	367	3,130	.05	.05	1.0	5
303	Portion——— 3 plums; 2 3/4 tbsp liquid.[36]	140	110	1	Trace	—	—	—	29	12	13	1.2	189	1,610	.03	.03	.5	3
	Prunes, dried, "softenized," with pits:																	
304	Uncooked——— 4 extra large or 5 large prunes.[36]	49	110	1	Trace	—	—	—	29	22	34	1.7	298	690	.04	.07	.7	1
305	Cooked, unsweetened, all sizes, fruit and liquid. 1 cup[35]	250	255	2	1	—	—	—	67	51	79	3.8	695	1,590	.07	.15	1.5	2
306	Prune juice, canned or bottled——— 1 cup———	256	195	1	Trace	—	—	—	49	36	51	1.8	602	—	.03	.03	1.0	5
	Raisins, seedless:																	
307	Cup, not pressed down——— 1 cup———	145	420	4	Trace	—	—	—	112	90	146	5.1	1,106	30	.16	.12	.7	1
308	Packet, 1/2 oz (1 1/2 tbsp)——— 1 packet———	14	40	Trace	Trace	—	—	—	11	9	14	.5	107	Trace	.02	.01	Trace	Trace
	Raspberries, red:																	
309	Raw, capped, whole——— 1 cup———	123	70	1	1	—	—	—	17	27	27	1.1	207	160	.04	.11	1.1	31
310	Frozen, sweetened, 10-oz container 1 container———	284	280	2	1	—	—	—	70	37	48	1.7	284	200	.06	.17	1.7	60
	Rhubarb, cooked, added sugar:																	
311	From raw——— 1 cup———	270	380	1	Trace	—	—	—	97	211	41	1.6	548	220	.05	.14	.8	16
312	From frozen, sweetened——— 1 cup———	270	385	1	Trace	—	—	—	98	211	32	1.9	475	190	.05	.11	.5	16

[27] Based on product with label claim of 100% of U.S. RDA in 6 fl oz.

[33] Weight includes rind. Without rind, the weight of the edible portion is 272 g for item 271 and 149 g for item 272.

[34] Represents yellow-fleshed varieties. For white-fleshed varieties, value is 50 International Units (I.U.) for 1 peach, 90 I.U. for 1 cup of slices.

[35] Value represents products without added ascorbic acid. For products with added ascorbic acid, value in milligrams is 116 for 1 peach, 103 for 1 cup.

[36] Weight includes pits. After removal of the pits, the weight of the edible portion is 258 g for item 302, 133 g for item 304, 43 g for item 303, and 213 g for item 305.

FRUITS AND FRUIT PRODUCTS—Con.

(A)	(B)	(Grams)	(C) Per-cent	(D) Cal-ories	(E) Grams	(F) Grams	(G) Grams	(H) Grams	(I) Grams	(J) Grams	(K) Milli-grams	(L) Milli-grams	(M) Milli-grams	(N) Milli-grams	(O) International units	(P) Milli-grams	(Q) Milli-grams	(R) Milli-grams	(S) Milli-grams
	Strawberries:																		
313	Raw, whole berries, capped------ 1 cup	149	90	55	1	1	—	—	—	13	31	31	1.5	244	90	0.04	0.10	0.9	88
	Frozen, sweetened:																		
314	Sliced, 10-oz container---- 1 container-----	284	71	310	1	1	—	—	—	79	40	48	2.0	318	90	.06	.17	1.4	151
315	Whole, 1-lb container (about 1 3/4 cups). 1 container----	454	76	415	1	1	—	—	—	107	59	73	2.7	472	140	.09	.27	2.3	249
316	Tangerine, raw, 2 3/8-in diam., size 176, without peel (about 4 per lb with peels and seeds). 1 tangerine-------	86	87	40	1	Trace	—	—	—	10	34	15	.3	108	360	.05	.02	.1	27
317	Tangerine juice, canned, sweetened. 1 cup-------	249	87	125	1	Trace	—	—	—	30	44	35	.5	440	1,040	.15	.05	.2	54
318	Watermelon, raw, 4 by 8 in wedge with rind and seeds (1/16 of 32 2/3-lb melon, 10 by 16 in). 1 wedge with rind and seeds[37]	926	93	110	2	1	—	—	—	27	30	43	2.1	426	2,510	.13	.13	.9	30

GRAIN PRODUCTS

(A)	(B)	(Grams)	(C) Per-cent	(D) Cal-ories	(E) Grams	(F) Grams	(G) Grams	(H) Grams	(I) Grams	(J) Grams	(K) Milli-grams	(L) Milli-grams	(M) Milli-grams	(N) Milli-grams	(O) International units	(P) Milli-grams	(Q) Milli-grams	(R) Milli-grams	(S) Milli-grams
	Bagel, 3-in diam.:																		
319	Egg------------------------ 1 bagel-------	55	32	165	6	2	0.5	0.9	0.8	28	9	43	1.2	41	30	.14	.10	1.2	0
320	Water---------------------- 1 bagel-------	55	29	165	6	1	.2	.4	.6	30	8	41	1.2	42	0	.15	.11	1.4	0
321	Barley, pearled, light, uncooked- 1 cup-------	200	11	700	16	2	.3	.2	.8	158	32	378	4.0	320	0	.24	.10	6.2	0
	Biscuits, baking powder, 2-in diam. (enriched flour, vegetable shortening):																		
322	From home recipe---------- 1 biscuit-----	28	27	105	2	5	1.2	2.0	1.2	13	34	49	.4	33	Trace	.08	.08	.7	Trace
323	From mix------------------ 1 biscuit-----	28	29	90	2	3	.6	1.1	.7	15	19	65	.6	32	Trace	.09	.08	.8	Trace
324	Breadcrumbs (enriched):[38] Dry, grated------------ 1 cup-------	100	7	390	13	5	1.0	1.6	1.4	73	122	141	3.6	152	Trace	.35	.35	4.8	Trace
	Soft. See White bread (items 349-350).																		
	Breads:																		
325	Boston brown bread, canned, slice, 3 1/4 by 1/2 in.[38] 1 slice-------	45	45	95	2	1	.1	.2	.2	21	41	72	.9	131	3[39]0	.06	.04	.7	0
	Cracked-wheat bread (3/4 enriched wheat flour, 1/4 cracked wheat):[38]																		
326	Loaf, 1 lb----------------- 1 loaf--------	454	35	1,195	39	10	2.2	3.0	3.9	236	399	581	9.5	608	Trace	1.52	1.13	14.4	Trace
327	Slice (18 per loaf)-------- 1 slice-------	25	35	65	2	1	.1	.2	.2	13	22	32	.5	34	Trace	.08	.06	.8	Trace
	French or Vienna bread, enriched:[38]																		
328	Loaf, 1 lb----------------- 1 loaf--------	454	31	1,315	41	14	3.2	4.7	4.6	251	195	386	10.0	408	Trace	1.80	1.10	15.0	Trace
	Slice:																		
329	French (5 by 2 1/2 by 1 in) 1 slice-------	35	31	100	3	1	.2	.4	.4	19	15	30	.8	32	Trace	.14	.08	1.2	Trace
330	Vienna (4 3/4 by 4 by 1/2 in). 1 slice-------	25	31	75	2	1	.2	.3	.3	14	11	21	.6	23	Trace	.10	.06	.8	Trace
	Italian bread, enriched:																		
331	Loaf, 1 lb----------------- 1 loaf--------	454	32	1,250	41	4	.6	.3	1.5	256	77	349	10.0	336	0	1.80	1.10	15.0	0
332	Slice, 4 1/2 by 3 1/4 by 3/4 in. 1 slice-------	30	32	85	3	Trace	Trace	Trace	.1	17	5	23	.7	22	0	.12	.07	1.0	0
	Raisin bread, enriched:[38]																		
333	Loaf, 1 lb----------------- 1 loaf--------	454	35	1,190	30	13	3.0	4.7	3.9	243	322	395	10.0	1,057	Trace	1.70	1.07	10.7	Trace
334	Slice (18 per loaf)-------- 1 slice-------	25	35	65	2	1	.2	.3	.2	13	18	22	.6	58	Trace	.09	.06	.6	Trace

NUTRITIVE VALUES OF THE EDIBLE PART OF FOODS - Continued

(Dashes (—) denote lack of reliable data for a constituent believed to be present in measurable amount)

Item No. (A)	Foods, approximate measures, units, and weight (edible part unless footnotes indicate otherwise) (B)	(g)	Water (C)	Food energy (D)	Protein (E)	Fat (F)	Fatty Acids Saturated (total) (G)	Unsaturated Oleic (H)	Linoleic (I)	Carbohydrate (J)	Calcium (K)	Phosphorus (L)	Iron (M)	Potassium (N)	Vitamin A value (O)	Thiamin (P)	Riboflavin (Q)	Niacin (R)	Ascorbic acid (S)
	Rye Bread:																		
	American, light (2/3 enriched wheat flour, 1/3 rye flour):																		
335	Loaf, 1 lb	454	36	1,100	41	5	0.7	0.5	2.2	236	340	667	9.1	658	0	1.35	0.98	12.9	0
336	Slice (4 3/4 by 3 3/4 by 7/16 in)	25	36	60	2	Trace	Trace	Trace	.1	13	19	37	.5	36	0	.07	.05	.7	0
	Pumpernickel (2/3 rye flour, 1/3 enriched wheat flour):																		
337	Loaf, 1 lb	454	34	1,115	41	5	.7	.5	2.4	241	381	1,039	11.8	2,059	0	1.30	.93	8.5	0
338	Slice (5 by 4 by 3/8 in)	32	34	80	3	Trace	.1	Trace	.2	17	27	73	.8	145	0	.09	.07	.6	0
	White bread, enriched:[38]																		
	Soft-crumb type:																		
339	Loaf, 1 lb	454	36	1,225	39	15	3.4	5.3	4.6	229	381	440	11.3	476	Trace	1.80	1.10	15.0	Trace
340	Slice (18 per loaf)	25	36	70	2	1	.2	.3	.3	13	21	24	.6	26	Trace	.10	.06	.8	Trace
341	Slice, toasted	22	25	70	2	1	.2	.3	.3	13	21	24	.6	26	Trace	.08	.06	.8	Trace
342	Slice (22 per loaf)	20	36	55	2	1	.2	.2	.2	10	17	19	.5	21	Trace	.08	.05	.7	Trace
343	Slice, toasted	17	25	55	2	1	.2	.2	.2	10	17	19	.5	21	Trace	.06	.05	.7	Trace
344	Loaf, 1 1/2 lb	680	36	1,835	59	22	5.2	7.9	6.9	343	571	660	17.0	714	Trace	2.70	1.65	22.5	Trace
345	Slice (24 per loaf)	24	36	75	2	1	.2	.3	.3	14	24	27	.7	29	Trace	.11	.07	.9	Trace
346	Slice, toasted	24	36	75	2	1	.2	.3	.3	14	24	27	.7	29	Trace	.09	.07	.9	Trace
347	Slice (28 per loaf)	24	36	65	2	1	.2	.3	.3	12	20	23	.6	25	Trace	.10	.06	.8	Trace
348	Slice, toasted	21	25	65	2	1	.2	.3	.3	12	20	23	.6	25	Trace	.08	.06	.8	Trace
349	Cubes	30	36	80	3	1	.3	.3	.3	15	25	29	.8	32	Trace	.12	.07	1.0	Trace
350	Crumbs	45	36	120	4	1	.3	.5	.5	23	38	44	1.1	47	Trace	.18	.11	1.5	Trace
	Firm-crumb type:																		
351	Loaf, 1 lb	454	35	1,245	41	17	3.9	5.9	5.2	228	435	463	11.3	549	Trace	1.80	1.10	15.0	Trace
352	Slice (20 per loaf)	23	35	65	2	1	.2	.3	.3	12	22	23	.6	28	Trace	.09	.06	.8	Trace
353	Slice, toasted	20	24	65	2	1	.2	.3	.3	12	22	23	.6	28	Trace	.07	.06	.8	Trace
354	Loaf, 2 lb	907	35	2,495	82	34	7.7	11.8	10.4	455	871	925	22.7	1,097	Trace	3.60	2.20	30.0	Trace
355	Slice (34 per loaf)	27	35	75	2	1	.2	.3	.3	14	26	28	.7	33	Trace	.11	.06	.9	Trace
356	Slice, toasted	23	24	75	2	1	.2	.3	.3	14	26	28	.7	33	Trace	.09	.06	.9	Trace
	Whole-wheat bread:																		
	Soft-crumb type:[38]																		
357	Loaf, 1 lb	454	36	1,095	41	12	2.2	2.9	4.2	224	381	1,152	13.6	1,161	Trace	1.37	.45	12.7	Trace
358	Slice (16 per loaf)	28	36	65	3	1	.1	.2	.2	14	24	71	.8	72	Trace	.09	.03	.8	Trace
359	Slice, toasted	24	24	65	3	1	.1	.2	.2	14	24	71	.8	72	Trace	.07	.03	.8	Trace
	Firm-crumb type:[38]																		
360	Loaf, 1 lb	454	36	1,100	48	14	2.5	3.3	4.9	216	449	1,034	13.6	1,238	Trace	1.17	.54	12.7	Trace
361	Slice (18 per loaf)	25	36	60	3	1	.1	.2	.3	12	25	57	.8	68	Trace	.06	.03	.7	Trace
362	Slice, toasted	21	24	60	3	1	.1	.2	.3	12	25	57	.8	68	Trace	.05	.03	.7	Trace
	Breakfast cereals:																		
	Hot type, cooked:																		
	Corn (hominy) grits, degermed:																		
363	Enriched	245	87	125	3	Trace	Trace	Trace	.1	27	2	25	.7	27	Trace[40]	.10	.07	1.0	0
364	Unenriched	245	87	125	3	Trace	Trace	Trace	.1	27	2	25	.2	27	Trace[40]	.05	.02	.5	0
365	Farina, quick-cooking, enriched	245	89	105	3	Trace	Trace	Trace	.1	22	147[41]	113[41]	(42)	25	0	.12	.07	1.0	0
366	Oatmeal or rolled oats	240	87	130	5	2	.4	.8	.9	23	22	137	1.4	146	0	.19	.05	.2	0
367	Wheat, rolled	240	80	180	5	1	—	—	—	41	19	182	1.7	202	0	.17	.07	2.2	0
368	Wheat, whole-meal	245	88	110	4	1	—	—	—	23	17	118	1.2	118	0	.15	.05	1.5	0
	Ready-to-eat:																		
369	Bran flakes (40% bran), added sugar, salt, iron, vitamins	35	3	105	4	1	—	—	—	28	19	125	15.6	137	1,650	.41	.49	4.1	12
370	Bran flakes with raisins, added sugar, salt, iron, vitamins	50	7	145	4	1	—	—	—	40	28	146	16.9	154	2,350	.58	.71	5.8	18

[37] Weight includes rind and seeds. Without rind and seeds, weight of the edible portion is 426 g.
[38] Made with vegetable shortening.
[39] Applies to product made with white cornmeal. With yellow cornmeal, value is 30 International Units (I.U.).
[40] Applies to white varieties. For yellow varieties, value is 150 International Units (I.U.).
[41] Applies to products that do not contain di-sodium phosphate. If di-sodium phosphate is an ingredient, value is 162 mg.
[42] Value may range from less than 1 mg to about 8 mg depending on the brand. Consult the label.

GRAIN PRODUCTS—Con.

(A)	(B)	Grams	(C) Per-cent	(D) Cal-ories	(E) Grams	(F) Grams	(G) Grams	(H) Grams	(I) Grams	(J) Grams	(K) Milli-grams	(L) Milli-grams	(M) Milli-grams	(N) Milli-grams	(O) Inter-national units	(P) Milli-grams	(Q) Milli-grams	(R) Milli-grams	(S) Milli-grams
	Breakfast cereals—Continued																		
	Ready-to-eat—Continued																		
	Corn flakes:																		
371	Plain, added sugar, salt, iron, vitamins. 1 cup	25	4	95	2	Trace	—	—	—	21	[43]	9	0.6	30	1,180	0.29	0.35	2.9	9
372	Sugar-coated, added salt, iron, vitamins. 1 cup	40	2	155	2	Trace	—	—	—	37	1	10	1.0	27	1,880	.46	.56	4.6	14
373	Corn, puffed, plain, added sugar, salt, iron, vita-mins. 1 cup	20	4	80	2	1	—	—	—	16	4	18	2.3	—	940	.23	.28	2.3	7
374	Corn, shredded, added sugar, salt, iron, thiamin, niacin. 1 cup	25	3	95	2	Trace	—	—	—	22	1	10	.6	—	0	.11	.05	.5	0
375	Oats, puffed, added sugar, salt, minerals, vitamins. 1 cup	25	3	100	3	1	—	—	—	19	44	102	2.9	—	1,180	.29	.35	2.9	9
	Rice, puffed:																		
376	Plain, added iron, thiamin, niacin. 1 cup	15	4	60	1	Trace	—	—	—	13	3	14	.3	15	0	.07	.01	.7	0
377	Presweetened, added salt, iron, vitamins. 1 cup	28	3	115	1	0	—	—	—	26	3	14	[43]1.1	43	1,250	.38	.43	5.0	[45]15
378	Wheat flakes, added sugar, salt, iron, vitamins. 1 cup	30	4	105	3	Trace	—	—	—	24	12	83	([43])	81	1,410	.35	.42	3.5	11
	Wheat, puffed:																		
379	Plain, added iron, thiamin, niacin. 1 cup	15	3	55	2	Trace	—	—	—	12	4	48	.6	51	0	.08	.03	1.2	0
380	Presweetened, added salt, iron, vitamins. 1 cup	38	3	140	3	Trace	—	—	—	33	7	52	[43]1.6	63	1,680	.50	.57	6.7	[45]20
381	Wheat, shredded, plain. 1 oblong biscuit or 1/2 cup spoon-size biscuits.	25	7	90	2	1	—	—	—	20	11	97	.9	87	0	.06	.03	1.1	0
382	Wheat germ, without salt and sugar, toasted. 1 tbsp	6	4	25	2	1	—	—	—	3	3	70	.5	57	10	.11	.05	.3	1
383	Buckwheat flour, light, sifted. 1 cup	98	12	340	6	1	0.2	0.4	0.4	78	11	86	1.0	314	0	.08	.04	.4	0
384	Bulgur, canned, seasoned. 1 cup	135	56	245	8	4	—	—	—	44	27	263	1.9	151	0	.08	.05	4.1	0
	Cake icings. See Sugars and Sweets (items 532-536).																		
	Cakes made from cake mixes with enriched flour:[46]																		
	Angelfood:																		
385	Whole cake (9 3/4-in diam. tube cake). 1 cake	635	34	1,645	36	1	—	—	—	377	603	756	2.5	381	0	.37	.95	3.6	0
386	Piece, 1/12 of cake. 1 piece	53	34	135	3	Trace	—	—	—	32	50	63	.2	32	0	.03	.08	.3	0
	Coffeecake:																		
387	Whole cake (7 3/4 by 5 5/8 by 1 1/4 in). 1 cake	430	30	1,385	27	41	11.7	16.3	8.8	225	262	748	6.9	469	690	.82	.91	7.7	1
388	Piece, 1/6 of cake. 1 piece	72	30	230	5	7	2.0	2.7	1.5	38	44	125	1.2	78	120	.14	.15	1.3	Trace
	Cupcakes, made with egg, milk, 2 1/2-in diam.:																		
389	Without icing. 1 cupcake	25	26	90	1	3	.8	1.2	.7	14	40	59	.3	21	40	.05	.05	.4	Trace
390	With chocolate icing. 1 cupcake	36	22	130	2	5	2.0	1.6	.6	21	47	71	.4	42	60	.05	.06	.4	Trace
	Devil's food with chocolate icing:																		
391	Whole, 2 layer cake (8- or 9-in diam.). 1 cake	1,107	24	3,755	49	136	50.0	44.9	17.0	645	653	1,162	16.6	1,439	1,660	1.06	1.65	10.1	1
392	Piece, 1/16 of cake. 1 piece	69	24	235	3	8	3.1	2.8	1.1	40	41	72	1.0	90	100	.07	.10	.6	Trace
393	Cupcake, 2 1/2-in diam. 1 cupcake	35	24	120	2	4	1.6	1.4	.5	20	21	37	.5	46	50	.03	.05	.3	Trace

TABLE A-7
NUTRITIVE VALUES OF THE EDIBLE PART OF FOODS - Continued
(Dashes (—) denote lack of reliable data for a constituent believed to be present in measurable amount)

NUTRIENTS IN INDICATED QUANTITY

Item No.	Foods, approximate measures, units, and weight (edible part unless footnotes indicate otherwise)	(grams)	Water	Food energy	Pro-tein	Fat	Fatty Acids Satu-rated (total)	Unsaturated Oleic	Lino-leic	Carbo-hydrate	Calcium	Phos-phorus	Iron	Potas-sium	Vitamin A value	Thiamin	Ribo-flavin	Niacin	Ascorbic acid
(A)	(B)		(C)	(D)	(E)	(F)	(G)	(H)	(I)	(J)	(K)	(L)	(M)	(N)	(O)	(P)	(Q)	(R)	(S)
	Gingerbread:																		
394	Whole cake (8-in square)------ 1 cake	570	37	1,575	18	39	9.7	16.6	10.0	291	513	570	8.6	1,562	Trace	0.84	1.00	7.4	Trace
395	Piece, 1/9 of cake---------- 1 piece	63	37	175	2	4	1.1	1.8	1.1	32	57	63	.9	173	Trace	.09	.11	.8	Trace
	White, 2 layer with chocolate icing:																		
396	Whole cake (8- or 9-in diam.)-- 1 cake	1,140	21	4,000	44	122	48.2	46.4	20.0	716	1,129	2,041	11.4	1,322	680	1.50	1.77	12.5	2
397	Piece, 1/16 of cake--------- 1 piece	71	21	250	3	8	3.0	2.9	1.2	45	70	127	.7	82	40	.09	.11	.8	Trace
	Yellow, 2 layer with chocolate icing:																		
398	Whole cake (8- or 9-in diam.)-- 1 cake	1,108	26	3,735	45	125	47.8	47.8	20.3	638	1,008	2,017	12.2	1,208	1,550	1.24	1.67	10.6	2
399	Piece, 1/16 of cake--------- 1 piece	69	26	235	3	8	3.0	3.0	1.3	40	63	126	.8	75	100	.08	.10	.7	Trace
	Cakes made from home recipes using enriched flour:[47]																		
	Boston cream pie with custard filling:																		
400	Whole cake (8-in diam.)------- 1 cake	825	35	2,490	41	78	23.0	30.1	15.2	412	553	833	8.2	[48]734	1,730	1.04	1.27	9.6	2
401	Piece, 1/12 of cake--------- 1 piece	69	35	210	3	6	1.9	2.5	1.3	34	46	70	.7	[48]61	140	.09	.11	.8	Trace
	Fruitcake, dark:																		
402	Loaf, 1-lb (7 1/2 by 2 by 1 1/2 in)-- 1 loaf	454	18	1,720	22	69	14.4	33.5	14.8	271	327	513	11.8	2,250	540	.72	.73	4.9	2
403	Slice, 1/30 of loaf--------- 1 slice	15	18	55	1	2	.5	1.1	.5	9	11	17	.4	74	20	.02	.02	.2	Trace
	Plain, sheet cake:																		
	Without icing:																		
404	Whole cake (9-in square)------ 1 cake	777	25	2,830	35	108	29.5	44.4	23.9	434	497	793	8.5	[48]614	1,320	1.21	1.40	10.2	2
405	Piece, 1/9 of cake---------- 1 piece	86	25	315	4	12	3.3	4.9	2.6	48	55	88	.9	[48]68	150	.13	.15	1.1	Trace
	With uncooked white icing:																		
406	Whole cake (9-in square)------ 1 cake	1,096	21	4,020	37	129	42.2	49.5	24.4	694	548	822	8.2	[48]669	2,190	1.22	1.47	10.2	2
407	Piece, 1/9 of cake---------- 1 piece	121	21	445	4	14	4.7	5.5	2.7	77	61	91	.8	[48]74	240	.14	.16	1.1	Trace
	Pound:[49]																		
408	Loaf, 8 1/2 by 3 1/2 by 3 1/4 in------ 1 loaf	565	16	2,725	31	170	42.9	73.1	39.6	273	107	418	7.9	345	1,410	.90	.99	7.3	0
409	Slice, 1/17 of loaf--------- 1 slice	33	16	160	2	10	2.5	4.3	2.3	16	6	24	.5	20	80	.05	.06	.4	0
	Spongecake:																		
410	Whole cake (9 3/4-in diam. tube cake)-- 1 cake	790	32	2,345	60	45	13.1	15.8	5.7	427	237	885	13.4	687	3,560	1.10	1.64	7.4	Trace
411	Piece, 1/12 of cake--------- 1 piece	66	32	195	5	4	1.1	1.3	.5	36	20	74	1.1	57	300	.09	.14	.6	Trace
	Cookies made with enriched flour:[50][51]																		
	Brownies with nuts:																		
	Home-prepared, 1 3/4 by 1 3/4 by 7/8 in:																		
412	From home recipe----------- 1 brownie	20	10	95	1	6	1.5	3.0	1.2	10	8	30	.4	38	40	.04	.03	.2	Trace
413	From commercial recipe------- 1 brownie	20	11	85	1	4	.9	1.4	1.3	13	9	27	.4	34	20	.03	.02	.2	Trace
414	Frozen, with chocolate icing,[52] 1 1/2 by 1 3/4 by 7/8 in.-- 1 brownie	25	13	105	1	5	2.0	2.2	.7	15	10	31	.4	44	50	.03	.03	.2	Trace
	Chocolate chip:																		
415	Commercial, 2 1/4-in diam., 3/8 in thick.-- 4 cookies	42	3	200	2	9	2.8	2.9	2.2	29	16	48	1.0	56	50	.10	.17	.9	Trace
416	From home recipe, 2 1/3-in diam.-- 4 cookies	40	3	205	2	12	3.5	4.5	2.9	24	14	40	.8	47	40	.06	.06	.5	Trace
417	Fig bars, square (1 5/8 by 1 5/8 by 3/8 in) or rectangular (1 1/2 by 1 3/4 by 1/2 in).-- 4 cookies	56	14	200	2	3	.8	1.2	.7	42	44	34	1.0	111	60	.04	.14	.9	Trace
418	Gingersnaps, 2-in diam., 1/4 in thick.-- 4 cookies	28	3	90	2	2	.7	1.0	.6	22	20	13	.7	129	20	.08	.06	.7	0
419	Macaroons, 2 3/4-in diam., 1/4 in thick.-- 2 cookies	38	4	180	2	9	—	—	—	25	10	32	.3	176	0	.02	.06	.2	0
420	Oatmeal with raisins, 2 5/8-in diam., 1/4 in thick.-- 4 cookies	52	3	235	3	8	2.0	3.3	2.0	38	11	53	1.4	192	30	.15	.10	1.0	Trace

[43] Value varies with the brand. Consult the label.
[44] Value varies with the brand. Consult the label.
[45] Applies to product with added ascorbic acid. Without added ascorbic acid, value is trace.
[47] Excepting angelfood cake, cakes were made from mixes containing vegetable shortening; icings, with butter.
[48] Applies to product made with a sodium aluminum-sulfate type baking powder. With a low-sodium type baking powder containing potassium, value would be about twice the amount shown.
[49] Excepting spongecake, vegetable shortening used for cake portion; butter, for icing. If butter or margarine used for cake portion, vitamin A values would be higher.
[49] Equal weights of flour, sugar, eggs, and vegetable shortening.
[50] Products are commercial unless otherwise specified.
[51] Made with enriched flour and vegetable shortening except for macaroons which do not contain flour or shortening.
[52] Icing made with butter.

(A)	(B)	Grams	(C) Per-cent	(D) Cal-ories	(E) Grams	(F) Grams	(G) Grams	(H) Grams	(I) Grams	(J) Grams	(K) Milli-grams	(L) Milli-grams	(M) Milli-grams	(N) Milli-grams	(O) Inter-national units	(P) Milli-grams	(Q) Milli-grams	(R) Milli-grams	(S) Milli-grams
	Cookies made with enriched flour:[50][51]—Continued																		
421	Plain, prepared from commercial chilled dough, 2 1/2-in diam., 1/4 in thick. 4 cookies	48	5	240	2	12	3.0	5.2	2.9	31	17	35	0.6	23	30	0.10	0.08	0.9	0
422	Sandwich type (chocolate or vanilla), 1 3/4-in diam., 3/8 in thick. 4 cookies	40	2	200	2	9	2.2	3.9	2.2	28	10	96	.7	15	0	.06	.10	.7	0
423	Vanilla wafers, 1 3/4-in diam., 1/4 in thick. 10 cookies	40	3	185	2	6	—	—	—	30	16	25	.6	29	50	.10	.09	.8	0
	Cornmeal:																		
424	Whole-ground, unbolted, dry form. 1 cup	122	12	435	11	5	.5	1.0	2.5	90	24	312	2.9	346	[53]620	.46	.13	2.4	0
425	Bolted (nearly whole-grain), dry form. 1 cup	122	12	440	11	4	.5	.9	2.1	91	21	272	2.2	303	[53]590	.37	.10	2.3	0
	Degermed, enriched:																		
426	Dry form 1 cup	138	12	500	11	2	.2	.4	.9	108	8	137	4.0	166	[53]610	.61	.36	4.8	0
427	Cooked 1 cup	240	88	120	3	Trace	Trace	.1	.2	26	2	34	1.0	38	[53]140	.14	.10	1.2	0
	Degermed, unenriched:																		
428	Dry form 1 cup	138	12	500	11	2	.2	.4	.9	108	8	137	1.5	166	[53]610	.19	.07	1.4	0
429	Cooked 1 cup	240	88	120	3	Trace	Trace	.1	.2	26	2	34	.5	38	[53]140	.05	.02	.5	0
	Crackers:[38]																		
430	Graham, plain, 2 1/2-in square 2 crackers	14	6	55	1	1	.3	.5	.3	10	6	21	.5	55	0	.02	.08	.5	0
431	Rye wafers, whole-grain, 1 7/8 by 3 1/2 in. 2 wafers	13	6	45	2	Trace	—	—	—	10	7	50	.5	78	0	.04	.03	.2	0
432	Saltines, made with enriched flour. 4 crackers or 1 packet	11	4	50	1	1	.3	.5	.4	8	2	10	.5	13	0	.05	.05	.4	0
	Danish pastry (enriched flour), plain without fruit or nuts:[54]																		
433	Packaged ring, 12 oz 1 ring	340	22	1,435	25	80	24.3	31.7	16.5	155	170	371	6.1	381	1,050	.97	1.01	8.6	Trace
434	Round piece, about 4 1/4-in diam. by 1 in. 1 pastry	65	22	275	5	15	4.7	6.1	3.2	30	33	71	1.2	73	200	.18	.19	1.7	Trace
435	Ounce 1 oz	28	22	120	2	7	2.0	2.7	1.4	13	14	31	.5	32	90	.08	.08	.7	Trace
	Doughnuts, made with enriched flour:[38]																		
436	Cake type, plain, 2 1/2-in diam., 1 in high. 1 doughnut	25	24	100	1	5	1.2	2.0	1.1	13	10	48	.4	23	20	.05	.05	.4	Trace
437	Yeast-leavened, glazed, 3 3/4-in diam., 1 1/4 in high. 1 doughnut	50	26	205	3	11	3.3	5.8	3.3	22	16	33	.6	34	25	.10	.10	.8	0
	Macaroni, enriched, cooked (cut lengths, elbows, shells):																		
438	Firm stage (hot): 1 cup	130	64	190	7	1	—	—	—	39	14	85	1.4	103	0	.23	.13	1.8	0
	Tender stage:																		
439	Cold macaroni 1 cup	105	73	115	4	Trace	—	—	—	24	8	53	.9	64	0	.15	.08	1.2	0
440	Hot macaroni 1 cup	140	73	155	5	1	—	—	—	32	11	70	1.3	85	0	.20	.11	1.5	0
	Macaroni (enriched) and cheese:																		
441	Canned[55] 1 cup	240	80	230	9	10	4.2	3.1	1.4	26	199	182	1.0	139	260	.12	.24	1.0	Trace
442	From home recipe (served hot)[56] 1 cup	200	58	430	17	22	8.9	8.8	2.9	40	362	322	1.8	240	860	.20	.40	1.8	Trace
	Muffins made with enriched flour:[38]																		
	From home recipe:																		
443	Blueberry, 2 3/8-in diam., 1 1/2 in high. 1 muffin	40	39	110	3	4	1.1	1.4	.7	17	34	53	.6	46	90	.09	.10	.7	Trace
444	Bran 1 muffin	40	35	105	3	4	1.2	1.4	.8	17	57	162	1.5	172	90	.07	.10	1.7	Trace
445	Corn (enriched degermed cornmeal and flour), 2 3/8-in diam., 1 1/2 in high. 1 muffin	40	33	125	3	4	1.2	1.6	.9	19	42	68	.7	54	[57]120	.10	.10	.7	Trace

TABLE A-7
NUTRITIVE VALUES OF THE EDIBLE PART OF FOODS - Continued

(Dashes (—) denote lack of reliable data for a constituent believed to be present in measurable amount)

NUTRIENTS IN INDICATED QUANTITY

Item No.	Foods, approximate measures, units, and weight (edible part unless footnotes indicate otherwise)	Water	Food energy	Protein	Fat	Fatty Acids Saturated (total)	Unsaturated Oleic	Linoleic	Carbohydrate	Calcium	Phosphorus	Iron	Potassium	Vitamin A value	Thiamin	Riboflavin	Niacin	Ascorbic acid
(A)	(B)	(C)	(D)	(E)	(F)	(G)	(H)	(I)	(J)	(K)	(L)	(M)	(N)	(O)	(P)	(Q)	(R)	(S)
446	Plain, 3-in diam., 1 1/2 in high — 1 muffin (40)	38	120	3	4	1.0	1.7	1.0	17	42	60	0.6	50	40	0.09	0.12	0.9	Trace
447	From mix, egg, milk: Corn, 2 3/8-in diam., 1 1/2 in high.[58] — 1 muffin (40)	30	130	3	4	1.2	1.7	.9	20	96	152	.6	44	[57]100	.08	.09	.7	Trace
448	Noodles (egg noodles), enriched, cooked — 1 cup (160)	71	200	7	2	—	—	—	37	16	94	1.4	70	110	.22	.13	1.9	0
449	Noodles, chow mein, canned — 1 cup (45)	1	220	6	11	—	—	—	26	—	—	—	—	—	—	—	—	—
450	Pancakes, (4-in diam.):[38] Buckwheat, made from mix (with buckwheat and enriched flours), egg and milk added. — 1 cake (27)	58	55	2	2	.8	.9	.4	6	59	91	.4	66	60	.04	.05	.2	Trace
451	Plain: Made from home recipe using enriched flour. — 1 cake (27)	50	60	2	2	.5	.8	.5	9	27	38	.4	33	30	.06	.07	.5	Trace
452	Made from mix with enriched flour, egg and milk added. — 1 cake (27)	51	60	2	2	.7	.7	.3	9	58	70	.3	42	70	.04	.06	.2	Trace
	Pies, piecrust made with enriched flour, vegetable shortening (9-in diam.): Apple:																	
453	Whole — 1 pie (945)	48	2,420	21	105	27.0	44.5	25.2	360	76	208	6.6	756	280	1.06	.79	9.3	9
454	Sector, 1/7 of pie — 1 sector (135)	48	345	3	15	3.9	6.4	3.6	51	11	30	.9	108	40	.15	.11	1.3	2
	Banana cream:																	
455	Whole — 1 pie (910)	54	2,010	41	85	26.7	33.2	16.2	279	601	746	7.3	1,847	2,280	.77	1.51	7.0	9
456	Sector, 1/7 of pie — 1 sector (130)	54	285	6	12	3.8	4.7	2.3	40	86	107	1.0	264	330	.11	.22	1.0	1
	Blueberry:																	
457	Whole — 1 pie (945)	51	2,285	23	102	24.8	43.7	25.1	330	104	217	9.5	614	280	1.03	.80	10.0	28
458	Sector, 1/7 of pie — 1 sector (135)	51	325	3	15	3.5	6.2	3.6	47	15	31	1.4	88	40	.15	.11	1.4	4
	Cherry:																	
459	Whole — 1 pie (945)	47	2,465	25	107	28.2	45.0	25.3	363	132	236	6.6	992	4,160	1.09	.84	9.8	Trace
460	Sector, 1/7 of pie — 1 sector (135)	47	350	4	15	4.0	6.4	3.6	52	19	34	.9	142	590	.16	.12	1.4	Trace
	Custard:																	
461	Whole — 1 pie (910)	58	1,985	56	101	33.9	38.5	17.5	213	874	1,028	8.2	1,247	2,090	.79	1.92	5.6	0
462	Sector, 1/7 of pie — 1 sector (130)	58	285	8	14	4.8	5.5	2.5	30	125	147	1.2	178	300	.11	.27	.8	0
	Lemon meringue:																	
463	Whole — 1 pie (840)	47	2,140	31	86	26.1	33.8	16.4	317	118	412	6.7	420	1,430	.61	.84	5.2	25
464	Sector, 1/7 of pie — 1 sector (120)	47	305	4	12	3.7	4.8	2.3	45	17	59	1.0	60	200	.09	.12	.7	4
	Mince:																	
465	Whole — 1 pie (945)	43	2,560	24	109	28.0	45.9	25.2	389	265	359	13.3	1,682	20	.96	.86	9.8	9
466	Sector, 1/7 of pie — 1 sector (135)	43	365	3	16	4.0	6.6	3.6	56	38	51	1.9	240	Trace	.14	.12	1.4	1
	Peach:																	
467	Whole — 1 pie (945)	48	2,410	24	101	24.8	43.7	25.1	361	95	274	8.5	1,408	6,900	1.04	.97	14.0	28
468	Sector, 1/7 of pie — 1 sector (135)	48	345	3	14	3.5	6.2	3.6	52	14	39	1.2	201	990	.15	.14	2.0	4
	Pecan:																	
469	Whole — 1 pie (825)	20	3,450	42	189	27.8	101.0	44.2	423	388	850	25.6	1,015	1,320	1.80	.95	6.9	Trace
470	Sector, 1/7 of pie — 1 sector (118)	20	495	6	27	4.0	14.4	6.3	61	55	122	3.7	145	190	.26	.14	1.0	Trace
	Pumpkin:																	
471	Whole — 1 pie (910)	59	1,920	36	102	37.4	37.5	16.6	223	464	628	7.3	1,456	22,480	.78	1.27	7.0	Trace
472	Sector, 1/7 of pie — 1 sector (130)	59	275	5	15	5.4	5.4	2.4	32	66	90	1.0	208	3,210	.11	.18	1.0	Trace
473	Piecrust (home recipe) made with enriched flour and vegetable shortening, 10-oz pkg. prepared and baked. — 1 pie shell, 9-in diam. (180)	15	900	11	60	14.8	26.1	14.9	79	25	90	3.1	89	0	.47	.40	5.0	0
474	Piecrust mix with enriched flour and vegetable shortening, baked. — Piecrust for 2-crust pie, 9-in diam. (320)	19	1,485	20	93	22.7	39.7	23.4	141	131	272	6.1	179	0	1.07	.79	9.9	0

[38] Made with vegetable shortening.
[50] Products are commercial unless otherwise specified.
[51] Made with enriched flour and vegetable shortening except for macaroons which do not contain flour or shortening.
[53] Applies to yellow varieties; white varieties contain only a trace.
[54] Contains vegetable shortening and butter.
[55] Made with corn oil.
[56] Made with regular margarine.
[57] Applies to product made with yellow cornmeal.
[58] Made with enriched degermed cornmeal and enriched flour.

(A)	(B)	Grams	(C) Per-cent	(D) Cal-ories	(E) Grams	(F) Grams	(G) Grams	(H) Grams	(I) Grams	(J) Grams	(K) Milli-grams	(L) Milli-grams	(M) Milli-grams	(N) Milli-grams	(O) Inter-national units	(P) Milli-grams	(Q) Milli-grams	(R) Milli-grams	(S) Milli-grams
475	Pizza (cheese) baked, 4 3/4-in sector; 1/8 of 12-in diam. pie.[9] — 1 sector	60	45	145	6	4	1.7	1.5	0.6	22	86	89	1.1	67	230	0.16	0.18	1.6	4
	Popcorn, popped:																		
476	Plain, large kernel — 1 cup	6	4	25	1	Trace	Trace	.1	.2	5	1	17	.2	—	—	—	.01	.1	0
477	With oil (coconut) and salt added, large kernel. — 1 cup	9	3	40	1	2	1.5	.2	.2	5	1	19	.2	—	—	—	.01	.2	0
478	Sugar coated — 1 cup	35	4	135	2	1	.5		.4	30	2	47	.5	—	0	—	.02	.4	0
	Pretzels, made with enriched flour:																		
479	Dutch, twisted, 2 3/4 by 2 5/8 in. — 1 pretzel	16	5	60	2	1				12	4	21	.2	21	0	.05	.04	.7	0
480	Thin, twisted, 3 1/4 by 2 1/4 by 1/4 in. — 10 pretzels	60	5	235	6	3				46	13	79	.9	78	0	.20	.15	2.5	0
481	Stick, 2 1/4 in long — 10 pretzels	3	5	10	Trace	Trace				2	1	4	Trace	4	0	.01	.01	.1	0
	Rice, white, enriched:																		
482	Instant, ready-to-serve, hot — 1 cup	165	73	180	4	Trace	Trace	Trace	Trace	40	5	31	1.3	—	0	.21	[59]	1.7	0
	Long grain:																			
483	Raw — 1 cup	185	12	670	12	1	.2	.2	.2	149	44	174	5.4	170	0	.81	.06	6.5	0
484	Cooked, served hot — 1 cup	205	73	225	4	Trace	.1	.1	.1	50	21	57	1.8	57	0	.23	.02	2.1	0
	Parboiled:																			
485	Raw — 1 cup	185	10	685	14	1	.2	.2	.2	150	111	370	5.4	278	0	.81	.07	6.5	0
486	Cooked, served hot — 1 cup	175	73	185	4	Trace	.1	.1	.1	41	33	100	1.4	75	0	.19	.02	2.1	0
	Rolls, enriched:[38]																			
	Commercial:																			
487	Brown-and-serve (12 per 12-oz pkg.), browned. — 1 roll	26	27	85	2	2	.4	.7	.5	14	20	23	.5	25	Trace	.10	.06	.9	Trace
488	Cloverleaf or pan, 2 1/2-in diam., 2 in high. — 1 roll	28	31	85	2	2	.4	.6	.4	15	21	24	.5	27	Trace	.11	.07	.9	Trace
489	Frankfurter and hamburger (8 per 11 1/2-oz pkg.). — 1 roll	40	31	120	3	2	.5	.8	.6	21	30	34	.8	38	Trace	.16	.10	1.3	Trace
490	Hard, 3 3/4-in diam., 2 in high. — 1 roll	50	25	155	5	2	.4	.6	.5	30	24	46	1.2	49	Trace	.20	.12	1.7	Trace
491	Hoagie or submarine, 11 1/2 by 3 by 2 1/2 in. — 1 roll	135	31	390	12	4	.9	1.4	1.4	75	58	115	3.0	122	Trace	.54	.32	4.5	Trace
	From home recipe:																			
492	Cloverleaf, 2 1/2-in diam., 2 in high. — 1 roll	35	26	120	3	3	.8	1.1	.7	20	16	36	.7	41	30	.12	.12	1.2	Trace
	Spaghetti, enriched, cooked:																			
493	Firm stage, "al dente," served hot. — 1 cup	130	64	190	7	1				39	14	85	1.4	103	0	.23	.13	1.8	0
494	Tender stage, served hot. — 1 cup	140	73	155	5	1				32	11	70	1.3	85	0	.20	.11	1.5	0
	Spaghetti (enriched) in tomato sauce with cheese:																			
495	From home recipe — 1 cup	250	77	260	9	9	2.0	5.4	.7	37	80	135	2.3	408	1,080	.25	.18	2.3	13
496	Canned — 1 cup	250	80	190	6	2	.5	.3	.4	39	40	88	2.8	303	930	.35	.28	4.5	10
	Spaghetti (enriched) with meat balls and tomato sauce:																			
497	From home recipe — 1 cup	248	70	330	19	12	3.3	6.3	.9	39	124	236	3.7	665	1,590	.25	.30	4.0	22
498	Canned — 1 cup	250	78	260	12	10	3.3	3.3	3.9	29	53	113	3.3	245	1,000	.15	.18	2.3	5
499	Toaster pastries — 1 pastry	50	12	200	3	6				36	54[60]	67[60]	1.9	74[60]	500	.16	.17	2.1	[60]
	Waffles, made with enriched flour, 7-in diam.:[38]																			
500	From home recipe — 1 waffle	75	41	210	7	7	2.3	2.8	1.4	28	85	130	1.3	109	250	.17	.23	1.4	Trace
501	From mix, egg and milk added — 1 waffle	75	42	205	7	8	2.8	2.9	1.2	27	179	257	1.0	146	170	.14	.22	.9	Trace

NUTRITIVE VALUES OF THE EDIBLE PART OF FOODS · Continued

(Dashes (—) denote lack of reliable data for a constituent believed to be present in measurable amount)

Item No. (A)	Foods, approximate measures, units, and weight (edible part unless footnotes indicate otherwise) (B)	Grams	Water (C) Percent	Food energy (D) Calories	Protein (E) Grams	Fat (F) Grams	Saturated (total) (G) Grams	Oleic (H) Grams	Linoleic (I) Grams	Carbohydrate (J) Grams	Calcium (K) Milligrams	Phosphorus (L) Milligrams	Iron (M) Milligrams	Potassium (N) Milligrams	Vitamin A value (O) International units	Thiamin (P) Milligrams	Riboflavin (Q) Milligrams	Niacin (R) Milligrams	Ascorbic acid (S) Milligrams
	Wheat flours:																		
	All-purpose or family flour, enriched:																		
502	Sifted, spooned — 1 cup	115	12	420	12	1	0.2	0.1	0.5	88	18	100	3.3	109	0	0.74	0.46	6.1	0
503	Unsifted, spooned — 1 cup	125	12	455	13	1	.2	.1	.5	95	20	109	3.6	119	0	.80	.50	6.6	0
504	Cake or pastry flour, enriched, sifted, spooned — 1 cup	96	12	350	7	1	.1	.1	.3	76	16	70	2.8	91	0	.61	.38	5.1	0
505	Self-rising, enriched, unsifted, spooned — 1 cup	125	12	440	12	1	.2	.1	.5	93	331	583	3.6	—	0	.80	.50	6.6	0
506	Whole-wheat, from hard wheats, stirred — 1 cup	120	12	400	16	2	.4	.2	1.0	85	49	446	4.0	444	0	.66	.14	5.2	0
	LEGUMES (DRY), NUTS, SEEDS; RELATED PRODUCTS																		
	Almonds, shelled:																		
507	Chopped (about 130 almonds) — 1 cup	130	5	775	24	70	5.6	47.7	12.8	25	304	655	6.1	1,005	0	.31	1.20	4.6	Trace
508	Slivered, not pressed down (about 115 almonds) — 1 cup	115	5	690	21	62	5.0	42.2	11.3	22	269	580	5.4	889	0	.28	1.06	4.0	Trace
	Beans, dry:																		
	Common varieties as Great Northern, navy, and others:																		
	Cooked, drained:																		
509	Great Northern — 1 cup	180	69	210	14	1	—	—	—	38	90	266	4.9	749	0	.25	.13	1.3	0
510	Pea (navy) — 1 cup	190	69	225	15	1	—	—	—	40	95	281	5.1	790	0	.27	.13	1.3	0
	Canned, solids and liquid:																		
	White with—																		
511	Frankfurters (sliced) — 1 cup	255	71	365	19	18	—	—	—	32	94	303	4.8	668	330	.18	.15	3.3	Trace
512	Pork and tomato sauce — 1 cup	255	71	310	16	7	2.4	2.8	.6	48	138	235	4.6	536	330	.20	.08	1.5	5
513	Pork and sweet sauce — 1 cup	255	66	385	16	12	4.3	5.0	1.1	54	161	291	5.9	—	—	.15	.10	1.3	—
514	Red kidney — 1 cup	255	76	230	15	1	—	—	—	42	74	278	4.6	673	10	.13	.10	1.5	—
515	Lima, cooked, drained — 1 cup	190	64	260	16	1	—	—	—	49	55	293	5.9	1,163	—	.25	.11	1.3	—
516	Blackeye peas, dry, cooked (with residual cooking liquid) — 1 cup	250	80	190	13	1	—	—	—	35	43	238	3.3	573	30	.40	.10	1.0	—
517	Brazil nuts, shelled (6-8 large kernels) — 1 oz	28	5	185	4	19	4.8	6.2	7.1	3	53	196	1.0	203	Trace	.27	.03	.5	—
518	Cashew nuts, roasted in oil — 1 cup	140	5	785	24	64	12.9	36.8	10.2	41	53	522	5.3	650	140	.60	.35	2.5	—
	Coconut meat, fresh:																		
519	Piece, about 2 by 2 by 1/2 in. — 1 piece	45	51	155	2	16	14.0	.9	.3	4	6	43	.8	115	0	.02	.01	.2	1
520	Shredded or grated, not pressed down — 1 cup	80	51	275	3	28	24.8	1.6	.5	8	10	76	1.4	205	0	.04	.02	.4	2
521	Filberts (hazelnuts), chopped (about 80 kernels) — 1 cup	115	6	730	14	72	5.1	55.2	7.3	19	240	388	3.9	810	—	.53	—	1.0	Trace
522	Lentils, whole, cooked — 1 cup	200	72	210	16	Trace	—	—	—	39	50	238	4.2	498	40	.14	.12	1.2	0
523	Peanuts, roasted in oil, salted (whole, halves, chopped) — 1 cup	144	2	840	37	72	13.7	33.0	20.7	27	107	577	3.0	971	—	.46	.19	24.8	0
524	Peanut butter — 1 tbsp	16	2	95	4	8	1.5	3.7	2.3	3	9	61	.3	100	—	.02	.02	2.4	0
525	Peas, split, dry, cooked — 1 cup	200	70	230	16	1	—	—	—	42	22	178	3.4	592	80	.30	.18	1.8	—
526	Pecans, chopped or pieces (about 120 large halves) — 1 cup	118	3	810	11	84	7.2	50.5	20.0	17	86	341	2.8	712	150	1.01	.15	1.1	2
527	Pumpkin and squash kernels, dry, hulled — 1 cup	140	4	775	41	65	11.8	23.5	27.5	21	71	1,602	15.7	1,386	100	.34	.27	3.4	—
528	Sunflower seeds, dry, hulled — 1 cup	145	5	810	35	69	8.2	13.7	43.2	29	174	1,214	10.3	1,334	70	2.84	.33	7.8	—
	Walnuts:																		
	Black:																		
529	Chopped or broken kernels — 1 cup	125	3	785	26	74	6.3	13.3	45.7	19	Trace	713	7.5	575	380	.28	.14	.9	—
530	Ground (finely) — 1 cup	80	3	500	16	47	4.0	8.5	29.2	12	Trace	456	4.8	368	240	.18	.09	.6	—
531	Persian or English, chopped (about 60 halves) — 1 cup	120	4	780	18	77	8.4	11.8	42.2	19	119	456	3.7	540	40	.40	.16	1.1	2

[19]Crust made with vegetable shortening and enriched flour.
[38]Made with vegetable shortening.
[59]Product may or may not be enriched with riboflavin. Consult the label.
[60]Value varies with the brand. Consult the label.

SUGARS AND SWEETS

(A)	(B)		(g)	(C)	(D)	(E)	(F)	(G)	(H)	(I)	(J)	(K)	(L)	(M)	(N)	(O)	(P)	(Q)	(R)	(S)
	Cake icings:																			
	Boiled, white:																			
532	Plain	1 cup	94	18	295	1	0	0	0	0	75	2	2	Trace	17	0	Trace	0.03	Trace	0
533	With coconut	1 cup	166	15	605	3	13	11.0	.9	Trace	124	10	50	0.8	277	0	0.02	.07	0.3	0
	Uncooked:																			
534	Chocolate made with milk and butter.	1 cup	275	14	1,035	9	38	23.4	11.7	1.0	185	165	305	3.3	536	580	.06	.28	.6	1
535	Creamy fudge from mix and water.	1 cup	245	15	830	7	16	5.1	6.7	3.1	183	96	218	2.7	238	Trace	.05	.20	.7	Trace
536	White	1 cup	319	11	1,200	2	21	12.7	5.1	.5	260	48	38	Trace	57	860	Trace	.06	Trace	Trace
	Candy:																			
537	Caramels, plain or chocolate	1 oz	28	8	115	1	3	1.6	1.1	.1	22	42	35	.4	54	Trace	.01	.05	.1	Trace
	Chocolate:																			
538	Milk, plain	1 oz	28	1	145	2	9	5.5	3.0	.3	16	65	65	.3	109	80	.02	.10	.1	Trace
539	Semisweet, small pieces (60 per oz).	1 cup or 6-oz pkg	170	1	860	7	61	36.2	19.8	1.7	97	51	255	4.4	553	30	.02	.14	.9	0
540	Chocolate-coated peanuts	1 oz	28	1	160	5	12	4.0	4.7	2.1	11	33	84	.4	143	Trace	.10	.05	2.1	Trace
541	Fondant, uncoated (mints, candy corn, other).	1 oz	28	8	105	Trace	1	.1	.3	.3	25	4	2	.3	1	0	Trace	Trace	Trace	0
542	Fudge, chocolate, plain	1 oz	28	8	115	Trace	3	1.3	1.4	.6	21	22	24	.3	42	Trace	.01	.03	.1	Trace
543	Gum drops	1 oz	28	12	100	Trace	Trace	—	—	—	25	2	Trace	.1	1	0	0	Trace	Trace	0
544	Hard	1 oz	28	1	110	0	Trace	—	—	—	28	6	2	.5	1	0	0	0	0	0
545	Marshmallows	1 oz	28	17	90	1	Trace	—	—	—	23	5	2	.5	2	0	0	Trace	Trace	0
	Chocolate-flavored beverage powders (about 4 heaping tsp per oz):																			
546	With nonfat dry milk	1 oz	28	2	100	5	1	.5	.3	Trace	20	167	155	.5	227	10	.04	.21	.2	1
547	Without milk	1 oz	28	1	100	1	1	.4	.2	Trace	25	9	48	.6	142	—	.01	.03	.1	Trace
548	Honey, strained or extracted	1 tbsp	21	17	65	Trace	0	0	0	0	17	1	1	.1	11	0	Trace	.01	.1	Trace
549	Jams and preserves	1 tbsp	20	29	55	Trace	Trace	—	—	—	14	4	2	.2	18	Trace	Trace	.01	Trace	Trace
550		1 packet	14	29	40	Trace	Trace	—	—	—	10	3	1	.1	12	Trace	Trace	Trace	Trace	Trace
551	Jellies	1 tbsp	18	29	50	Trace	Trace	—	—	—	13	4	1	.3	14	Trace	Trace	.01	Trace	Trace
552		1 packet	14	29	40	Trace	Trace	—	—	—	10	3	1	.2	11	Trace	Trace	Trace	Trace	1
	Sirups:																			
	Chocolate-flavored sirup or topping:																			
553	Thin type	1 fl oz or 2 tbsp	38	32	90	1	1	.5	.3	Trace	24	6	35	.6	106	Trace	.01	.03	.2	0
554	Fudge type	1 fl oz or 2 tbsp	38	25	125	2	5	3.1	1.6	.1	20	48	60	.5	107	60	.02	.08	.2	Trace
	Molasses, cane:																			
555	Light (first extraction)	1 tbsp	20	24	50	—	—	—	—	—	13	33	9	.9	183	—	.01	.01	Trace	—
556	Blackstrap (third extraction)	1 tbsp	20	24	45	—	—	—	—	—	11	137	17	3.2	585	—	.02	.04	.4	—
557	Sorghum	1 tbsp	21	23	55	—	—	—	—	—	14	35	5	2.6	—	—	—	.02	Trace	—
558	Table blends, chiefly corn, light and dark.	1 tbsp	21	24	60	0	0	0	0	0	15	9	3	.8	1	0	0	—	0	0
	Sugars:																			
559	Brown, pressed down	1 cup	220	2	820	0	0	0	0	0	212	187	42	7.5	757	0	.02	.07	.4	0
	White:																			
560	Granulated	1 cup	200	1	770	0	0	0	0	0	199	0	0	.2	6	0	0	0	0	0
561		1 tbsp	12	1	45	0	0	0	0	0	12	0	0	Trace	Trace	0	0	0	0	0
562		1 packet	6	1	23	0	0	0	0	0	6	0	0	Trace	Trace	0	0	0	0	0
563	Powdered, sifted, spooned into cup.	1 cup	100	1	385	0	0	0	0	0	100	0	0	.1	3	0	0	0	0	0

TABLE A-7

NUTRITIVE VALUES OF THE EDIBLE PART OF FOODS · Continued

(Dashes (—) denote lack of reliable data for a constituent believed to be present in measurable amount)

Item No. (A)	Foods, approximate measures, units, and weight (edible part unless footnotes indicate otherwise) (B)		Water (C) Per-cent	Food energy (D) Cal-ories	Pro-tein (E) Grams	Fat (F) Grams	Fatty Acids Satu-rated (total) (G) Grams	Unsaturated Oleic (H) Grams	Unsaturated Lino-leic (I) Grams	Carbo-hydrate (J) Grams	Calcium (K) Milli-grams	Phos-phorus (L) Milli-grams	Iron (M) Milli-grams	Potas-sium (N) Milli-grams	Vitamin A value (O) Inter-national units	Thiamin (P) Milli-grams	Ribo-flavin (Q) Milli-grams	Niacin (R) Milli-grams	Ascorbic acid (S) Milli-grams
	VEGETABLE AND VEGETABLE PRODUCTS		Grams																
	Asparagus, green:																		
	Cooked, drained:																		
	Cuts and tips, 1 1/2- to 2-in lengths:																		
564	From raw	1 cup	145 94	30	3	Trace	—	—	—	5	30	73	0.9	265	1,310	0.23	0.26	2.0	38
565	From frozen	1 cup	180 93	40	6	Trace	—	—	—	6	40	115	2.2	396	1,530	.25	.23	1.8	41
	Spears, 1/2-in diam. at base:																		
566	From raw	4 spears	60 94	10	1	Trace	—	—	—	2	13	30	.4	110	540	.10	.11	.8	16
567	From frozen	4 spears	60 92	15	2	Trace	—	—	—	2	13	40	.7	143	470	.10	.08	.7	16
568	Canned, spears, 1/2-in diam. at base.	4 spears	80 93	15	2	Trace	—	—	—	3	15	42	1.5	133	640	.05	.08	.6	12
	Beans:																		
	Lima, immature seeds, frozen, cooked, drained:																		
569	Thick-seeded types (Fordhooks)	1 cup	170 74	170	10	Trace	—	—	—	32	34	153	2.9	724	390	.12	.09	1.7	29
570	Thin-seeded types (baby limas)	1 cup	180 69	210	13	Trace	—	—	—	40	63	227	4.7	709	400	.16	.09	2.2	22
	Snap:																		
	Green:																		
	Cooked, drained:																		
571	From raw (cuts and French style).	1 cup	125 92	30	2	Trace	—	—	—	7	63	46	.8	189	680	.09	.11	.6	15
	From frozen:																		
572	Cuts	1 cup	135 92	35	2	Trace	—	—	—	8	54	43	.9	205	780	.09	.12	.5	7
573	French style	1 cup	130 92	35	2	Trace	—	—	—	8	49	39	1.2	177	690	.08	.10	.4	9
574	Canned, drained solids (cuts).	1 cup	135 92	30	2	Trace	—	—	—	7	61	34	2.0	128	630	.04	.07	.4	5
	Yellow or wax:																		
	Cooked, drained:																		
575	From raw (cuts and French style).	1 cup	125 93	30	2	Trace	—	—	—	6	63	46	.8	189	290	.09	.11	.6	16
	From frozen:																		
576	Cuts	1 cup	135 92	35	2	Trace	—	—	—	8	47	42	.9	221	140	.09	.11	.5	8
577	Canned, drained solids (cuts).	1 cup	135 92	30	2	Trace	—	—	—	7	61	34	2.0	128	140	.04	.07	.4	7
	Beans, mature. See Beans, dry (items 509-515) and Blackeye peas, dry (item 516).																		
	Bean sprouts (mung):																		
578	Raw	1 cup	105 89	35	4	Trace	—	—	—	7	20	67	1.4	234	20	.14	.14	.8	20
579	Cooked, drained	1 cup	125 91	35	4	Trace	—	—	—	7	21	60	1.1	195	30	.11	.13	.9	8
	Beets:																		
	Cooked, drained, peeled:																		
580	Whole beets, 2-in diam	2 beets	100 91	30	1	Trace	—	—	—	7	14	23	.5	208	20	.03	.04	.3	6
581	Diced or sliced	1 cup	170 91	55	2	Trace	—	—	—	12	24	39	.9	354	30	.05	.07	.5	10
	Canned, drained solids:																		
582	Whole beets, small	1 cup	160 89	60	2	Trace	—	—	—	14	30	29	1.1	267	30	.02	.05	.2	5
583	Diced or sliced	1 cup	170 89	65	2	Trace	—	—	—	15	32	31	1.2	284	30	.02	.05	.2	5
584	Beet greens, leaves and stems, cooked, drained.	1 cup	145 94	25	2	Trace	—	—	—	5	144	36	2.8	481	7,400	.10	.22	.4	22
	Blackeye peas, immature seeds, cooked and drained:																		
585	From raw	1 cup	165 72	180	13	1	—	—	—	30	40	241	3.5	625	580	.50	.18	2.3	28
586	From frozen	1 cup	170 66	220	15	1	—	—	—	40	43	286	4.8	573	290	.68	.19	2.4	15
	Broccoli, cooked, drained:																		
	From raw:																		
587	Stalk, medium size	1 stalk	180 91	45	6	1	—	—	—	8	158	112	1.4	481	4,500	.16	.36	1.4	162
588	Stalks cut into 1/2-in pieces	1 cup	155 91	40	5	Trace	—	—	—	7	136	96	1.2	414	3,880	.14	.31	1.2	140
	From frozen:																		
589	Stalk, 4 1/2 to 5 in long	1 stalk	30 91	10	1	Trace	—	—	—	1	12	17	.2	66	570	.02	.03	.2	22
590	Chopped	1 cup	185 92	50	5	1	—	—	—	9	100	104	1.3	392	4,810	.11	.22	.9	105
	Brussels sprouts, cooked, drained:																		
591	From raw, 7-8 sprouts (1 1/4- to 1 1/2-in diam.).	1 cup	155 88	55	7	1	—	—	—	10	50	112	1.7	423	810	.12	.22	1.2	135
592	From frozen	1 cup	155 89	50	5	Trace	—	—	—	10	33	95	1.2	457	880	.12	.16	.9	126

VEGETABLE AND VEGETABLE PRODUCTS—Con.

(A)	(B)		(C)	(D)	(E)	(F)	(G)	(H)	(I)	(J)	(K)	(L)	(M)	(N)	(O)	(P)	(Q)	(R)	(S)
	Cabbage:																		
	Common varieties:																		
	Raw:																		
593	Coarsely shredded or sliced	1 cup	70	15	1	Trace	—	—	—	4	34	20	0.3	163	90	0.04	0.04	0.02	33
594	Finely shredded or chopped	1 cup	90	20	1	Trace	—	—	—	5	44	26	.4	210	120	.05	.05	.3	42
595	Cooked, drained	1 cup	145	30	2	Trace	—	—	—	6	64	29	.4	236	190	.06	.06	.4	48
596	Red, raw, coarsely shredded or sliced	1 cup	70	20	1	Trace	—	—	—	5	29	25	.6	188	30	.06	.04	.3	43
597	Savoy, raw, coarsely shredded or sliced.	1 cup	70	15	2	Trace	—	—	—	3	47	38	.6	188	140	.04	.06	.2	39
598	Cabbage, celery (also called pe-tsai or wongbok), raw, 1-in pieces.	1 cup	75	10	1	Trace	—	—	—	2	32	30	.5	190	110	.04	.03	.5	19
599	Cabbage, white mustard (also called bokchoy or pakchoy), cooked, drained.	1 cup	170	25	2	Trace	—	—	—	4	252	56	1.0	364	5,270	.07	.14	1.2	26
	Carrots:																		
	Raw, without crowns and tips, scraped:																		
600	Whole, 7 1/2 by 1 1/8 in, or strips, 2 1/2 to 3 in long.	1 carrot or 18 strips	72	30	1	Trace	—	—	—	7	27	26	.5	246	7,930	.04	.04	.4	6
601	Grated	1 cup	110	45	1	Trace	—	—	—	11	41	40	.8	375	12,100	.07	.06	.7	9
602	Cooked (crosswise cuts), drained	1 cup	155	50	1	Trace	—	—	—	11	51	48	.9	344	16,280	.08	.08	.8	9
	Canned:																		
603	Sliced, drained solids	1 cup	155	45	1	Trace	—	—	—	10	47	34	1.1	186	23,250	.03	.05	.6	3
604	Strained or junior (baby food)	1 oz (1 3/4 to 2 tbsp)	28	10	Trace	Trace	—	—	—	2	7	6	.1	51	3,690	.01	.01	.1	1
	Cauliflower:																		
605	Raw, chopped	1 cup	115	31	3	Trace	—	—	—	6	29	64	1.3	339	70	.13	.12	.8	90
	Cooked, drained:																		
606	From raw (flower buds)	1 cup	125	30	3	Trace	—	—	—	5	26	53	.9	258	80	.11	.10	.8	69
607	From frozen (flowerets)	1 cup	180	30	3	Trace	—	—	—	6	31	68	.9	373	50	.07	.09	.7	74
	Celery, Pascal type, raw:																		
608	Stalk, large outer, 8 by 1 1/2 in, at root end.	1 stalk	40	5	Trace	Trace	—	—	—	2	16	11	.1	136	110	.01	.01	.1	4
609	Pieces, diced	1 cup	120	20	1	Trace	—	—	—	5	47	34	.4	409	320	.04	.04	.4	11
	Collards, cooked, drained:																		
610	From raw (leaves without stems)	1 cup	190	65	7	1	—	—	—	10	357	99	1.5	498	14,820	.21	.38	2.3	144
611	From frozen (chopped)	1 cup	170	50	5	1	—	—	—	10	299	87	1.7	401	11,560	.10	.24	1.0	56
	Corn, sweet:																		
	Cooked, drained:																		
612	From raw, ear 5 by 1 3/4 in	1 ear[6 1]	140	70	2	1	—	—	—	16	2	69	.5	151	[6 2]310	.09	.08	1.1	7
	From frozen:																		
613	Ear, 5 in long	1 ear[6 1]	229	120	4	1	—	—	—	27	4	121	1.0	291	[6 2]440	.18	.10	2.1	9
614	Kernels	1 cup	165	130	5	1	—	—	—	31	5	120	1.3	304	[6 2]580	.15	.10	2.5	8
	Canned:																		
615	Cream style	1 cup	256	210	5	2	—	—	—	51	8	143	1.5	248	[6 2]840	.08	.13	2.6	13
	Whole kernel:																		
616	Vacuum pack	1 cup	210	175	5	1	—	—	—	43	6	153	1.1	204	[6 2]740	.06	.13	2.3	11
617	Wet pack, drained solids	1 cup	165	140	4	1	—	—	—	33	8	81	.8	160	[6 2]580	.05	.08	1.5	7
	Cowpeas. See Blackeye peas. (Items 585-586).																		
	Cucumber slices, 1/8 in thick (large, 2 1/8-in diam.; small, 1 3/4-in diam.):																		
618	With peel	6 large or 8 small slices	28	5	Trace	Trace	—	—	—	1	7	8	.3	45	70	.01	.01	.1	3

TABLE A-7

NUTRITIVE VALUES OF THE EDIBLE PART OF FOODS - Continued

(Dashes (—) denote lack of reliable data for a constituent believed to be present in measurable amount)

Item No. (A)	Foods, approximate measures, units, and weight (edible part unless footnotes indicate otherwise) (B)		Water (C)	Food energy (D)	Pro-tein (E)	Fat (F)	Fatty Acids Satu-rated (total) (G)	Unsaturated Oleic (H)	Lino-leic (I)	Carbo-hydrate (J)	Calcium (K)	Phos-phorus (L)	Iron (M)	Potas-sium (N)	Vitamin A value (O)	Thiamin (P)	Ribo-flavin (Q)	Niacin (R)	Ascorbic acid (S)
619	Without peel—	6 1/2 large or 9 small pieces.	28	96	5	Trace	Trace	—	—	—	1	5	5	0.1	45	Trace	0.01	0.01	0.1	3
620	Dandelion greens, cooked, drained—	1 cup	105	90	35	2	1	—	—	—	7	147	44	1.9	244	12,290	.14	.17	—	19
621	Endive, curly (including escarole), raw, small pieces.	1 cup	50	93	10	1	Trace	—	—	—	2	41	27	.9	147	1,650	.04	.07	.3	5
	Kale, cooked, drained:																			
622	From raw (leaves without stems and midribs).	1 cup	110	88	45	5	1	—	—	—	7	206	64	1.8	243	9,130	.11	.20	1.8	102
623	From frozen (leaf style)—	1 cup	130	91	40	4	1	—	—	—	7	157	62	1.3	251	10,660	.08	.20	.9	49
	Lettuce, raw: Butterhead, as Boston types:																			
624	Head, 5-in diam.	1 head[63]	220	95	25	2	Trace	—	—	—	4	57	42	3.3	430	1,580	.10	.10	.5	13
625	Leaves	1 outer or 2 inner or 3 heart leaves.	15	95	Trace	Trace	Trace	Trace	—	—	Trace	5	4	.3	40	150	.01	.01	Trace	1
	Crisphead, as Iceberg:																			
626	Head, 6-in diam	1 head[64]	567	96	70	5	1	—	—	—	16	108	118	2.7	943	1,780	.32	.32	1.6	32
627	Wedge, 1/4 of head—	1 wedge	135	96	20	2	Trace	—	—	—	4	27	30	.7	236	450	.08	.08	.4	8
628	Pieces, chopped or shredded—	1 cup	55	96	5	Trace	Trace	—	—	—	2	11	12	.3	96	180	.03	.03	.2	3
629	Looseleaf (bunching varieties including romaine or cos), chopped or shredded pieces.	1 cup	55	94	10	1	Trace	—	—	—	2	37	14	.8	145	1,050	.03	.04	.2	10
630	Mushrooms, raw, sliced or chopped—	1 cup	70	90	20	2	Trace	—	—	—	3	4	81	.6	290	Trace	.07	.32	2.9	2
631	Mustard greens, without stems and midribs, cooked, drained.	1 cup	140	93	30	3	1	—	—	—	6	193	45	2.5	308	8,120	.11	.20	.8	67
632	Okra pods, 3 by 5/8 in, cooked—	10 pods	106	91	30	2	Trace	—	—	—	6	98	43	.5	184	520	.14	.19	1.0	21
	Onions: Mature: Raw:																			
633	Chopped—	1 cup	170	89	65	3	Trace	—	—	—	15	46	61	.9	267	[65]Trace	.05	.07	.3	17
634	Sliced—	1 cup	115	89	45	2	Trace	—	—	—	10	31	41	.6	181	[65]Trace	.03	.05	.2	12
635	Cooked (whole or sliced), drained.	1 cup	210	92	60	3	Trace	—	—	—	14	50	61	.8	231	[65]Trace	.06	.06	.4	15
636	Young green, bulb (3/8 in diam.) and white portion of top.	6 onions	30	88	15	Trace	Trace	—	—	—	3	12	12	.2	69	Trace	.02	.01	.1	8
637	Parsley, raw, chopped—	1 tbsp	4	85	Trace	Trace	Trace	Trace	—	—	Trace	7	2	.2	25	300	Trace	.01	Trace	6
638	Parsnips, cooked (diced or 2-in lengths).	1 cup	155	82	100	2	1	—	—	—	23	70	96	.9	587	50	.11	.12	.2	16
	Peas, green: Canned:																			
639	Whole, drained solids—	1 cup	170	77	150	8	1	—	—	—	29	44	129	3.2	163	1,170	.15	.10	1.4	14
640	Strained (baby food)—	1 oz (1 3/4 to 2 tbsp)	28	86	15	1	Trace	—	—	—	3	3	18	.3	28	140	.02	.03	.3	3
641	Frozen, cooked, drained—	1 cup	160	82	110	8	Trace	—	—	—	19	30	138	3.0	216	960	.43	.14	2.7	21
642	Peppers, hot, red, without seeds, dried (ground chili powder, added seasonings).	1 tsp	2	9	5	Trace	Trace	—	—	—	1	5	4	.3	20	1,300	Trace	.02	.2	Trace
	Peppers, sweet (about 5 per lb, whole), stem and seeds removed:																			
643	Raw—	1 pod	74	93	15	1	Trace	—	—	—	4	7	16	.5	157	310	.06	.06	.4	94
644	Cooked, boiled, drained—	1 pod	73	95	15	1	Trace	—	—	—	3	7	12	.4	109	310	.05	.05	.4	70
	Potatoes, cooked:																			
645	Baked, peeled after baking (about 2 per lb, raw).	1 potato	156	75	145	4	Trace	—	—	—	33	14	101	1.1	782	Trace	.15	.07	2.7	31
	Boiled (about 3 per lb, raw):																			
646	Peeled after boiling—	1 potato	137	80	105	3	Trace	—	—	—	23	10	72	.8	556	Trace	.12	.05	2.0	22
647	Peeled before boiling—	1 potato	135	83	90	3	Trace	—	—	—	20	8	57	.7	385	Trace	.12	.05	1.6	22
	French-fried, strip, 2 to 3 1/2 in long:																			
648	Prepared from raw—	10 strips	50	45	135	2	7	1.7	1.2	3.3	18	8	56	.7	427	Trace	.07	.04	1.6	11
649	Frozen, oven heated—	10 strips	50	53	110	2	4	1.1	.8	2.1	17	5	43	.9	326	Trace	.07	.01	1.3	11
650	Hashed brown, prepared from frozen.	1 cup	155	56	345	3	18	4.6	3.2	9.0	45	28	78	1.9	439	Trace	.11	.03	1.6	12
	Mashed, prepared from— Raw:																			
651	Milk added—	1 cup	210	83	135	4	2	.7	.4	Trace	27	50	103	.8	548	40	.17	.11	2.1	21

[61]Weight includes cob. Without cob, weight is 77 g for item 612, 126 g for item 613.
[62]Based on yellow varieties. For white varieties, value is trace.
[63]Weight includes refuse of outer leaves and core. Without these parts, weight is 163 g.
[64]Weight includes core. Without core, weight is 539 g.
[5]Value based on white-fleshed varieties. For yellow-fleshed varieties, value in International Units (i.U.) is 70 for item 633, 50 for item 634, and 80 for item 635.

VEGETABLE AND VEGETABLE PRODUCTS—Con.

(A)	(B)	Grams	(C) Per cent	(D) Calories	(E) Grams	(F) Grams	(G) Grams	(H) Grams	(I) Grams	(J) Grams	(K) Milligrams	(L) Milligrams	(M) Milligrams	(N) Milligrams	(O) International units	(P) Milligrams	(Q) Milligrams	(R) Milligrams	(S) Milligrams
	Potatoes, cooked—Continued																		
	Mashed, prepared from—Continued																		
	Raw—Continued																		
652	Milk and butter added------ 1 cup	210	80	195	4	9	5.6	2.3	0.2	26	50	101	0.8	525	360	0.17	0.11	2.1	19
653	Dehydrated flakes (without milk), water, milk, butter, and salt added. 1 cup	210	79	195	4	7	3.6	2.1	.2	30	65	99	.6	601	270	.08	.08	1.9	11
654	Potato chips, 1 3/4 by 2 1/2 in oval cross section. 10 chips	20	2	115	1	8	2.1	1.4	4.0	10	8	28	.4	226	Trace	.04	.01	1.0	3
655	Potato salad, made with cooked salad dressing. 1 cup	250	76	250	7	7	2.0	2.7	1.3	41	80	160	1.5	798	350	.20	.18	2.8	28
656	Pumpkin, canned------- 1 cup	245	90	80	2	1				19	61	64	1.0	588	15,680	.07	.12	1.5	12
657	Radishes, raw (prepackaged) stem ends, rootlets cut off. 4 radishes	18	95	5	Trace	Trace				1	5	6	.2	58	Trace	.01	.01	.1	5
658	Sauerkraut, canned, solids and liquid. 1 cup	235	93	40	2	Trace				9	85	42	1.2	329	120	.07	.09	.5	33
	Southern peas. See Blackeye peas (items 585-586).																		
	Spinach:																		
659	Raw, chopped------- 1 cup	55	91	15	2	Trace				2	51	28	1.7	259	4,460	.06	.11	.3	28
	Cooked, drained:																		
660	From raw------- 1 cup	180	92	40	5	1				6	167	68	4.0	583	14,580	.13	.25	.9	50
	From frozen:																		
661	Chopped------- 1 cup	205	92	45	6	1				8	232	90	4.3	683	16,200	.14	.31	.8	39
662	Leaf------- 1 cup	190	92	45	6	1				7	200	84	4.8	688	15,390	.15	.27	1.0	53
663	Canned, drained solids------- 1 cup	205	91	50	6	1				7	242	53	5.3	513	16,400	.04	.25	.6	29
	Squash, cooked:																		
664	Summer (all varieties), diced, drained. 1 cup	210	96	30	2	Trace				7	53	53	.8	296	820	.11	.17	1.7	21
665	Winter (all varieties), baked, mashed. 1 cup	205	81	130	4	1				32	57	98	1.6	945	8,610	.10	.27	1.4	27
	Sweetpotatoes:																		
	Cooked (raw, 5 by 2 in; about 2 1/2 per lb):																		
666	Baked in skin, peeled------- 1 potato	114	64	160	2	1				37	46	66	1.0	342	9,230	.10	.08	.8	25
667	Boiled in skin, peeled------- 1 potato	151	71	170	3	1				40	48	71	1.1	367	11,940	.14	.09	.9	26
668	Candied, 2 1/2 by 2-in piece--- 1 piece	105	60	175	1	3	2.0	.8	.1	36	39	45	.9	200	6,620	.06	.04	.4	11
	Canned:																		
669	Solid pack (mashed)------- 1 cup	255	72	275	5	1				63	64	105	2.0	510	19,890	.13	.10	1.5	36
670	Vacuum pack, piece 2 3/4 by 1 in. 1 piece	40	72	45	1	Trace				10	10	16	.3	80	3,120	.02	.02	.2	6
	Tomatoes:																		
671	Raw, 2 3/5-in diam. (3 per 12 oz pkg.). 1 tomato[66]	135	94	25	1	Trace				6	16	33	.6	300	1,110	.07	.05	.9	[6,7]28
672	Canned, solids and liquid------- 1 cup	241	94	50	2	Trace				10	[6,8]14	46	1.2	523	2,170	.12	.07	1.7	41
673	Tomato catsup------- 1 cup	273	69	290	5	1				69	60	137	2.2	991	3,820	.25	.19	4.4	41
674	------- 1 tbsp	15	69	15	Trace	Trace				4	3	8	.1	54	210	.01	.01	.2	2
	Tomato juice, canned:																		
675	Cup------- 1 cup	243	94	45	2	Trace				10	17	44	2.2	552	1,940	.12	.07	1.9	39
676	Glass (6 fl oz)------- 1 glass	182	94	35	2	Trace				8	13	33	1.6	413	1,460	.09	.05	1.5	29
677	Turnips, cooked, diced------- 1 cup	155	94	35	1	Trace				8	54	37	.6	291	Trace	.06	.08	.5	34
	Turnip greens, cooked, drained:																		
678	From raw (leaves and stems)--- 1 cup	145	94	30	3	Trace				5	252	49	1.5	—	8,270	.15	.33	.7	68
679	From frozen (chopped)------- 1 cup	165	93	40	4	Trace				6	195	64	2.6	246	11,390	.08	.15	.7	31
680	Vegetables, mixed, frozen, cooked-- 1 cup	182	83	115	6	1				24	46	115	2.4	348	9,010	.22	.13	2.0	15

TABLE A-7
NUTRITIVE VALUES OF THE EDIBLE PART OF FOODS - Continued

(Dashes (—) denote lack of reliable data for a constituent believed to be present in measurable amount)

NUTRIENTS IN INDICATED QUANTITY

Item No. (A)	Foods, approximate measures, units, and weight (edible part unless footnote: indicate otherwise) (B)		Water (C)	Food energy (D)	Protein (E)	Fat (F)	Saturated (total) (G)	Oleic (H)	Linoleic (I)	Carbohydrate (J)	Calcium (K)	Phosphorus (L)	Iron (M)	Potassium (N)	Vitamin A value (O)	Thiamin (P)	Riboflavin (Q)	Niacin (R)	Ascorbic acid (S)
	MISCELLANEOUS ITEMS																		
	Baking powders for home use:																		
	Sodium aluminum sulfate:																		
681	With monocalcium phosphate monohydrate.	1 tsp---- 3.0	2	5	Trace	Trace	0	0	0	1	58	87	—	5	0	0	0	0	0
682	With monocalcium phosphate monohydrate, calcium sulfate.	1 tsp---- 2.9	1	5	Trace	Trace	0	0	0	1	183	45	—	—	0	0	0	0	0
683	Straight phosphate.	1 tsp---- 3.8	2	5	Trace	Trace	0	0	0	1	239	359	—	6	0	0	0	0	0
684	Low sodium.	1 tsp---- 4.3	2	5	Trace	Trace	0	0	0	2	207	314	—	471	0	0	0	0	0
685	Barbecue sauce.	1 cup---- 250	81	230	4	17	2.2	4.3	10.0	20	53	50	2.0	435	900	.03	.03	.8	13
686	Beverages, alcoholic: Beer.	12 fl oz---- 360	92	150	1	0				14	18	108	Trace	90	—	.01	.11	2.2	—
	Gin, rum, vodka, whisky:																		
687	80-proof.	1 1/2-fl oz jigger---- 42	67	95	—	—	0	0	0	Trace	—	—	—	1	—	—	—	—	—
688	86-proof.	1 1/2-fl oz jigger---- 42	64	105	—	—	0	0	0	Trace	—	—	—	1	—	—	—	—	—
689	90-proof.	1 1/2-fl oz jigger---- 42	62	110	—	—	0	0	0	Trace	—	—	—	1	—	—	—	—	—
	Wines:																		
690	Dessert.	3 1/2-fl oz glass---- 103	77	140	Trace	0	0	0	0	8	8	—	—	77	—	.01	.02	.2	—
691	Table.	3 1/2-fl oz glass---- 102	86	85	Trace	0	0	0	0	4	9	10	.4	94	—	Trace	.01	.1	—
	Beverages, carbonated, sweetened, nonalcoholic:																		
692	Carbonated water.	12 fl oz---- 366	92	115	0	0	0	0	0	29	—	—	—	—	0	0	0	0	0
693	Cola type.	12 fl oz---- 369	90	145	0	0	0	0	0	37	—	—	—	—	0	0	0	0	0
694	Fruit-flavored sodas and Tom Collins mixer.	12 fl oz---- 372	88	170	0	0	0	0	0	45	—	—	—	—	0	0	0	0	0
695	Ginger ale.	12 fl oz---- 366	92	115	0	0	0	0	0	29	—	—	—	0	0	0	0	0	0
696	Root beer.	12 fl oz---- 370	90	150	0	0	0	0	0	39	—	—	—	0	0	0	0	0	0
	Chili powder. See Peppers, hot, red (item 642).																		
	Chocolate:																		
697	Bitter or baking.	1 oz---- 28	2	145	3	15	8.9	4.9	.4	8	22	109	1.9	235	20	.01	.07	.4	0
	Semisweet, see Candy, chocolate (item 539).																		
698	Gelatin, dry.	1 7-g envelope---- 7	13	25	6	Trace	0	0	0	0	—	—	—	—	—	—	—	—	—
699	Gelatin dessert prepared with gelatin dessert powder and water.	1 cup---- 240	84	140	4	0	0	0	0	34	—	—	—	—	—	—	—	—	—
700	Mustard, prepared, yellow.	1 tsp or individual serving pouch or cup. 5	80	5	Trace	Trace	—	—	Trace	Trace	4	4	.1	7	—	—	—	—	—
	Olives, pickled, canned:																		
701	Green.	4 medium or 3 extra large or 2 giant.[69] 16	78	15	Trace	2	.2	1.2	.1	Trace	8	2	.2	7	40	—	—	—	—
702	Ripe, Mission.	3 small or 2 large[69]---- 10	73	15	Trace	2	.2	1.2	.1	Trace	9	1	.1	2	10	—	—	—	—
	Pickles, cucumber:																		
703	Dill, medium, whole, 3 3/4 in long, 1 1/4-in diam.	1 pickle---- 65	93	5	Trace	Trace				1	17	14	.7	130	70	Trace	.01	Trace	4
704	Fresh-pack, slices 1 1/2-in diam., 1/4 in thick.	2 slices---- 15	79	10	Trace	Trace				3	5	4	.3	—	20	Trace	Trace	Trace	1
705	Sweet, gherkin, small, whole, about 2 1/2 in long, 3/4-in diam.	1 pickle---- 15	61	20	Trace	Trace				5	2	2	.2	—	10	Trace	Trace	Trace	1
706	Relish, finely chopped, sweet.	1 tbsp---- 15	63	20	Trace	Trace				5	3	2	.1	—	—	—	—	—	—
	Popcorn. See items 476-478.																		
707	Popsicle, 3-fl oz size.	1 popsicle---- 95	80	70	0	0	0	0	0	18	0	—	Trace	—	0	0	0	0	0

[66] Weight includes cores and stem ends. Without these parts, weight is 123 g.
[67] Based on year-round average. For tomatoes marketed from November through May, value is about 12 mg; from June through October, 32 mg.
[68] Applies to product without calcium salts added. Value for products with calcium salts added may be as much as 63 mg for whole tomatoes, 241 mg for cut forms.
[69] Weight includes pits. Without pits, weight is 13 g for item 701, 9 g for item 702.

(A)	(B)		(C)	(D)	(E)	(F)	(G)	(H)	(I)	(J)	(K)	(L)	(M)	(N)	(O)	(P)	(Q)	(R)	(S)
		Grams	Per cent	Calories	Grams	Grams	Grams	Grams	Grams	Grams	Milligrams	Milligrams	Milligrams	Milligrams	International units	Milligrams	Milligrams	Milligrams	Milligrams
	MISCELLANEOUS ITEMS—Con.																		
	Soups:																		
	Canned, condensed:																		
	Prepared with equal volume of milk:																		
708	Cream of chicken------- 1 cup	245	85	180	7	10	4.2	3.6	1.3	15	172	152	0.5	260	610	0.05	0.27	0.7	2
709	Cream of mushroom----- 1 cup	245	83	215	7	14	5.4	2.9	4.6	16	191	169	.5	279	250	.05	.34	.7	1
710	Tomato---------------- 1 cup	250	84	175	7	7	3.4	1.7	1.0	23	168	155	.8	418	1,200	.10	.25	1.3	15
	Prepared with equal volume of water:																		
711	Bean with pork-------- 1 cup	250	84	170	8	6	1.2	1.8	2.4	22	63	128	2.3	395	650	.13	.08	1.0	3
712	Beef broth, bouillon, consomme. 1 cup	240	96	30	5	0	0	0	0	3	Trace	31	.5	130	Trace	Trace	.02	1.2	
713	Beef noodle----------- 1 cup	240	93	65	4	3	.6	.7	.8	7	7	48	1.0	77	50	.05	.05	1.0	
714	Clam chowder, Manhattan type (with tomatoes, without milk). 1 cup	245	92	80	2	3	.5	.4	1.3	12	34	47	1.0	184	880	.02	.02	1.0	Trace
715	Cream of chicken------ 1 cup	240	92	95	3	6	1.6	2.3	1.1	8	24	34	.5	79	410	.02	.05	.5	Trace
716	Cream of mushroom----- 1 cup	240	90	135	2	10	2.6	1.7	4.5	10	41	50	.5	98	70	.02	.12	.7	Trace
717	Minestrone------------ 1 cup	245	90	105	5	3	.7	.9	1.3	14	37	59	1.0	314	2,350	.07	.05	1.0	
718	Split pea------------- 1 cup	245	85	145	9	3	1.1	1.2	.4	21	29	149	1.5	270	440	.25	.15	1.5	1
719	Tomato---------------- 1 cup	245	91	90	2	3	.5	.5	1.0	16	15	34	.7	230	1,000	.05	.05	1.2	12
720	Vegetable beef-------- 1 cup	245	92	80	5	2				10	12	49	.7	162	2,700	.05	.05	1.0	
721	Vegetarian------------ 1 cup	245	92	80	2	2				13	20	39	1.0	172	2,940	.05	.05		
	Dehydrated:																		
722	Bouillon cube, 1/2 in- 1 cube	4	4	5	1	Trace				Trace				4					
	Mixes:																		
	Unprepared:																		
723	Onion----------------- 1 1/2-oz pkg	43	3	150	6	5	1.1	2.3	1.0	23	42	49	.6	238	30	.05	.03	.3	6
	Prepared with water:																		
724	Chicken noodle-------- 1 cup	240	95	55	2	1				8	7	19	.2	19	50	.07	.05	.5	Trace
725	Onion----------------- 1 cup	240	96	35	1	1				6	10	12	.2	58	Trace	Trace	Trace	Trace	2
726	Tomato vegetable with noodles. 1 cup	240	93	65	1	1				12	7	19	.2	29	480	.05	.02	.5	5
727	Vinegar, cider-------- 1 tbsp	15	94	Trace	Trace	0	0	0	0	1	1	1	.1	15					
728	White sauce, medium, with enriched flour. 1 cup	250	73	405	10	31	19.3	7.8	.8	22	288	233	.5	348	1,150	.12	.43	.7	2
	Yeast:																		
729	Baker's, dry, active-- 1 pkg	7	5	20	3	Trace				3	3	90	1.1	140	Trace	.16	.38	2.6	Trace
730	Brewer's, dry--------- 1 tbsp	8	5	25	3	Trace				3	[7]17	140	1.4	152	Trace	1.25	.34	3.0	Trace

[7]Value may vary from 6 to 60 mg.

(Courtesy of United States Department of Agriculture)

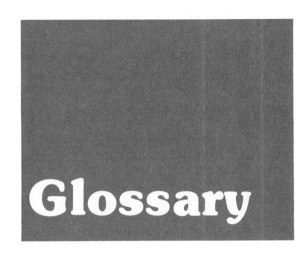

Glossary

abrasive—substance with rough surface

absorption—taking in of nutrients

abstinence—avoidance

accompaniment dish—dish served in addition to, and with, the main course

acid-ash foods—foods that leave an acid ash after oxidation; meats, cereals, legumes and cranberries, plums and prunes

acidosis—condition in which excess acids accumulate or there is a loss of base in the body

acute—sudden but short-lived

adapt—change to suit specific requirements

adipose tissue—fatty tissue

a la king—served in a white sauce with bits of green pepper and pimiento. A common example is chicken a la king.

alkaline-ash foods—foods that leave an alkaline ash after oxidation; fruits, vegetables (except corn and lentils), milk and cream

alkalosis—condition in which excess base accumulates in, or acids are lost from, the body

allergen—substance causing allergy

allergic reaction—adverse physical reaction to specific substance(s)

allergy—sensitivity to specific substance(s)

ambulatory—able to walk

amenorrhea—the stoppage of the monthly menstrual flow

amino acids—nitrogen-containing chemical compounds of which protein is composed

amniocentesis—testing of the baby in utero

amphetamines—drugs intended to inhibit appetite

anabolism—the creation of new compounds during metabolism

angina pectoris—pain in the heart muscle due to inadequate blood supply

anorexia—lack of appetite

anorexia nervosa—psychologically induced lack of appetite

antibiotic therapy—drug treatment with antibiotics

antibodies—substances produced by body in reaction to foreign substance; neutralize toxins from foreign bodies

anticoagulant—drug used to thin the blood

anxiety—apprehension

arterial—referring to the arteries

arteriosclerosis—generic term for thickened arteries

arthritis—chronic disease involving the joints

ascites—abnormal collection of fluid in the abdomen

ascorbic acid—vitamin C

aseptic—sterile

aspartame—artificial sweetener made from protein; does not require insulin for metabolism

aspic—highly seasoned jelly made from broth, stock, or tomato juice. An example is tomato aspic.

aspirated—inhaled or suctioned

asymptomatic—without symptoms

atherosclerosis —a form of arteriosclerosis affecting the intima (inner lining) of the artery walls

au gratin —prepared in white sauce with cheese added. Potatoes au gratin are an example.

average weight —normal weight for a particular size

avitaminosis —without vitamins

azotemia —abnormally large amounts of nitrogen in the blood

bacteria —microorganism that may or may not cause disease

bake —cook in the oven as is done with cakes and cookies

balanced diet —one that includes all the essential nutrients in appropriate amounts

barbecue —to bake or roast over coals or on a spit, basting with spicy sauce, as is done with chicken and pork ribs

basal metabolism rate (BMR) —the rate at which energy is needed for body maintenance

Basic Four food groups —simplified method of maintaining a balanced diet that divides foods into 4 groups: meats, vegetables and fruits, dairy foods and breads and cereals

baste —to brush or pour hot fat on cooking foods, as is done with roasting poultry

beat —to combine with air by mixing vigorously; this is often done with eggs

beriberi —deficiency disease caused by a lack of vitamin B_1 (thiamin)

beverage —a drink

bile —secretion of the liver, stored in the gallbladder; essential for the digestion of fats

biotin —a B vitamin; necessary for metabolism

blanch —to plunge into boiling water and then into cold water. This may be done with almonds to remove their brown skins.

bland —mild or soothing

bland diet —diet containing only mild-flavored foods with soft textures

blemish —mark

blend —to mix thoroughly, as is done when combining ingredients for cakes and cookies

blood plasma —fluid part of the blood

boil —to cook in liquid at 100°C (212°F) as is indicated when bubbles break on the surface of the liquid

bone marrow —soft tissue in the bone center

botulism —deadliest of food poisonings; caused by bacteria named *Clostridium botulinum*

boullion —clear soup broth

braise —to cook in a covered container with a small amount of liquid, as is done with less tender cuts of meat

bran —outer covering of grain kernels

brine —water/salt solution

broil —to cook under or over direct heat. Tender meats can be broiled.

broth —liquid part of soup

brush —to spread a thin amount of sauce, oil, or egg over food as is commonly done with yeast breads

bubbled —burped, to get rid of stomach gas

buttermilk —milk made from the addition of harmless bacteria to skim milk; also a byproduct of buttermaking

cachexia —severe malnutrition and body wasting caused by chronic disease

caffeine —stimulant in coffee, tea, and many cola beverages

calipers —mechanical device used to measure percentage of body fat

caloric requirement —number of kcal required by the body each day

calorie —the unit used to measure the fuel value of foods

calorimeter —device used to scientifically determine the kcal value of foods

capillaries —tiny blood vessels connecting veins and arteries

carbohydrate —the energy nutrient providing the greatest amount of energy in the average diet

carcinogen —cancer-causing substance

cardiac disease —heart disease

cardiovascular —pertaining to the heart and entire circulatory system

cardiovascular disease—disease affecting heart and blood vessels

carotene—provitamin A

carrier—one who is capable of transmitting an infectious organism

casserole—a combination of foods providing a meal in one dish or the dish in which the casserole is served

catabolism—the breakdown of compounds during metabolism

catalyst—a substance that causes another substance to react

cataracts—a clouding of the lens of the eye, obstructing sight

cellulose—indigestible carbohydrate; necessary for providing fiber in the diet

centi—prefix meaning one hundred

cerebral accident—stroke; occlusion of artery in the brain

certified milk—milk that has been handled according to health regulations

cheilosis—condition caused by riboflavin deficiency; characterized by cracks and sores on the lips

chemical digestion—chemical changes in foods during digestion caused by hydrolysis

chemical method of regulation—very conservative approach to the dietary treatment of diabetes mellitus; means food must be weighed, urine tests made frequently, and insulin amounts adjusted throughout the day.

chemotherapy—treatment with drugs

cholecalciferol—the form of vitamin D that is formed in humans from cholesterol in the skin

cholecystectomy—removal of the gallbladder

cholecystitis—inflammation of the gallbladder

cholelithiasis—gallstones

cholesterol—fat-like substance that is a constituent of body cells; it is synthesized in the liver; also available in animal foods

chop—to cut into small, irregular pieces, as is done with onions, celery, hard-cooked eggs, and nuts

chyme—the food mass as it has been mixed with gastric juices

circulation—the body process whereby the blood is moved throughout the body

cirrhosis—generic term for liver disease characterized by cell loss

citrus fruit—oranges, grapefruit, lemons, and limes (all rich in vitamin C)

clear liquid diet—diet that includes only liquids containing primarily carbohydrates and water; nutritionally inadequate

clinical method of regulation—very liberal approach to the dietary treatment of diabetes mellitus; patients are allowed to choose foods, except for sugar; if the diet cannot control the disease, insulin is prescribed.

coagulate—to thicken

coarse foods—foods containing fiber

cobalamins—group of organic compounds known as vitamin B_{12}

coenzyme—an active part of an enzyme

collagen—protein substance that holds body cells together

combine—to mix together

compensated heart disease—heart disease in which the heart is able to maintain circulation to all body parts

complete protein—proteins that contain all nine essential amino acids

compote—fruit in syrup; also, the long-stemmed dish in which it may be served

condiment—"extra" food such as catsup, pickles, relish, etc.

congestive heart failure—a form of decompensated heart disease

consistency—texture

constipation—difficulty in evacuating feces; characterized by dry, hard stool

consumer—one who makes purchases and uses commerical products

convalescent—in a state of recovery or the convalescent diet that is also called the "light" diet

convenience food—food that has been partially

prepared commercially and consequently is quickly and easily completed at home

coordination—integration of various procedures

coronary occlusion—blockage of a coronary artery

crash reducing diets—fad-type diet intended to reduce weight very quickly; in fact reduces water, not fat tissue

craving—abnormal desire

cream—to mix with beaters or the back of a spoon until food is smooth and creamy in consistency; done to mix shortening and sugar for cakes and cookies

creatinine—an end (waste) product of protein metabolism

croquette—combination of finely chopped food and white sauce shaped in a ball or cone, rolled in egg and crumbs, and fried in deep fat. An example might be chicken croquettes.

cube—to dice or cut into small, regular squares, as may be done with cheese

cuisine—style of cooking or preparing food

culinary—referring to cooking

cultural—relating to one's background

custom—habit

cut in—to blend shortening with flour using two knives or a pastry blender

cystine—a nonessential amino acid

cysts—growths

decaffeinated—having had caffeine removed almost completely

decompensated heart disease—heart disease in which the heart is unable to maintain circulation to all body parts

deficiency—a lack

deficiency disease—disease caused by the lack of a specific nutrient

dehydrated—having lost large amounts of water

density—compactness; the mass of substance per unit of volume

deodorize—to remove odor by cleaning

depression—an indentation; or feelings of sadness

desensitize—to gradually reduce the body's sensitivity (allergic reaction) to specific items

desired weight—average weight for body size

deviled—highly seasoned. An example might be deviled eggs.

dextrin—the intermediate product in starch digestion; before it changes to maltose and ultimately, glucose

diabetes mellitus—chronic disease in which the body lacks the normal ability to metabolize glucose

diabetic coma—unconsciousness caused by a state of acidosis due to too much sugar or too little insulin

dialysis—mechanical filtration of the blood; used when the kidneys are no longer able to perform normally

diaphragm—thin membrane or partition

diarrhea—loose bowel movement

dice—to cube or cut into very small, regular squares

dietary guidelines—guides for planning a healthy diet

dietary laws—rules to be followed in meal planning in some religions

dietician—person planning therapeutic diets

diet therapy—treatment of a disease through diet

digestion—breakdown of food in the body in preparation for absorption

disaccharides—double sugars that are reduced by hydrolysis to monosaccharides. Examples are sucrose, maltose, and lactose

diuretics—substances used to increase the amount of urine excreted

diverticulitis—inflammation of the diverticula

diverticulosis—intestinal disorder characterized by little pockets forming in the sides of the intestines; pockets are called diverticula

dredge—to coat heavily with flour, as is sometimes done before browning meat; or to coat with sugar, as may be done with some cookie dough just before baking

dried milk—milk with water removed

duodenum—first (and smallest) section of the small intestine

duodenal ulcer—ulcer occurring in the duodenum

durability—strength

dust—to sprinkle lightly with flour or sugar, as may be done to the top of baked products.

dwarfism—condition of stunted growth

dysentery—disease caused by microorganism; characterized by diarrhea

dyspepsia—gastrointestinal discomfort of vague origin

early dumping syndrome—nausea and diarrhea caused by food moving too quickly from the stomach to the small intestine

eclamptic stage—convulsive stage of toxemia

economic status—status as determined by income

edema—the abnormal retention of fluid and sodium by the body

edible portion—that part of the food that can be eaten

efficiency—effective use of time and energy

eggnog—milk, egg, sugar beverage; similar to milkshake

elective surgery—surgery performed at patient's choice

elimination—evacuation of wastes

elimination diets—limited diets in which only certain foods are allowed; intended to find the food allergen causing reaction

emotional bond—loving attachment

emotional stress—strain caused by anxiety

emulsified fats—finely divided fat, held in suspension by another liquid

endocardium—the lining of the heart

endocrine glands—ductless glands that secrete hormones directly into the blood stream

endocrine system—the ductless glands

endogenous insulin—insulin produced within the body

endosperm—the inner part of the kernel of grain; contains the carbohydrate

English system of weights and measures—includes inch, foot, yard, cup, pound, quart, etc., as opposed to the metric system which is based on the number 10

energy imbalance—either eating too much or too little for the amount of energy expended

energy value—the kcal content of specific foods

enriched foods—foods to which nutrients, usually B vitamins and iron, have been added to improve their nutritional value

enteral feeding—feeding by tube directly into the patient's stomach or intestine

enterostomies—surigcal openings into the stomach or intestinal wall

environment—surroundings

enzyme—organic substances that cause changes in other substances

ergocalciferol—the form of vitamin D found in plants

esophagus—tube leading from the mouth to the stomach; part of the gastrointestinal system

equivalent—equal

evaporated milk—milk that has had 60 percent of its water removed

Exchange lists—lists of foods with interchangeable nutrient and kcal contents; used in specific forms of diet therapy

exogenous insulin—insulin injected into the body

fad diets—currently popular and usually reducing diets; usually nutritionally inadequate and not useful, permanent, methods of weight reduction

fast foods—restaurant food that is ready to serve before orders are taken

fats—highest calorie energy nutrient

fat soluble—can be dissolved in fat

fatty acids—a component of fats that determines the classification of the fat

fecal matter—solid waste from large intestine

feces—solid waste from the large intestine

Federal Food, Drug, and Cosmetic Act—law requiring that food shipped from one state to another be pure, safe to eat, and prepared under sanitary conditions. It also requires ingredients and weight on the label.

fetus—infant in utero

fever—hypermetabolic state with raised body temperature; commonly due to infection

fiber—indigestible, edible parts of plants

fibrosis—development of tough, stringy tissue

fillet—thin strip of meat or fish

filtrate—the substance to be filtered

flake—to separate gently with a fork, as may be

done to fish

flatulence—gas in the intestinal tract

flatware—knives, forks and spoons

flavor—taste

fold—to blend very gently with a down, across, up, and over motion to retain air in a mixture, as is done when combining heavy mixtures with light, whipped ingredients

folic acid—a form of vitamin B, also called folacin; essential for metabolism

food additives—chemical substances added to foods during processing

food customs—food habits

food faddists—people who have certain beliefs about particular foods or diets

food residue—that part of the food that is indigestible

fortified foods—foods that have had vitamins and minerals added

fortified margarine—margarine that has had specific nutrients added

free diet—the liberal approach to the dietary treatment of diabetes mellitus; see *clinical method of regulation*

freeze-dried foods—foods that have been frozen rapidly and then dehydrated

fructose—the simple sugar (monosaccharide) found in fruit and honey

fry—to cook in hot fat, as may be done with potatoes or chicken

full liquid diet—diet consisting of liquids and food that is liquid at body temperature

fundus (of the stomach)—upper part of the stomach

galactose—the simple sugar (monosaccharide) to which lactose is broken down during digestion

galactosemia—inherited error in metabolism that prevents normal metabolism of lactose

galactosuria—galactose in the urine

gallbladder—the organ located next to the liver; stores the bile produced by the liver & subsequently releases it as needed for the digestion of fats

garnish—to trim or decorate food; the trimmings. Such trimmings should harmonize in color, flavor, and shape with the dish it decorates. Examples are parsley, egg slices, pickles, carrot curls.

gastric bypass—surgical reduction of the stomach area

gastric juices—the digestive secretions of the stomach

gastric lipase—enzyme secreted by the stomach to aid in the digestion of fats

gastric ulcer—ulcer in the stomach

gastrointestinal—pertaining to the digestive system

genetic predisposition—inherited tendency

geriatrics—the branch of medicine involved with diseases of the elderly

germ—embryo or tiny life center of each kernel of grain

gerontology—the study of aging

glomerulonephritis—inflammation of the glomeruli of the kidneys

glomerulus—filtering unit in the kidneys

glossitis—inflammation of the tongue

glucose—the simple sugar to which carbohydrate must be broken down for absorption

glycogen—glucose as stored in the liver and muscles

glycosuria—excess sugar in the urine

goiter—enlarged tissue of the thyroid gland due to a deficiency of iodine

gout—inherited error of metabolism causing pain in the joints of fingers and toes

grade stamps—the purple stamp on meats indicating quality

grams—small unit of measurement of weight in the metric system; 30 grams equal one ounce

grate—to rub on a rough surface, producing small particles, as is done with onions, lemons, and oranges

grill—to broil

hematuria—blood in the urine

hemoglobin—the red coloring matter in the blood

hemolysis—the destruction of red blood cells

hemorrhage—unusually heavy bleeding

hiatus hernia—condition wherein part of the

stomach protrudes through the diaphragm into the chest cavity

hollow-calorie foods—foods that provide large amounts of kcal in the form of carbohydrates and fats, but very few vitamins, minerals, or proteins

homogenized milk—whole milk processed to break fat into small drops that do not separate

homous—form of serving chick peas common to Middle Easterners

hormone—substance secreted by the endocrine glands

hydrochloric acid—gastric secretion necessary for the digestion of protein and some minerals

hydrogenation—the combining of fat with hydrogen, thereby making it a saturated fat

hydrolysis—the addition of water resulting in the breakdown of the molecule

hyperalimentation—highly concentrated intravenous feeding

hypercholesteremia—unusually high levels of cholesterol in blood

hypoglycemic agents—oral drugs that stimulate the pancreas to produce insulin

hyperglycemia—excessive amounts of sugar in the blood

hyperkalemia—excessive amounts of potassium in the blood

hyperlipidemia—excessive amounts of fats in the blood

hypermetabolic—higher than normal rate of metabolism

hypersensitivity—abnormally strong sensitivity to certain substance(s)

hypertension—higher than normal blood pressure

hyperthyroidism—condition in which the thyroid gland secretes too much thyroxine and T_3; the body's rate of metabolism is unusually high

hypervitaminosis—condition caused by excessive ingestion of one or more vitamins

hypoalbuminemia—abnormally low amounts of protein in the blood

hypocalcemia—abnormally low amount of calcium in the blood

hypoglycemia—subnormal levels of blood sugar

hypogonadism—subnormal development of male sex organs

hypothyroidism—condition in which the thyroid gland secretes too little thyroxine and T_3; body metabolism is slower than normal

IDDM—insulin-dependent diabetes mellitus

ideal weight—average

ileum—last part of the small intestine

immunity—ability to resist certain diseases

impulsive shopper—one who buys in accordance with the desires of the moment

incomplete protein—protein that does not contain all of the nine essential amino acids

infectious—contagious; communicable

insecticide—chemical used to kill insects

insulin—secretion of the Islets of Langerhans in the pancreas gland, essential for the proper metabolism of glucose

insulin coma—unconsciousness caused by too much insulin or too little food

insulin reaction—hypoglycemia leading to insulin coma caused by too much insulin or too little food

International Units (IU)—units of measurment of some vitamins

intima—lining of arteries

iodized salt—salt that has had the mineral iodine added for the prevention of goiter

irradiate—expose to ultraviolet light

iron—mineral essential to the blood

islets of Langerhans—part of the pancreas gland from which insulin is secreted

isoleucine—amino acid

invisible fats—fats that are not immediately noticeable such as those in egg yolk, cheese, cream, salad dressings, etc.

jejunoileal bypass—surgical procedure in which the jejunum of the small intestine is attached to a very small section of the ileum in an effort to reduce the amount of absorptive surface

jejunum—the middle section comprising about two-fifths of the small intestine

jellied fruit—fruit combined with gelatin

joule—unit used to measure the energy value of

food in the metric system; 4.184 kjoules equal 1 kcal.

julienne—to cut into thin strips, as may be done with meat used in salads and vegetables

junket—milk pudding

kcal intake—number of kcal taken in

ketones—substances to which fatty acids are broken down in the liver

ketonuria—ketone bodies in the urine

kilogram—unit of measurement of weight in the metric system; 1 kilogram equals 2.2 pounds

kilojoule—unit used to measure the energy value of food in the metric system; 4.184 kilojoules equal 1 kcal.

knead—to mix by folding and squeezing with the hands, as in mixing yeast bread doughs

kwashiorkor—deficiency disease caused by extreme lack of protein

lactase—enzyme secreted by the small intestine for the digestion of lactose

lactation—the period during which the mother is nursing the baby

lacteals—lymphatic vessels in the small intestine that absorb fatty acids and glycerol

lactose—the sugar in milk; a disaccharide

lacto-vegetarians—vegetarians who eat dairy products

leavened bread—bread that contains a leavening agent

legumes—plant food that is grown in a pod, for example, beans and peas

leucine—an amino acid

light diet—also called the convalescent diet; very close to the regular diet but more advanced than the soft diet

lipid—fat

lipoproteins—carriers of fat in the blood

liter—unit of volume measurement in the metric system. The approximate equivalent of one quart in the English system

lumen—the hollow area in a tube

macrominerals—those minerals that are required in relatively large amounts

malignant—life threatening

malnutrition—poor nutrition

maltase—enzyme secreted by the small intestine essential for the digestion of maltose

maltose—the double sugar (disaccharide) occurring as a result of the digestion of grain

maple syrup urine disease—disease caused by an inborn error of metabolism in which the body cannot metabolize certain amino acids

marasmus—severe wasting caused by lack of protein and all nutrients, or faulty absorption

marinade—distinctive liquid or sauce in which some foods are kept for a specified time to alter their original flavors

marinate—to let stand in a marinade

meat alternates—substitute food for meat such as cheese, eggs, fish

meat analogs—substances made to imitate meat; usually of soybean origin

meat thermometer—special thermometer for checking internal temperature of meat during cooking

mechanical digestion—that part of digestion that requires certain mechanical movement such as chewing, swallowing, and peristalsis

mechanical-soft diet—soft diet for people who cannot chew; all meats are ground and fruits and vegetables are pureed

megaloblastic anemia—anemia in which the red blood cells are unusually large and are not completely mature

menaquinones—the form of vitamin K found in bacteria, animals, and humans

menses—menustruation

mental retardation—below normal intellectual capacity

meringue—egg white and sugar mixture

metabolism—the use of the food by the body after digestion resulting in energy

metastasize—movement of cancer cells through the blood from one organ to another

meter—metric unit of measurement of length; approximate equivalent of 1 yard

metric system—system of measurement based on the number 10

micro- (a prefix)—very small

microminerals—those minerals that are required

in minute amounts

microorganisms —microscopic organisms such as bacteria or viruses

milli- (a prefix) —a measurement of one-thousandth of a particular item

milliliter —used to measure volume; one-thousandth of a liter; equivalent of 1 cubic centimeter

mince —to chop as finely as possible, as may be done with celery, onions, or parsley

milling —the grinding of grain

mineral —one of many inorganic substances essential to life and classified generally as minerals

minimum-residue diet —diet severely restricted in food residue; nutritionally inadequate

mocha —combination of coffee and chocolate flavors. An example is mocha icing.

monosaccharides —simplest carbohydrates; sugars that cannot be further reduced by hydrolysis. Examples are glucose, fructose, and galactose

monounsaturated fats —fats that are neither saturated nor polyunsaturated and are thought to play little part in atherosclerosis

morning sickness —early morning nausea common to some pregnancies

mortality rate —rate of death

MSG —monosodium glutamate; a form of spice containing large amounts of sodium

mucous membrane —lining of body passages that open to the outside such as the alimentary, genitourinary, and respiratory tracts

mutations —changes

myocardial infarction —heart attack; caused by the blockage of an artery leading to the heart

myocardium —middle muscular layer of the heart wall

nasogastric tube —tube leading from the nose to the stomach for tube feeding

nausea —the urge to vomit

necrosis —tissue death due to lack of blood supply

neoplasm —new growth; refers to cancerous tumors

neoplasia —cancer

nephritic —pertaining to the kidneys

nephritis —inflammatory disease of the kidneys

nephrolithiasis —kidney stones

nephron —unit of the kidney containing a glomerulus

nephrosclerosis —hardening of renal arteries

niacin —B vitamin

niacin equivalent (NE) —unit of measuring niacin; 1 NE equals 1 mg niacin or 60 mg tryptophan

NIDDM —non-insulin dependent diabetes mellitus

nitrogen —chemical element found only in protein; essential to life

normal weight —average weight for size and age

nourish —to provide with materials necessary to promote and sustain life

nutrient —chemical substance found in food that is necessary for good health

nutrient content —the amount of nutrients contained in a food or beverage

nutrient requirement —specific amount of specific nutrient needed by the body at a certain age

nutrient supplement —nutrients supplied in addition to normal diet; can be supplied orally, in tablets, or liquids, or parenterally

nutrition —the result of those processes whereby the body takes in and uses food for growth, development, and the maintenance of health.

nutrition labeling —specific labeling required by the FDA for foods making nutritional claims

nutritional anemia —anemia caused by insufficient iron in the diet

nutritional edema —edema caused by lack of protein

nutritionally adequate —contains recommended amounts of essential nutrients

nutritional status —state of one's nutrition

nutritional value —the nutrient content of foods and beverages

obesity —excessive body fat, 20 percent above average

obstetrician —doctor who cares for the mother during pregnancy and delivery

on demand —feeding infants as they desire

opaque —neither transparent nor translucent

osmosis—movement of substances through a semi-permeable membrane

osteomalacia—a condition in which bones become soft, usually in older people, because of calcium loss

osteoporosis—condition in which bones become brittle because there have been insufficient mineral deposits

overweight—weight 10—20 percent above average

ovo-lacto-vegetarians—vegetarians who will eat dairy products and eggs

oxidation—the process of combining substances with oxygen

pan-broil—to fry, pouring off fat as it accumulates, as may be done when cooking bacon

pancreas—gland that secretes enzymes essential for digestion, and insulin, which is essential for glucose metabolism

pancreatic amylase—the enzyme secreted by the pancreas gland that is essential for the digestion of starch

pancreatic lipase—the enzyme secreted by the pancreas gland that is essential for the digestion of fat

pancreatic protease—the enzyme secreted by the pancreas that is essential for the digestion of protein

pancreatitis—inflammation of the pancreas

pantothenic acid—a B vitamin

paralysis—inability to move

parasite—organism that is completely dependent on another organism for its existence

parboil—to partially cook by boiling or simmering, as may be done to julienne potatoes before frying

parenteral—feeding through a blood vessel

pasteurization—process in which harmful micro-organisms are killed

pastry blender—small utensil with 5 or 6 cutting edges for rapid mixing of solid fat with flour as, for example, in pastry making

pediatrician—doctor specializing in the health problems of children

peer group—group of people approximately one's own age

peer pressure—pressure of one's friends and colleagues of the same age

pellagra—deficiency disease caused by a lack of niacin

pepsin—an enzyme secreted by the stomach that is essential for the digestion of proteins

peptic ulcers—ulcer of the stomach or duodenum

peptidases—enzymes secreted by the small intestine that are essential for the digestion of protein

Perfringens—type of bacteria that can cause food poisoning

pericardium—outer covering of the heart

peridontal disease—disease of the mouth and gums

peristalsis—rhythmical movement of the intestinal tract, moving the chyme along

pernicious anemia—severe, chronic anemia caused by a deficiency of vitamin B_{12}. Usually due to the body's inability to absorb B_{12}

phenylalanine—amino acid

phenylalanine hydroxylase—liver enzyme necessary to metabolize the amino acid, phenylalanine

phenylketonuria—condition caused by an inborn error of metabolism in which the infant lacks an enzyme necessary to metabolize the amino acid, phenylalanine

phlebitis—inflammation of a vein

phylloquinone—vitamin K as found in green plants

physical disability—physical lack or handicap

physical stress—bodily strain

pica—abnormal craving for non-food substance

pigmentation—coloring matter in the skin

placenta—maternal organ in which the fetus develops and derives its nourishment

poach—to cook in liquid just below the boiling point, as may be done with eggs, fish, or chicken

polluted water—water contaminated with toxins

polycystic kidney disease—rare, hereditary kidney disease causing cysts or growths on the kidneys that can ultimately cause kidney failure in middle age

polydipsia—abnormal thirst

polyphagia—abnormally increased appetite

polysaccharides—complex carbohydrates containing combinations of monosaccharides. Examples include starch, dextrin, cellulose and glycogen

polyunsaturated fats—fats whose carbon atoms contain only limited amounts of hydrogen and consequently do not contribute to heart disease

polyuria—excessive secretion of urine

postoperative—after surgery

posture—body position

precursor—something that comes before something else; in vitamins it is also called a provitamin, something from which the body can synthesize the specific vitamin

preeclampsia—toxemia; characterized by edema, high blood pressure, and protein in the urine

process cheese—made from natural cheese, spices, and liquid

prohormone—substance that precedes the hormone and from which the body can synthesize the hormone

proteases—enzymes secreted by the pancreas gland; essential for the digestion of protein

protein—the only one of the six essential nutrients containing nitrogen

proteinuria—protein in the urine

protozoa—type of microorganism that can cause dysentery

provitamin—see precursor

psychological development—development of the psyche

ptyalin—also called *salivary amylase*; it is the digestive secretion of the salivary glands

puree—to press through a strainer to remove fiber; the food that has been pressed through the strainer. An example is puree of spinach.

purines—end products of nucleoprotein metabolism

pylorus—the end of the stomach nearest the intestine

pyridoxal—see pyridoxine

pyridoxamine—see pyridoxine

pyridoxine—one of the three vitaminers of vitamin B_6; see also pyridoxal and pyridoxamine

rate of growth—the speed at which one grows

raw milk—milk that has not been processed in any way; may contain harmful microorganisms

RDAs—recommended daily dietary allowances as determined by the Food and Nutrition Board of the National Academy of Science

refined foods—foods that have been processed to remove most or all naturally occurring fiber

regurgitation—vomiting

renal—refers to kidneys

renal calculi—kidney stones

rennin—enzyme secreted by the stomach necessary for the digestion of proteins in milk

resection—reduction

respiration—breathing

restored foods—those foods to which manufacturers have returned the naturally occurring nutrients

retardation—slowing

retinol—the preformed vitamin A

Retinol Equivalent (RE)—the equivalent of 3.33 IU of vitamin A

riboflavin—the name for vitamin B_2

rickets—deficiency disease caused by the lack of vitamin D; causes malformed bones and pain in infants

roughage—fiber; the apple skin, grain bran, etc.

saccharin—artificial sweetener

saliva—secretion of the salivary glands

salivary amylase—also called *ptyalin*; it is the enzyme secreted by the salivary glands to act on starch

salmonella—form of food poisoning caused by bacteria of the same name; Salmonellosis is formal name

sanitation—cleanliness

satiety—feeling of satisfaction; fullness

saturated fats—fats whose carbon atoms contain all of the hydrogen atoms they can; considered a contributory factor in atherosclerosis

saute—to fry slowly in a small amount of fat, as may be done with onions, peppers, or eggs

score—to make shallow, even cuts on the surface; often done with ham that is to be baked

scald—to bring a liquid just to the boiling point and immediately remove it from the heat, as may be done with milk

scurvy—a deficiency disease caused by a lack of vitamin C

sear—to brown quickly at a high temperature, as is sometimes done with meat

seasonal—sold as the product is ripe, according to the growing season

secretions—liquid emissions

self-esteem—feelings of self-worth

shoyu—Japanese form of Soy sauce

shred—to tear, or rub, or cut into thin pieces, as is done with lettuce and cabbage

sift—to put dry ingredients through a sieve to remove lumps, as is done with flour

simmer—to cook in liquid just below the boiling point; indicated by tiny bubbles breaking just beneath the surface of the liquid

Sippy Diet—conservative treatment of peptic ulcers; not commonly used, contains only milk and antacids

skeletal system—body's bone structure

skewer—a metal or wooden pick for fastening foods, or to fasten foods with such a pick

skim milk—milk with fat removed

skin tests—allergy tests using potential allergens on scratches on the skin

social status—one's social class

sodium chloride—table salt

soft diet—one of the basic hospital diets; contains only foods with soft textures

souffle—light, fluffy dish having eggs as the main ingredient. Examples are cheese and chocolate souffles.

stamina—strength

standard hospital diets—basic diets used by most hospitals; can be modified in texture, kcal content, and nutrient content.

standard weight—average weight for height and age

staphylococcus—form of bacteria causing food poisoning called "staph" or "staphylococcal poisoning"

staple food—foods commonly used and kept on hand, such as flour or potatoes in the U.S.

stasis—stoppage or slowing

steam—to cook in covered container over but not touching boiling water, as done with vegetables, shellfish, and some quick breads

steak—cut of meat or fish across the flesh of the animal

steatorrhea—abnormal amounts of fat in the feces

steep—to let stand in hot liquid for a specified time, as is done with tea

sterile—free of infectious organisms

sterilizing process—process used to clean item of infectious organisms

stew—to cook slowly in liquid or a mixture of meat and vegetables cooked by this method. An example is beef and vegetable stew.

stimulant—substance that increases heart rate, such as caffeine

stock—liquid in which foods have been cooked. Examples are meat or vegetable stocks.

stunted growth—growth that did not reach its full potential

sucrase—enzyme secreted by the small intestine to aid in digestion of sucrose

sucrose—a double sugar or disaccharide; examples are granulated, powdered, or brown sugar.

sweetbreads—edible animal glands

sweetened condensed milk—milk that has had water removed and sugar added

synthesize—to make a substance from other substances

synthetic—human-made

tamales—Mexican bread made of cornmeal

tempura—fried foods, Japanese style

terminal—situation in which death is unavoidable

tetany—involuntary muscle movement

texture—consistency

textured protein—meat analogs; imitation meat products

therapeutic diets—diets used in treatment of disease

thiamin—vitamin B_1

thrombosis—blockage, as a blood clot

thyroid gland—controls body metabolism; secretes thyroxine and T_3

thyroxine—secretion of the thyroid gland

timbale—finely chopped foods combined with eggs and baked in a mold. Examples are chicken timbales.

tocopherols—vitamers of vitamin E

tortillas—Mexican bread made of cornmeal

toxemia—a condition characterized by high blood pressure, edema, and protein in the urine. Can occur in pregnancy

toxin—poison

TPN—total parenteral nutrition

trace element—minerals that are essential, but only in very small amounts

transferase—a liver enzyme necessary for the metabolism of galactose

trauma—stress to the body

trichinosis—disease caused by the parasite Trichinella spiralis; can be transmitted through undercooked pork

triglycerides—combinations of fatty acids and glycerol

triiodothyronine (T_3)—secretion of the thyroid gland

trimester—three-month period; commonly used to denote periods of pregnancy

tryptophan—an amino acid and a precursor of niacin

ulcerative colitis—disease of the colon characterized by numerous ulcerated areas

underweight—weight that is 10—15 percent below average

unpalatable—inedible

urea—chief nitrogenous waste product of protein metabolism

uremia—condition in which protein wastes are circulating in the blood

ureters—tubes leading from the kidneys to the bladder

uric acid—one of the nitrogenous waste products of protein metabolism

urticaria—hives; common allergic reaction

valine—amino acid

vascular disease—disease of the blood vessels

vascular system—circulatory system

vegans—vegetarians who avoid all animal foods

venison—meat from deer

villi—the tiny, hair-like structures in the small intestines through which nutrients are absorbed

visible fats—fats in foods that are easily seen, such as on meat, or in butter

vitamers—different chemical forms of a vitamin that serve the same purpose in the body

vitamin supplements—concentrated forms of vitamins; may be in tablet or liquid form

vitamin—organic substances necessary for life although they do not, independently, provide energy

volume—amount in terms of space consumed

water soluble—soluble in water

weaning—training the infant to drink from the cup instead of the nipple

weighed diet—used in the conservative dietary treatment of diabetes mellitus; requires actual weighing of food portions to balance with the amount of insulin injected

whip—to beat rapidly, introducing air, as may be done to egg whites or heavy cream

wok—common form of frying pan used for Oriental cooking

xerophthalmia—serious eye disease characterized by dry mucous membranes of the eye, caused by a deficiency of vitamin A

xerostomia—sore, dry mouth caused by a reduction of salivary secretions. May be caused by radiation for treatment of cancer.

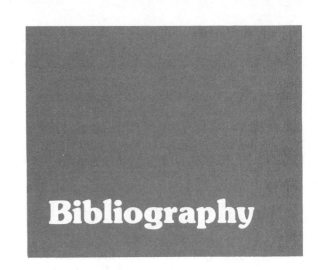

Bibliography

BOOKS

American Diabetes Association and American Dietetic Association. *Family Cookbook*. Englewood Cliffs, N.J.: Prentice-Hall Inc. 1980.

American Dietetic Association. *Handbook of Clinical Dietetics*. New Haven: Yale University. 1981.

American Home Economics Association. *Handbook of Food Preparation*. Washington, D.C.: American Home Economics Association. 1975.

Anderson, Jean. *Jean Anderson's Processor Cooking*. New York: William Morrow & Co., Inc. 1979.

Anderson, Jean, and Elaine Hanna. *The Doubleday Cookbook*. Garden City, N.Y.: Doubleday and Co., Inc. 1975.

Anderson, Linnea *et al. Nutrition in Health and Disease*, 17th ed. Philadelphia: J.B. Lippincott Company. 1982.

Atkins, Robert C. *Dr. Atkins' Diet Revolution*. Bantam Books. 1972.

Bennion, Marion. *Introductory Foods*, 7th ed. New York: Macmillan Publishing Company. 1980.

Bland, Jeffrey ed. *Medical Applications of Clinical Nutrition*. New Canaan, Ct.: Keats Publishing Co. 1983.

Bodinski, Lois H. *The Nurse's Guide to Diet Therapy*. New York: John Wiley & Sons. 1982.

Briggs, George M., and Doris H. Calloway. *Bogert's Nutrition and Physical Fitness*, 10th ed. Philadelphia: W.B. Saunders Co. 1979.

Charley, Helen. *Food Science*, 2nd ed. New York: John Wiley & Sons. 1982.

Corbin, Cheryl. *Nutrition*. New York: Holt Rinehart & Winston. 1980.

Department of Foods and Nutrition, College of Home Economics Kansas State University. *Practical Cookery*. New York: John Wiley & Sons, Inc. 1975.

Eschleman, Marian M. *Introductory Nutrition and Diet Therapy*. Philadelphia: J. B. Lippincott Co. 1984.

Garrison, Carolyn, and Ruth E. Brasher. *Modern Household Equipment*. New York: Macmillan Publishing Company. 1982.

Goodhart, R. S., M.D., and Maurice E. Shils, M.D. *Modern Nutrition in Health and Disease*. Philadelphia: Lea & Febiger. 1980.

Gray, Henry. *Gray's Anatomy*. New York: Bounty Books. 1977.

Green, Marilyn L., and Joann Harry. *Nutrition in Contemporary Nursing Practice*. New York: John Wiley & Sons. 1981.

Greenwood, M.R.C., ed. *Obesity*. New York: Churchill Livingstone Inc. 1983.

Howard, Roseanne B., and Nancie H. Herbold. *Nutrition in Clinical Care*, 2nd ed. New York: McGraw Hill Book Company. 1982.

Howe, Phyllis Sullivan. *Basic Nutrition in Health and Disease*. Philadelphia: W.B. Saunders Co. 1981.

Hui, Y.H. *Human Nutrition and Diet Therapy*. Monterey Calif.: Wadsworth Health Sciences Division of Wadsworth Inc. 1983.

Iowa Dietetic Association. *Simplified Diet Manual with Meal Patterns*, 5th ed. Ames: Iowa State University Press. 1984.

Kerschner, Velma L. *Nutrition and Diet Therapy*. Philadelphia: F.A. Davis Co. 1983.

Kinder, Faye, Nancy Green, and Natholyn Harris. *Meal Management*, 6th ed., New York: Macmillan Publishing Company. 1984.

Krause, Marie V, and L. Kathleen Mahan. *Food, Nutrition and Diet Therapy*, 6th ed. Philadelphia: W.B. Saunders Co., 1979.

Long, Patricia J., and Barbara Shannon. *Focus on Nutrition*. Englewood Cliffs, N.J.: Prentice-Hall Inc. 1983.

Luke, Barbara. *Maternal Nutrition*. Boston: Little Brown & Co. 1979.

Luke, Barbara. *Principles of Nutrition and Diet Therapy*. Boston: Little Brown & Co. 1984.

Mahan, L.K., and J.M. Rees. *Nutrition in Adolescence*. St. Louis: Times Mirror/ Mosby College Publishing. 1984.

Massachusetts General Hospital Dietary Department. *Diet Manual*. Boston: Little, Brown & Company. 1976.

Mayo Clinic, Rochester Methodist Hospital and St. Mary's Hospital. *Mayo Clinic Diet Manual, a Handbook of Dietary Practices*. Philadelphia: W. B. Saunders Co. 1981.

McWilliams, M. *Nutrition for the Growing Years*, 2nd ed. New York: John Wiley & Sons. 1975.

National Research Council, National Academy of Sciences. *Recommended Dietary Allowances*, 9th ed. Washington, D.C. 1980.

Peckham, Gladys, and Jeanne Freeland-Graves. *Foundations of Food Preparation*, 4th ed. New York: Macmillan Publishing Company. 1979.

Pipes, Peggy L. *Nutrition in Infancy and Childhood*, 2nd ed. St. Louis: C. V. Mosby Co. 1981.

Poleman, Charlotte M., and Christine Locastro Capra. *Shackelton's Nutrition Essentials and Diet Therapy*, 5th ed. Philadelphia: W.B. Saunders Co. 1984.

Roberts, Bonnie S. Worthington, Joyce Vermeersch, and Sue Rodwell Williams.

Nutrition in Pregnancy and Lactation, 2nd ed. St. Louis: C.V. Mosby Co. 1981.

Robinson, Corinne H. *Basic Nutrition and Diet Therapy*, 4th ed. New York: Macmillan Publishing Company. 1980.

Robinson, Corinne H. *Fundamentals of Normal Nutrition*, 3rd ed. New York: Macmillan Publishing Company. 1978.

Robinson, Corinne H., and Marilyn R. Lawler. *Normal and Therapeutic Nutrition*, 16th ed. New York: MacMillan Publishing Company. 1982.

Spock, Dr. Benjamin. *Baby and Child Care*. New York: Pocket Books, 1977.

Suitor, Carol W., and Merrily F. Crowley. *Nutrition Principles and Application in Health Promotion*. Philadelphia: J.B. Lippincott Co. 1984.

Thiele, Victoria. *Clinical Nutrition*, 2nd ed. St. Louis: C.V. Mosby Co. 1980.

Turner, Dorothea. *Handbook of Diet Therapy*, 5th ed. Chicago: University of Chicago Press, 1970.

U.S. Department of Agriculture. *Composition of Food*. 1963, 1975.

University of Iowa Hospitals and Clinics. *Recent Advances in Therapeutic Diets*. Iowa City: Iowa State University Press. 1979.

White, Marlene Boskind, and William C. White, Jr. *Bulimarexia*. New York: W. W. Norton & Co. 1983.

Whitney, Eleanor Noss. *Nutrition Concepts and Controversies*, 2nd ed. St. Paul: West Publishing Company. 1982.

Whitney, Eleanor Noss, and Corinne Balog Cataldo. *Understanding Normal and Clinical Nutrition*. St. Paul: West Publishing Co. 1983.

Whitney, Eleanor Noss, and Eva May Nunnelley Hamilton. *Understanding Nutrition*, 3rd ed. St. Paul: West Publishing Co. 1984.

Williams, Sue Rodwell. *Essentials of Nutrition and Diet Therapy*, 3rd ed. St. Louis: C.V. Mosby Co. 1982.

Williams, Sue Rodwell. *Mowry's Basic Nutrition and Diet Therapy*, 7th ed. St. Louis: C.V. Mosby Co. 1984.

Williams, Sue Rodwell. *Nutrition and Diet Therapy*, 4th ed. St. Louis: C.V. Mosby Co. 1981.

Wilson, Eva D. et al. *Principles of Nutrition*, 3rd ed. New York: John Wiley & Sons, Inc. 1975.

Winick, Myron. *Nutrition in Health and Disease*. New York: John Wiley & Sons, 1980.

PERIODICALS AND PUBLICATIONS

American Diabetes Association Inc., and the American Dietetic Association

American Diabetes Association Inc., and the American Dietetic Association. *Exchange Lists for Meal Planning*. New York, New York. 1976.

American Diabetes Association Inc. and the American Dietetic Association. *Principles of Nutrition and Dietary Recommendations for Individuals with Diabetes Mellitus. 1979.* Diabetes, Vol. 28, November, 1979

American Heart Association

American Heart Association. *Your Mild Sodium-Restricted Diet* (revised). Dallas, Texas. 1969.

American Heart Association. *Your 1000 Milligram Sodium Diet* (revised). Dallas, Texas. 1969.

American Heart Association. *Your 500 Milligram Sodium Diet* (revised). Dallas, Texas. 1968.

American Heart Association. *The Way to a Man's Heart.* Dallas, Texas. 1968.

American Heart Association, Subcommittee on Diet and Hyperlipidemia, Council on Arteriosclerosis. *A Maximal Approach to the Dietary Treatment of the Hyper-lipidemias*, Diets A—D. Dallas, Texas. 1973.

_____. *Rationale of the Diet-Heart Statement of the American Heart Association.* Report of Nutrition Committee. 1982.

_____. *Diet and Coronary Heart Disease.* The Nutrition Committee of the Steering Committee for Medical and Community Programs of the A.H.A. 1978.

_____. *Diet in the Healthy Child.* Task Force Committee of the Nutrition Committee and the Cardiovascular Disease in the Young Council of the A.H.A. 1983.

_____. *The Value and Safety of Diet Modification to Control Hyperlipidemia in Childhood and Adolescence.* A Statement for Physicians. An ad hoc committee of the Steering Committee for Medical and Community Program of the A.H.A. Reprinted from *Circulation* (58:381A, 1978).

American Medical Association

The American Medical Association. *Your Age and Your Diet.* 1981.

American Medical Association. *Sodium and Your Health.* 1982.

_____. *Vitamin-Mineral Supplements and their Correct Use.* 1981.

_____. *The Science of Infant Nutrition and the Art of Infant Feeding.* Journal of the American Medical Association. Aug. 18, 1978. Vol. 240, No. 7.

_____. *The Beverly Hills Diet. Dangers of the Newest Weight Loss Fad.* JAMA, Nov. 13, 1981. Vol. 246, No. 19.

_____. *Nutrition and the New Health Awareness.* JAMA, June 1982. Vol. 247.

_____. *Single Nutrient Effects on Immunologic Functions.* Report of a Workshop Sponsored by the Dept. of Food and Nutrition and its Nutrition Advisory Group of the AMA. JAMA January 1981. Vol. 245, No. 1.

_____. *The Dilemma of Morbid Obesity.* JAMA. August 1981. Vol. 246, No. 9.

_____. *AMA Concepts of Nutrition and Health*—Council on Scientific Affairs. JAMA November 1979. Vol. 242, No. 21.

_____. *Nutritional Care of the Cancer Patient*. JAMA. July, 1980. Vol. 244, No. 4.

_____. *Enteral and Parenteral Nutrition in the Care of the Cancer Patient*. JAMA. October 1981. Vol. 245, No. 15.

Department of Health and Human Services

Department of Health and Human Services. *More Than You Ever Thought You Would Know About Food Additives*. HHS Publication NO. (FDA) 82-2160. Washington, D.C. 1982.

_____. *What About Nutrients in Fast Foods?* HHS Publication No. (FDA) 83-2172. Washington, D.C. 1983.

_____. *Some Facts and Myths About Vitamins*. HHS Publication No. (FDA) 79-2117. Washington, D.C. 1982.

_____. *The Confusing World of Health Foods*. HHS Publication No. (FDA) 79-2108. Washington, D.C. 1983.

_____. *A Consumer's Guide to Food Labels*. HHS Publication No. (FDA) 77-2083. Washington, D.C. 1983.

_____. *A Primer on Dietary Minerals*. HHS Publication No. (FDA) 77-2070. Washington, D.C. 1982.

_____. *Grandma Called It Roughage*. HHS Publication No. (FDA) 78-2087. Washington, D.C. 1982.

_____. *Can Your Kitchen Pass the Food Storage Test?* HHS Publication (FDA) 74-2052. Washington, D.C. 1982.

Miscellaneous

National Live Stock and Meat Board. *Lessons on Meat*. Chicago. 1974.

National Academy of Sciences

National Academy of Sciences, Committee on Nutrition Misinformation. *Hazards of Overuse of Vitamin D*. Washington, D. C., November 1974.

National Academy of Sciences, Committee on Nutrition Misinformation. *Selenium and Human Health*. Sept. 1976.

National Academy of Sciences. Food and Nutrition Board, Division of Biological Sciences, Assembly of Life Sciences, National Research Council. *Toward Healthful Diets*. Washington, D.C. 1980.

National Research Council. Committee on Nutrition of the Mother and Preschool Child. Food and Nutrition Board, Assembly of Life Sciences. *Nutritional Services in Perinatal Care*. National Academy Press. Washington, D.C. 1981.

National Academy of Sciences, Commitee on Nutrition of the Mother and Preschool Child, Food and Nutrition Board, National Research Council. *Laboratory Indices of Nutritional Status in Pregnancy.* Summary Report. Washington, D.C. 1977.

_____. *Fetal and Infant Nutrition and Susceptibility to Obesity.* Washington, D.C. 1978.

National Academy of Sciences. *Vegetarian Diets.* A Statement of the Food and Nutrition Board Division of Biological Sciences, Assembly of Life Sciences, National Research Council. Prepared by the Committee on Nutritional Misinformation. National Academcy of Sciences. May, 1974.

National Academy of Sciences. Food and Nutrition Board, Division of Biological Sciences, Assembly of Life Sciences, National Research Council. *Toward Healthful Diets.* Washington, D.C. 1980.

New York City Department of Health

Bureau of Nutrition, Department of Health, City of New York. *The Prudent Diet.* 1981.

Bureau of Nutrition, Department of Health, City of New York. *Fats and Fatty Acids.* 1982.

United States Department of Agriculture

United States Department of Agriculture. *Keeping Food Safe to Eat.* Home and Garden Bulletin No. 162. Washington, D.C. 1980.

United States Department of Agriculture. *Nutritive Value of Foods.* Home and Garden Bulletin No. 72. Washington, D.C. 1981.

United States Department of Agriculture. *Food Safety for the Family.* Washington, D.C. 1980.

United States Department of Agriculture. *Nutrition and Your Health. Dietary Guide for Americans.* Home and Garden Bulletin No. 232. 1980.

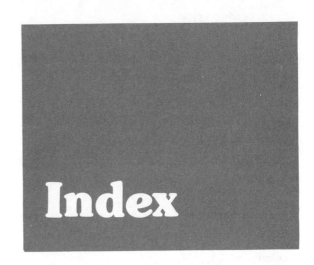

Index